Nursing Ethics
Communities in Dialogue

Rose Mary Volbrecht, PhD
Nursing Ethics Instructor
Health Care Ethics Consultant
Associate Professor of Philosophy
Gonzaga University
Spokane, Washington

Content Consultant
Karen Groth, RN, ARNP, MSN, CS, FNP
Cancer Care Northwest PS

Editorial Consultant
Patti Cleary

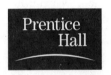
Prentice
Hall

Upper Saddle River, New Jersey 07458

Library of Congress Cataloging-in-Publication Data

Volbrecht, Rose Mary.
  Nursing ethics : communities in dialogue / Rose Mary Volbrecht.
    p. ; cm.
  Includes bibliographical references.
  ISBN 0-13-030521-9
  1. Nursing ethics.   2. Community health nursing.   3. Transcultural nursing.   I. Title.
  [DNLM: 1. Ethics, Nursing. 2. Community Health Nursing. 3. Cultural Diversity.
  4. Transcultural Nursing. WY 85 V899n 2001}
  RT85. V65 2001
  174'.2—dc21   2001021471

Publisher: *Julie Alexander*
Executive Editor: *Maura Conner*
Acquisitions Editor: *Nancy Anselment*
Editorial Assistant: *Mary Ellen Ruitenberg*
Director of Production and Manufacturing: *Bruce Johnson*
Managing Production Editor: *Patrick Walsh*
Manufacturing Manager: *Ilene Sanford*
Creative Director: *Cheryl Asherman*
Design Coordinator: *Maria Guglielmo*
Cover Designer: *Gary J. Sella*
Marketing Manager: *Nicole Benson*
Editorial Consultant: *Patti Cleary, San Francisco, CA*
Composition: *Rainbow Graphics*
Printing and Binding: *Hamilton Printing*

Pearson Education LTD
Pearson Education Australia PTY, Limited
Pearson Education Singapore, Pte. Ltd
Pearson Education North Asia Ltd
Pearson Education Canada, Ltd
Pearson Educación de Mexico, S.A. de C.V.
Pearson Education—Japan
Pearson Education Malaysia, Pte. Ltd

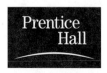

10 9 8 7 6 5 4 3 2 1
0-13-030521-9

For my pack:

Alpha One, Kenzie, Derrick, and Ridley

Contents

Chapter 3   Applying Rule Ethics   65

Chapter 4   Virtue Ethics: Character, Judgment, and Community   93

Chapter 5   Applying Virtue Ethics   131

Chapter 6   Feminist Ethics: Reconstructing the Community   159

Chapter 7   Applying Feminist Ethics   205

Chapter 8   Care for the Frail Elderly: A Comparative Analysis   237

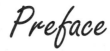

Preface

Introduction to the Text's Rationale

In many ways a book represents an invitation to the reader to engage in a dialogue with the author. Often, when we meet someone for the first time, we try to develop a sense of "where that person is coming from." The following introduction aims to open the author–reader dialogue and to give the reader a sense of where the author is coming from by presenting this book's rationale.

Dynamism of Health Care and Nursing

Health care, in general, and nursing, in particular, are in a critical period of transition. More than ever, the boundaries of health care are subject to challenge and revision. Scrutiny of health care priorities and delivery methods raises key ethical questions. Relationships between health care institutions and the communities they serve as well as among those who practice within this dynamic sphere are also increasingly a focus of reevaluation. Economic pressures and rapid technological developments further complicate the dynamic context of health care and nursing. Within this context, nurses and the communities they serve must engage in reflection and dialogue about the values that should guide the restructuring of health care.

Ethics consists of an ongoing dialogue about what communities value and what they should do in light of these values. This text seeks to prepare nurses to become active participants in communal dialogues about values in health care.

Key Role of Nursing

The dialogue about health care values and their impact on approaches to practice extends beyond an internal exchange among health care professionals. The general public as well as governmental, educational, commercial, and social institutions are also heavily invested in this dialogue process. Nursing can and must play a vital role in this dialogue. The wealth of their experience as patient educators and advocates positions them to be key players in this complex reshaping of health care. Because they serve on the front lines of care, nurses offer a unique perspective: they see the needs, the gaps, and the shortcomings as well as the achievements of our health care system. Nurses are also afforded the unique position of mediator on behalf of patients and families in an increasingly complex health care system.

The public typically entrusts nurses to represent their interests and relies on them to translate "medicalese." Nurses are increasingly called on to educate organizations and decision makers about patient needs. They must also increase their efforts to educate the public about nursing's unique roles within the health care milieu.

The Dialogue of Ethics Is Contextual

As participants in discussions about ethics within multiple contexts, nurses discover that individuals and communities draw upon a variety of languages, concepts, and ethical traditions as they take positions on ethical issues. Thus, the dialogue of ethics is contextual: Ethics begins with critical reflection on a community's moral experiences within concrete contexts. In the United States and Canada, as well as in other parts of the world, the contexts of ethical dialogue encompass diverse cultures and ideas. This diversity and the dynamism of health care makes imperative the conscious and systemic reflection on moral beliefs in order to understand multiple ethical positions and to articulate one's own.

Diversity of Ethical Theories

Within the Western discipline of ethics, on which this text will focus, many different ethical traditions exist. Most ethics texts that focus on nursing or other health care disciplines rely primarily on one of these ethical perspectives—rule ethics. This text introduces this important ethical theory as well as two others: virtue ethics and feminist ethics.

Because these three ethical theories have significantly shaped the current dialogue in health care ethics, nurses need to understand how each theory (1) frames primary questions of ethics and (2) approaches decision making to address these questions.

The application of Virtue Ethics and Feminist Ethics to nursing ethics has not been well articulated in the nursing literature. One of the distinguishing contributions of this text is the development of a nursing virtue ethics and a nursing feminist ethics.

Historical, Cultural Contexts

Understanding how ethical theories have developed helps guide us to apply them. Ethics is a dynamic conversation among people who live together in community. Although communities share many common challenges, each community confronts unique issues that shape what they perceive as the basic questions of ethics and the appropriate process for addressing them. The presentation of rule ethics, virtue ethics, and feminist ethics in this text includes an exploration of the particular historical, cultural contexts from which each theory emerged. Consideration of these contexts helps us to understand the concepts and principles emphasized by each theory and reminds us that ethical theories are dynamic and may need modification to accommodate changes in context.

Nursing Ethics as Applied Ethics

This is a text in applied ethics. Applied ethics is the process of interpreting and adapting moral concepts and values in order to solve emerging moral problems. The changing health care environment requires nurses to be able to think critically and to apply ethical theories to new contexts. This degree of competence requires more than the knowledge of a handful of moral concepts and rules. Ethically competent nursing requires the ability to explain and justify certain ethical concepts and rules and to apply them to concrete and ever-changing contexts.

Overview of the Text's Structure

This text is organized into eight chapters. Chapter 1 provides an introduction to ethics in nursing. It presents general concepts of ethics, examines the pluralistic nature of ethics, and introduces a five-step framework for ethical analysis.

Chapters 2 through 6 present three ethical perspectives: rule ethics, virtue ethics, and feminist ethics. For each perspective, a theoretical chapter presents concepts and a companion chapter guides the reader through an application of the theory that follows the five-step framework for ethical analysis. Application chapters conclude with suggestions for additional areas of application of the relevent ethical perspective. All chapters include questions for further reflection and discussion. A number of case studies throughout the text encourage the reader to apply the ethical theories to particular contexts. Experiential accounts introduce the theory chapters and "Communities in Dialogue" cases address ethical issues that require broader, community-wide consideration.

The final chapter compares the three theoretical perspectives through the examination of ethical issues related to the increasing dependence of the frail elderly on formal and informal care in the community. Nursing codes of ethics and a guide to Internet resources relevant to nursing ethics are presented in the appendices.

Acknowledgments

Many nurses and other health care professionals have helped to shape the dialogue of this text. I wish to thank the nurses who as my students have taught me about the work they do with incomparable passion and commitment. In particular, I thank the students at Gonzaga University who reviewed sections of this text and provided excellent feedback. I am also grateful to the members of the Holy Family Hospital Ethics Committee with whom I have enjoyed an extended dialogue about health care values. Thanks to this committee and the members of the Visiting Nurses Association Ethics Committee who read and discussed Chapter 5 in connection with a workshop on applications of virtue ethics in health care.

I am grateful to those nurses who contributed case material for allowing me to draw upon their experiences. Thanks to Terry Buxton, Diane Goedde, Mark Polakoff, Karen Groth, Molly Liter, Elizabeth McDonald, and Gail Peterson. At several key stages, Karen Groth shared her extensive clinical expertise and provided suggestions that served to enhance content presentation.

At Gonzaga University, Susan Norwood and David Calhoun, chairpersons of the Nursing and Philosophy Departments, provided encouragement and support. Cheryl Lepper shared her artistic expertise as well as her unique brand of humor. Jane Rinehart, who offered invaluable support throughout, provided helpful guidance with the presentation of feminist ethics and insightful comments on Chapter 6.

I wish to thank nursing faculty whose reviews of the manuscript helped to improve it and Nancy Anselment at Prentice Hall for her support of this project.

I have been extraordinarily fortunate to have the guidance and companionship of my editorial consultant, Patti Cleary. Her ability to provide detailed criticism while continuing to focus on broad themes is remarkable. She challenged and encouraged me, and what you will read is much better for her efforts.

Finally, I wish to thank those friends whose support and patience have been inestimable: Kathie; my parents, Effie and Marshall; my sister, Kathy; Pat; Elaine; Gena; Val; and Alice. Without good friends, why would anyone care about ethics?

Reviewers

Janet H. Robinson, PhD, RN
Professor and Associate Dean, Graduate Program
Medical College of Ohio
School of Nursing
Toledo, Ohio

Eileen Kohlenburg, PhD, RN, CNAA
UNCG School of Nursing
Greensboro, North Carolina

1

Ethics as Communal Dialogue

CHAPTER OUTLINE

*E*thics, a process of reflecting consciously on our moral beliefs, consists of an ongoing dialogue about what communities value and what they should do in light of these values. The goal of this text is to prepare nurses to become active participants in community dialogues about health care values. Communities that engage in dialogues relevant to the practice of nursing include patients, their families and their caregivers, professional nursing groups, health care organizations and work units, and the larger communities nurses serve. Ethics, a dynamic process of conversation and action, is sensitive to the constantly changing context of health care. In order to participate effectively in the continuing conversations of their communities, nurses need to understand the concepts and language used, the issues that are discussed, and the ways various theoretical perspectives shape how participants contribute to these conversations.

In this chapter, as we explore key concepts of ethics, we'll examine the pluralistic nature of ethics and the attendant implications for contemporary nursing. The chapter concludes with the presentation of a five-step framework for ethical analysis.

What Is Nursing Ethics?

Nursing ethics refers to the analysis of ethical issues that emerge in the practice of nursing. These issues are considered in light of ideal norms intended to guide nurses, including values, principles, and virtues of the nursing profession. *Values* are beliefs or attitudes about the worth of a goal, an object, or a behavior. Values refer to things that are desirable in themselves and not simply as a means to other things. What we value is what we care about, prize, and desire to promote. Health is the most obvious value in nursing, but other values include respect, truth, and justice. *Principles* are the most fundamental guiding precepts of action from which more specific rules may be derived. Respect for the inherent dignity and worth of every human being is an example of a fundamental principle of nursing ethics. *Virtues* are defining qualities or strengths of character that promote the development of a desired kind of person or community, such as the professional nursing community. Compassion and trustworthiness are examples of nursing virtues.

The term *nursing ethics* also describes what nurses actually believe about what is right, wrong, good, and bad. In contrast to ideal norms about how nurses *ought* to act or the qualities that ought to define a good nurse, *moral beliefs* refer to the beliefs and norms that actually guide nurses in their everyday practice. *Morality* is the term that most accurately refers to this set of actual beliefs, though the terms *morality* and *ethics* are often used interchangeably. *Nursing ethics* refers also to the discipline that analyzes the values and norms that guide nursing. As a discipline, ethics is related to but distinct from values clarification, which has been central to nursing education. Values clarification, a process of becoming more aware of one's personal values and moral beliefs and those of one's patients and their families, is a key component of individualized nursing care.

The discipline of ethics goes beyond values clarification to the systematic study of how ethical norms are expressed within a variety of ethical traditions. In short, the discipline of ethics strives to articulate the why behind ethical norms. Why should we live by this set of norms rather than another? How are these norms justified? Are there other sets of norms that can be justified and, if so, why should we prefer one group of norms over others?

Ethics is a dynamic process. It is not a matter of discovering immutable laws of nature but "a continuing negotiation *among* people" who join together to live in and develop a community (Walker, 1998). *Ethics,* an ongoing conversation among members of a community, is a dialogue about what values and principles are needed to make our society and our lives as civilized and fruitful as possible (MacIntyre, 1984; Solomon, 1993; Wallace; 1988). Through the process of conversation, members of a community who generally share moral beliefs refine their understanding of these beliefs, develop consensus on fundamental values/principles, and extend their applications to analogous situations as they arise. Determining ethical actions, however, is not the only reason we study ethics. Examining our system of ethics also helps us to understand who we and others are as revealed by the values that distinguish us. We also learn to whom we are accountable, what responses to people and their actions are appropriate, and what warrants our passion and our efforts (Walker, 1998).

Nursing ethics is part of the broader discipline of bioethics. *Bioethics,* the study of the ethics of health care and the biological sciences, addresses ethical issues that emerge in health care disciplines as well as ethical concerns in research on human and nonhuman subjects. Bioethics is a multidisciplinary project; it includes work by philosophers, theologians, health care professionals, lawyers, social scientists, biological scientists, and economists. The bulk of work in contemporary bioethics has focused on medical ethics. Clearly, there are interconnections between nursing ethics and medical ethics, yet insofar as nurses are guided by unique goals and philosophy, nursing ethics is a discipline distinct from medical ethics.

History of Nursing Ethics

The long history of nursing ethics reaches back to nursing's inception in Anglo-American cultures in the late 1800s. Ethics has been an integral part of nursing education and practice throughout its history. Nurses may be motivated to enter nursing for practical, moral, or spiritual reasons, but regardless of individual motivations, nursing is inherently a moral enterprise. "Nursing encompasses the prevention of illness, the alleviation of suffering, and the protection, promotion and restoration of health in the care of individuals, families, groups, and communities" (American Nurses Association [ANA], 2000). The commitment to care for and about people, often in their most vulnerable moments, has been the persistent and foundational value of the nursing profession. Throughout its history, the profession has provided moral guidance to practicing nurses.

Early nursing ethics focused on the appropriate character of nurses and the virtues that were seen as essential to the profession. Although early ethics texts and journal articles are sometimes dismissed as mere discussions of professional etiquette, these early writers saw clearly that professional behavior could not be separated from nurses' moral character. It is also noteworthy that these early writers recognized that nursing ethics was not only about the interactions of nurses with individual patients. From its inception, the nursing profession has been conscious of its social responsibilities as well (Fowler, 1997). The focus on character and virtues is reflected in the ANA codes of nursing ethics until 1968, when the language shifts to a duty-based ethics. Discussion of character and virtues are once again included in the most recent revision of the ANA code (ANA, 2000).

While the basic goals and values of nursing have been fairly constant in the last 100-plus years of its professional history, the focus of nursing ethics has varied over time to respond to the changing contexts of nursing practice. In the 1960s, for instance, nursing ethics reflects the changing role of women in society and nursing's evolving conception of itself as a collaborative profession rather than one subordinate to medicine. As nursing roles have been reconceived and the domain of nursing responsibilities has expanded in the past decade, nursing ethics has addressed new issues such as the delegation of traditional nursing functions to non-nursing care-givers. Similarly, discussion of nursing's social responsibilities has shifted from child labor laws and the needs of immigrants to issues of poverty and civil rights, intimate partner violence, and the effects of managed care.

Today, as members of a variety of oversight and policy-making bodies, nurses contribute significantly. These include organizational ethics committees, patient rights task forces, and human subjects review boards. They also include many com-mittees, task forces, and advisory boards at the community, state, national, and international level that develop and review policies with significant ethical implica-tions.

Nursing Codes of Ethics

Soon after the birth of the Anglo-American nursing profession, nurses expressed their desire for some professional statement of the principles of nursing ethics. The desire for a code of ethics reflected nurses' need for an explicit public statement of the goals and values that defined their newly organized profession as well as guidance in mak-ing ethical decisions in their practice. The ANA did not approve an official code of ethics until 1950, although earlier versions were drafted in 1926, 1940, and 1949. In 1954, the Canadian Nurses Association (CNA) adopted the International Council of Nurses (ICN) Code of Ethics (1953) as its first official code, and it was not until 1980 that it adopted its own unique code (CNA, 1997). The Nightingale Pledge, written in 1893, was never adopted as an official code of ethics for the nursing pro-fession. It held significant meaning for many nurses, however, and filled a critical gap in the absence of any official professional codes (Fowler, 1997).

Codes of ethics are an important expression of the communal dialogue within professional communities. A professional code of ethics represents a public statement of a profession's agreement with the society within which it practices. The *Code for Nurses: Ethical Concepts Applied to Nursing* (International Council of Nurses, 2000) provides a public declaration at the international level (see Appendix A). The *Code for Nurses with Interpretative Statements* (ANA, 1985) (Appendix B) and the *Code of Ethics for Registered Nurses* (CNA, 1997) (Appendix C) are examples of professional declarations.

Nursing codes state what communities of nurses *profess*, that is, the goals and val-ues they are committed to and the responsibilities they accept. Thus, codes of ethics provide a public identity for professions and acknowledge the special commitment they make to their societies. The nursing profession commits to serve communities by providing individualized nursing care and by promoting the health interests of the larger society. Nursing codes of ethics guide nurses in ethical decision making and provide an important means for them to exercise professional self-regulation.

Nursing codes of ethics are dynamic documents. They are revised periodically to address changes in society's needs and values and to reflect changes in how the profession of nursing defines itself. The process of revising these codes is as important as the documents produced. Each revision requires extended conversations within the profession, which provide opportunities for its members to affirm or modify its moral commitments. This process of reflection and dialogue forms the heart of ethics, and without it codes of ethics become historical documents rather than expressions of living traditions.

Nursing codes do not eliminate the need for ethical decision making. They are intended to summarize the moral commitments of nursing. In order to provide a succinct statement of these commitments, they must be fairly general. A code cannot speak to every possible ethical situation that may arise in nursing practice. The more extensive interpretive statements of the ANA code provide greater specificity to guide practice and are more frequently revised to respond to the changing social context of nursing. These more extensive statements, however, cannot be entirely comprehensive. Regardless how explicit and comprehensive a code may be, morally responsible nurses must be prepared to support the ethical decisions they make. Nursing codes provide a meaningful starting point for reflection on particular ethical issues, and all nurses are accountable for understanding and conducting themselves in accordance with them. Yet nurses who adhere to professional codes of ethics must still be prepared to give reasons for the decisions they make. Following a code of ethics is not sufficient; nurses must personally examine the values and goals of their profession and be morally accountable for their choices and for the professional life that they create.

Law and Ethics

Nursing practice is also governed by law. The requirements of nursing codes may exceed those of the law, just as ethical responsibilities in general may do so. Ethics and law both result from communal conversations about basic values and guidelines that support community living. Law and ethics overlap in their prescriptions, but they do not always concur. Persons of good conscience, including nurses, may conclude in some situations that an action is legal but unethical. Nurses may believe, for instance, that the practice of denying health care insurance to persons with chronic illnesses is unethical even though it is often legal. Conversely, some nurses may believe that certain illegal actions are ethical; for example, that the use of euthanasia is ethical in some instances. These potential conflicts reinforce the need for nurses to understand how ethical concepts can illuminate and support ethical decisions.

A society's moral beliefs provide the reasons underlying laws such as those regarding murder, child abuse, or rape and the sanctions that authorize punishment of those who violate these laws. But the law also regulates individual and organizational behavior in areas that involve pragmatic rather than moral issues, including laws such as "drive on the right side of the road" and "all government offices shall be closed on Thanksgiving."

Religion, Spirituality, and Ethics

Ethics has evolved from both theological and philosophical traditions. Theologians explore the spiritual and religious foundations of morality in order to articulate and apply ethical theories based on these foundations. In philosophical ethics, reasons are offered to support moral beliefs that can be shared by all members of a community whether they believe in God or not.

Religious beliefs and traditions are a rich source of insight regarding morality. People from these traditions should share their wisdom with their larger communities, while respecting the fact that not everyone in these communities will share their religious background. When people assert that their moral views are the right ones because they come from God, they inhibit communal dialogue. Alternatively, people help to foster communal dialogue when they share what they have learned from their spiritual and religious traditions and look for ways in which people from other traditions (religious or not) might find common ground with them.

Although philosophical ethics appeals to nonreligious sources of morality, it does not exclude consideration of the spiritual aspect of human lives. Spirituality refers to the animating life force or essence of being that permeates human life. People's experience of this life force contributes to their sense of meaning and purpose. Spirituality is experienced and expressed in relations with self, other, nature, God, or some other higher power. All human beings have spiritual as well as physical and mental dimensions. Some people express their spiritual beliefs primarily through institutionalized religious practices, while others do not.

Nursing is committed to holistic care that is responsive to the physiological, psychosocial, and spiritual dimensions of human life. In order to provide guidance for our individual and communal lives, philosophical ethics must also be attentive to each of these aspects of human life. For some nurses, spirituality or religious beliefs form an important aspect of their identity; for others they do not. But all nurses will interact with a variety of people from many different backgrounds. It is critical that nurses are able to speak about ethics in language that helps them to interact effectively with all patients and to participate in public conversations in which many perspectives will be represented.

Changing Landscape of Nursing

Change is a persistent fact of health care. Technological developments, increasing economic pressures, and restructuring of nursing roles are among the changes that affect nursing ethics. Changes such as these often outpace the ethical consensus of society, producing many ethical challenges for health care professionals. Ethics helps us to think critically and systematically about these new challenges.

Health care ethics has often focused on dramatic developments in medical technology that dominate headlines. Yet the enormous impact of technology on nursing and health care is undeniable. New technology has expanded our ability to extend human life, to create new life, and even to alter the genetic structure of human organisms. Accompanying these expanded possibilities is increasing ethical uncertainty. As technology has steadily pushed back the point of viability, for instance, many low-birth-weight babies who previously would not have survived are rescued through intensive medical efforts. At the same time, many of these infants die after months of expensive treatment and many of those who survive leave the neonatal intensive care unit with significant health problems. Genetic engineering offers the possibility to correct or eliminate genetic disorders in embryos before implantation or in fetuses in utero. But intertwined with the potential to reduce disability and illness are fundamental ethical concerns about our conceptions of disability, possible misuse of genetic information, and long-term effects of genetic engineering. The study of ethics can provide nurses with the foundation and skills needed to face these and related challenges.

Economic analysts and ordinary consumers alike frequently refer to the economic crisis in health care. Despite the sometimes drastic measures of managed care to control escalating health care costs, they continue to rise at five times the rate of inflation. The American health care system is the most technologically advanced and the most expensive system in the world. Nearly a fifth of the nonelderly population in the United States lack health care insurance and millions of others lack adequate coverage. Meanwhile, federal and state governments struggle to meet the costs of publicly funded health care programs. Cuts in Medicare and Medicaid reimbursements have had substantial effects on physicians, health care organizations, and their staffs, including nurses. Canadians have more successfully addressed the issue of equal access to health care, but they also face continuing pressures created by increasing costs of health care.

Changes in the health care environment continue to influence the reconfiguration of staff composition and settings in which nurses practice. This restructuring has resulted in an increasing patient-to-nurse ratio and greater utilization of unlicensed assistive personnel (UAP). While UAP provide critical support services to registered nurses, there is widespread concern that UAP in multiple health care settings are inappropriately performing functions that are within the legal practice of nursing (ANA, 1992). The situation of understaffing and the inappropriate utilization of UAP present ethical challenges for nurses as they make difficult judgments about patient safety, acceptance of responsibilities, and the delegation of tasks to others.

Cultural Values and Health Care

Another factor that makes nursing ethics particularly challenging today is the increasingly pluralistic nature of Western societies whose members reflect diverse cultures. Culture is the sum of beliefs, customs, values, practices, likes and dislikes, rituals, and so on that are created over time, shared, and passed on to others through socialization (Newman, 1995; Spector, 2000). Culture is the "design of living" that distinguishes one society from another. If we think of culture as a society's personality (Newman, 1995), we must recognize that the United States reflects multiple personalities. Until recently, many Americans were encouraged to assume that these multiple cultures would eventually assimilate into a common culture. The ideal of the American melting pot, however, is now widely acknowledged to be a myth. Although assimilation has been the goal of some immigrant groups, distinct cultural differences have always existed in North American society. Many now believe that cultural differences should be embraced rather than eliminated. Differences among people are often significant and shape what people believe and how they conduct their everyday lives.

Culturally Based Beliefs About Health and Illness

Cultural diversity creates many challenges for health care professionals who must appreciate the influence of cultural beliefs and values on patient perceptions of health and illness in order to provide effective care. Cultures vary widely in their beliefs about what causes illness, how to prevent and treat it, how to maintain health, how to express pain and suffering, and so forth (Spector, 2000).

Cultures also differ widely in their value systems. When diverse cultures interact within the health care system, profound value conflicts may emerge. Values regarding family relations and roles, sexuality, individual and family privacy, gender roles, and religious and spiritual beliefs will shape patient and health care provider perceptions of their moral responsibilities in response to illness and health promotion. Cultural differences often contribute to conflict over such issues as birth control, use of blood and blood products, organ donations, the use of surgical or pharmacological interventions, and the use of traditional methods of health restoration such as cupping, herbal treatments, or purging.

The application of ethical responsibilities will also be shaped by diverse cultural values. In Western health care, self-determination and autonomy are emphasized, and health care professionals have a duty to provide information to the individual patient who (if competent) makes decisions and gives informed consent for treatment. In more group-oriented cultures, patients and their families may suffer unnecessary stress if information regarding the outcomes of tests, surgeries, or medical results is not shared with patients and their families simultaneously. In some cultures individual patients may defer to a community leader or spiritual elder who will hear information, make decisions, and decide what information should be conveyed to the patient and family. Ignoring this role of the community leader can have significant consequences in certain Southeast Asian and Native American cultures that believe that the act of telling itself may cause the death of a person with a serious illness (Crow, Matheson, and Steed, 2000).

Clashing Values and Moral Judgments

The Hmong are a Southeast Asian mountain people who allied themselves with the United States during the Vietnam War. Thousands of Hmong families were airlifted to the United States after the war; most settled in or near Fresno, California. The Hmong are shamanistic animists, believing the world is inhabited by spirits and that interacting with them shapes human lives.

Anne Fadiman, in *The Spirit Catches You and You Fall Down*, insightfully presents the experiences of a Hmong family, the Lees, as they interact with Western medical institutions in seeking help for their daughter Lia. This tragic story, presented in Box 1–1, illustrates how conflicting cultural value systems create difficult ethical dilemmas for health care professionals and the patients/families who seek their help (Fadiman, 1997).

Box 1–1   A Little Medicine and a Little Neeb

Lia was diagnosed at age eight months with a severe seizure disorder. The Lees believed that Lia's soul fled her body and became lost following a frightening episode at age three months. Her seizures, they believed, were caused by a soul-stealing *dab* spirit that periodically caught hold of Lia and threw her to the ground.

As is characteristic of Hmong parents, the Lees were devoted to Lia and extremely attentive to her needs. Their attitudes toward Lia's seizures were conflicted, however. Epileptics have a special status in Hmong culture; they are believed to embody special spirits and often become shamans. Although most of the time the Lees hoped that their daughter's illness could be healed, they also considered it an honor. Their attitudes about Western medicine were also conflicted. When three of their other children had been seriously ill in a refugee camp, they were treated by Western physicians as well as through traditional Hmong methods. All three recovered and the Lees concluded that it was sometimes acceptable for Western medicine to supplement—but never to replace—traditional treatments. Thus, the Lees' approach to Lia's treatment was "a little medicine and a little *neeb* [a healing spirit]" (Fadiman, 1997, p. 106).

Lia's seizure disorder, unusually severe and difficult to control, over a four-year period required her to be hospitalized seventeen times and seen in the emergency room and as an outpatient on more than 100 occasions. Two dedicated pediatricians, Neil Ernst and Peggy Philp, supervised her care at the county hospital. During this same time, the Lees also tried a host of traditional therapies, including amulets, cupping, and animal sacrifices. Lia's condition worsened, and her physicians attributed this deterioration to the parents' failure to give Lia all of the drugs they prescribed. The parents, on the other hand, attributed her worsening condition to the effects of the drugs, which had serious and long-lasting side effects. Eventually, Lia suffered irreversible brain damage.

Drs. Ernst and Philp prided themselves on uncompromising care for all of their patients, including those like Lia whose care was Medicaid funded. Lia did not respond to the usual drug treatment for grand mal seizures, so her physicians searched relentlessly for an effective alternative. Because Lia's condition was progressive and unstable, they believed that constant fine-tuning of her drug regimen was necessary, and Lia's prescriptions changed 23 times in four years, involving varying combinations, amounts, and times of day.

continues

Box 1–1   A Little Medicine and a Little Neeb (cont.)

The treatment complexity alone would have overwhelmed most parents, but the added problems of illiteracy and communication barriers made the drug regimen nearly impossible to implement. The Lees frequently modified dosages and sometimes refused to give Lia her medications, believing they were making her seizures worse and changing her personality.

Eventually, the clash of values led to a legal battle over custody of Lia. When Lia was two years old, Drs. Ernst and Philp regarded the Lees' lack of compliance with their medical prescriptions as child neglect and petitioned Child Protective Services to remove Lia from her parents' care. They felt that this was the only chance to halt the steady decline in Lia's intellectual capacity and prevent irreversible brain damage. Despite the assessment by social workers that the Lees were loving and attentive caretakers, Lia was removed from their care for several months. Her condition continued to deteriorate. Six months after returning to her home, Lia developed septic shock and experienced extended grand mal seizures, which left her in a persistent vegetative state. Her parents took her home and continued to care for her.

Fadiman wonders if Lia might have been better served if, rather than insisting on finding the "optimal" treatment, her physicians had chosen a simpler drug regimen and attempted to tailor treatment in such a way that the family would have been more likely to comply with it. She notes that despite their dedication to Lia's care, Drs. Ernst and Philp made no real attempts to understand how the Lees perceived the cause and nature of Lia's illness or their reasons for altering her drug regimen (Fadiman, 1997).

Clashes between parents and representatives of Western medicine about the treatment of children are some of the most difficult ethical dilemmas that arise when value systems of different cultures conflict. Such disputes have occurred with American Jehovah's Witnesses, Christian Scientists, and fundamentalist Christians who refuse treatments prescribed by Western medical professionals that conflict with their value systems. It is presumptuous for Western health care professionals to assume that their understanding of what is the best treatment for these children should always be preferred. The reality of diverse and conflicting value systems raises critical questions about the objectivity of moral judgments in health care ethics. Box 1–2 highlights some of these questions.

Cross-Cultural Moral Standards

There are significant differences in values and moral beliefs across cultures. Some traditions view honor killings as not only accepted but also expected. A brother may kill his sister-in-law who has an extramarital affair in order to avenge his brother's honor. American street gangs support similar codes of conduct. The use of all but natural means of birth control is contrary to Mormon and Roman Catholic moral beliefs, while many other cultures encourage the use of various birth control methods.

Cultures differ widely in their moral beliefs about issues such as sex, marriage, gender roles, child rearing, and responsibilities to one's elders. These differences of moral beliefs exist not only in distinct cultures separated geographically and politically but also within geopolitical cultures such as the United States. A nurse in the United States may care for a Sudanese woman suffering from chronic pelvic infection and intractable dysmenorrhea resulting from genital infibulation (a clitoridectomy followed by suturing of labia to prevent intercourse) performed when she was eight years old. Female circumcision is practiced today in 26 African countries. The influx of refugees and immigrants from these countries has challenged Western health professionals who attempt to provide appropriate care for circumcised women.

Respect for each individual and a commitment to deliver nursing services without prejudice or judgment of personal beliefs, lifestyle, or values is fundamental to nursing practice. The importance of this moral value to nursing practice cannot be overstated. At the same time, conflicts of moral values and beliefs will occur in nursing practice. How should nurses approach moral differences across cultures? Is there a single, universal moral truth beneath the often perplexing diversity of culturally influenced beliefs? Or are moral beliefs and values merely subjective opinions of individuals and the cultures to which they belong? How can moral judgments be made across cultures with different value systems?

Diversity exists within the discipline of ethics itself. The discipline of Western ethics, which supports many different theories of ethics, is subject to the same sort of questions related to its diversity. Does one of these ethical theories represent the best way to think about ethics? Or will another theory that has yet to emerge offer the best approach? How does a person or a community choose an ethical theory to live by—is it simply a matter of subjective preference? Is the choice of an ethical theory a rational process independent of cultural context? Is the choice influenced by cultural context but more than a matter of preference?

Ethical Pluralism

These are difficult questions to answer. When we consider questions about moral truth in diverse cultures, we are actually theorizing about ethical theories. In pluralistic cultures such as the United States, people who discuss ethical issues draw upon many different cultural value systems and varied ethical theories. How can we make moral judgments that will be valid across these different cultures? Philosophers have developed several perspectives to address this question. One of these, ethical pluralism, is the approach of this text. *Ethical pluralism* is the view that culturally diverse societies reflect multiple moral standards, which may result in conflicting moral truths. These ideas about what is moral, however, are not purely subjective; to be considered as standards, they must be justified. The position of ethical pluralism does not rule out the possibility that a consensus on moral standards could emerge across cultures. But it does not assume that compatibility among moral standards necessarily exists or that compatibility is required to formulate moral judgments within and across diverse cultures (Hinman, 1998; Kekes, 1993; Wolf, 1992).

The pluralist perspective appreciates divergence in values and recognizes that genuine differences in moral standards exist across cultural boundaries. Pluralism considers diversity to be a potential resource. Yet pluralists do not believe that "anything goes." Pluralism recognizes the existence of multiple moral standards—it does not suggest that there are no standards or that the multiple standards are arbitrary. Standards of morality must be justified; communities must give a reasonable account of why and how they have arrived at their values. Arguments can be assessed as better or worse. Some arguments will be incoherent, inconsistent, or illogical. Others may be logically consistent but not persuasive.

FALSE PROMISES OF ETHICAL RELATIVISM

Ethical pluralism rejects the view of *ethical relativism,* a position that maintains that moral judgments can be evaluated as right or wrong relative only to the dominant preferences of a particular culture. This view proposes that what is right is always relative to a particular culture's values so that whatever a community accepts as moral determines what is moral in that community. If a majority of people in a culture believe that honor killings are morally justified, then they are moral in that culture. Any judgment about this practice that originates outside of this culture is invalid.

Ethical relativism claims to promote tolerance with its insistence that no culture has the right to assert that its values are better than any other culture's. This tolerance of diverse moral beliefs may resonate with the commitment nurses are expected to make to be nonjudgmental. But nurses regularly encounter people from cultures in which the majority do not accept an obligation to be tolerant of all other people. These include members of the Aryan Nation, who do not believe they should tolerate Jews or persons of color; some anti-abortionists, whose intolerance is used to justify violent attacks on abortion clinics; and persons who do not tolerate homosexuals because they believe them to be a violation of the laws of nature and/or God.

The most critical problem with ethical relativism is that it provides us with no guidance when cultures conflict as in the Lia Lee case summarized in Box 1–1. If, as ethical relativism asserts, moral judgments can be assessed only within a particular culture, then how do we assess judgments when cultures overlap? Each of us, in fact, belongs to multiple cultures. Our individual identity is defined by the multiple cultures of which we are a part, including ethnic, religious, family, work, professional, and educational cultures. We will share one culture with some people and another with others. No two people can claim the same cultural heritage or identity. If moral judgments can be evaluated as right or wrong relative only to a particular culture, then one might argue that each individual's values and standards can be judged relative only to his or her own unique, individual culture. This extreme form of individual ethical relativism is often expressed in the statement "Everything is relative, so we each have to do what we believe is right." Many believe that ethical relativism must inevitably collapse into this realm of the individual in which all values and moral standards are relative to each person. Ethical relativism is thus counterproductive to the kind of communal dialogue that is so essential in health care ethics.

While ethical relativism purports to promote respect for and tolerance of diverse moral beliefs, in practice it seems to encourage a kind of moral isolation. Retreating to "it's all relative" or "but this is just my opinion" may be a way of avoiding criticism of one's own beliefs. There is an implicit agreement that if I don't push you to defend your beliefs, you won't push me to defend mine. Rather than promoting tolerance of diverse beliefs, however, this seems to encourage withdrawal from thoughtful conversation and critical reflection on conflicting moral beliefs. This withdrawal may be motivated by a fear of examining one's own beliefs, intellectual laziness, or moral indifference—not caring what other people think. None of these attitudes promote genuine respect and tolerance for diverse moral beliefs.

ETHICS AS COMMUNAL DIALOGUE

Ethical pluralism, in contrast, promotes an ongoing dialogue among members of a community in which they carefully reflect on their moral beliefs and standards. One component of this dialogue is to uncover and clarify a community's shared moral understandings. What is expected of whom and why? Another part of the dialogue is more critical and involves asking how well a community's shared values and principles make life in this community fulfilling. Much of this work of critical reflection will be comparative, asking whether this community's shared values and principles promote a way of life that is better or worse than others that are known or imagined (Walker, 1998).

All ethical theories are the result of critical reflection by theorists, their critics, and their advocates about their own moral experiences within their historical–social contexts. As this text examines three ethical theories, rule ethics, virtue ethics, and feminist ethics, we will pay careful attention to the historical–social contexts from which each emerged. We will note how this context shapes what each perceives to be the primary questions of ethical theory, what gets prioritized in the theory, and how these questions and priorities shape the decision processes for each theory. The contextual influence of these theories does not invalidate them or make them less applicable to other contexts. An ideal ethical theory is not one that is without context; it is one that critically reflects on its context in light of ongoing experience and cross-cultural dialogue.

Seeking Moral Truth

The contextual, dialogic view of ethical pluralism deviates from the perspective of most traditional ethical theories, which have asserted that in order to resolve moral conflicts between cultures, we must appeal to some standard *outside* of these individual cultures. This assertion, referred to as ***ethical objectivism,*** claims that moral truths are objective and universal, applying to all cultures at all times. Morality is objective, not relative to what a particular culture or individual thinks is right. In order to be objective, moral truths must be based on something that is external to individuals or cultures. Thus, ethical objectivists believe that moral standards are based on something that is public and knowable by everyone. This foundation for moral standards must transcend particular cultures so that moral truths apply universally across all cultures and all time periods.

Transcendent or Contextual Truths?

Objectivists note that there will always be areas of moral judgment that produce disagreement among thoughtful, conscientious people. Yet there are situations in which we must be able to say a resounding "No, you cannot do that—that action is immoral regardless of your culture." Genocide is wrong, rape is wrong, and killing another human being because you don't like him or her is wrong. We do not need a poll of a culture's personal preferences to determine the morality of these actions. They are so obviously harmful to human beings that they must be considered morally wrong everywhere regardless of the opinion of the majority of people in a specific culture.

Objectivists believe that the people in one culture can be justified in making these moral judgments about the actions of people in other cultures only if moral truth transcends or stands outside of particular cultures. This outside standard applies universally to all contexts in which human beings interact. Thus, genocide is morally wrong regardless of whether it takes place in Nazi Germany, Rwanda, Bosnia, or the nineteenth-century American frontier. Without such transcendent moral standards, objectivists assert that cross-cultural moral judgments cannot be made at all.

On the other hand, pluralism does not seek foundations for moral judgments that are independent of all cultures or the particularities of human experience. Instead, pluralism views moral standards as emerging from the experiences of concrete people who interact, form relationships, and build a common life together. We are all born into particular communities that share beliefs about how people should treat one another and how responsibilities are assigned and distributed. These moral beliefs and standards are constructed and sustained by people who share their lives with one another. Morality is in this sense essentially collaborative. It cannot be discovered alone through abstract reasoning; it is created (Walker, 1998; Wallace, 1988).

Objectivists assume that moral truths must be based on something "outside" of all cultural contexts. The presumption is that personal experiences and relationships always bias or distort our knowing. We hear echoes of this view in everyday life. In the selection of a jury for an assault case, prospective jurors may be asked whether they or anyone close to them has experienced a violent attack. A person who answers yes is generally eliminated from the jury pool. The assumption is that this person, biased by previous experience, could not be objective. Being objective is envisioned as the process of putting aside all personal or cultural identity, stripping down to pure reasoning that is untainted by any particular context. In order for moral judgments to be objective, they must be based on transcendent values or standards, that is, on something that is outside of all contexts. A moral judgment will be correct, according to ethical objectivism, when it measures up to this objective, independent standard.

Obviously, bias can be a bad thing. Campaign finance reform has become a pressing concern as the contributions to political campaigns have increased dramatically. It is hard to believe that a senator who receives millions of dollars from the pharmaceutical industry will not be biased when considering legislation intended to control rising prescription prices. The biases of racism and sexism lead to unfair discrimination in workplaces, education, and politics. But the fact that people can be inappropriately biased does not mean that we must escape all contexts in order to make good moral judgments. It is impossible to view the world and human actions outside of all contexts, nor should we necessarily try to escape them in order "to see the truth."

DIVERSE EXPERIENCES AS RESOURCES

Pluralists do not regard people's individual and cultural experiences as liabilities that undermine objectivity. They perceive diversity as a strength; our particular identities and cultures are resources for seeing our lives and our worlds from diverse points of view. Individuals experience the world, even within a single community, from different points of view and different positions. Because of their unique identities and histories, individual members of a community will face different moral challenges and they will face shared moral challenges in different ways. They will have various understandings of the benefits, costs, and risks of social policies and practices. They will develop diverse strategies for resolving problems because of their distinct contexts and conditions. These personal experiences and perspectives offer the community multiple insights and resources for conceptualizing problems and generating solutions. They may also alert the community to the fact that some responsibilities are unfairly distributed and some positions are not freely chosen. These insights are critical for the process of improving and recreating the moral standards of a community.

It makes little sense to assume that we can "take off" our personal identity and history as we can remove tinted glasses that color our perception. On the other hand, if people do not reflect on how their particular experiences differ from those of others, then they will mistakenly believe that everyone perceives the world as they do. Pluralism recognizes that everyone has a unique perspective and encourages individuals and groups to become aware of how their unique and shared identities affect their perceptions. Each perspective offers the community potentially new insights about how to develop a fruitful community life.

RESPONDING TO MORAL DISAGREEMENT

The goal of pluralism is to appreciate and learn from multiple perspectives, while continually searching for ways to resolve conflicts and to develop a shared way of life. Pluralism recognizes that serious moral disagreements do occur both within and across cultures. We can respect differences while also strongly disagreeing with others. Pluralists recognize that we are all fallible and must be open to revising our moral beliefs and ethical theories when our positions are shown to be logically inconsistent or when we recognize that certain practices do not promote human welfare in the ways that we thought they did (Hinman, 1998). This attitude of fallibility does not mean that pluralists do not care intensely about their moral values or that they should not advocate for their acceptance by others. If, after responsibly thinking through an ethical issue, an individual or a community believes they have good reasons to support their conclusions, it would be odd if they did not advocate this position and seek to persuade others to adopt it. We can never be certain that we are right, but moral judgments must be made and we must make them based on our best thinking and wisdom.

At the same time, pluralists recognize that other cultures may have clearly different moral standards and beliefs. It would be arrogant and insensitive to presume that our moral views should be adopted by others. The reasons that justify our coming to certain conclusions may not apply in the same way to other cultures. We may not share enough background assumptions about the world, other moral beliefs, or social contexts for our reasons to be persuasive in another culture. We may not share enough to be able to draw the same moral conclusions (Walker, 1998).

Does this mean that we have no obligations to act when we have good reasons to believe that vulnerable people are being harmed in other societies? Pluralists believe that in some cases we are obligated to help protect people from the aggression of others in their communities, particularly when these vulnerable people request outside help. We may also have obligations to assist people in other cultures to change situations that they find oppressive. But outsiders must be cautious in presuming that they are in a position to judge that the social structures in radically different moral cultures are morally unacceptable and justify outside intervention.

Sherwin suggests that in evaluating community standards the important considerations are (1) how standards are reached, (2) whose interests they serve, and (3) what procedures exist for reevaluating them. Clearly, moral standards that are enforced through direct violence and slaughter are not justified. But standards may also be set by more subtle means of coercion, exploitation, manipulation, and ignorance. These processes may be difficult to understand without detailed study of the social structures and relationships in particular societies (Sherwin, 1992).

Framework for Ethical Analysis

Three ethical theories will be presented and applied in this text. Rule ethics, virtue ethics, and feminist ethics were chosen because they have each significantly shaped how Western cultures think about morality. Perspectives other than these three have been influential in Western cultures or have shaped non-Western cultures. Rule ethics and virtue ethics, however, have been the primary philosophical ethical theories shaping ethical discussions in the context of health care in Western cultures. Feminist ethics, a more recent voice in these discussions, is significant because it teaches us to be aware that some voices have dominated these conversations and others have been silenced or marginalized. These three ethical theories are reflected in the newly revised ANA code (ANA, 2000).

Each of these ethical theories contributes distinct insights to our moral understandings. Although these theories complement one another by offering diverse points of view, they cannot be neatly synthesized into one comprehensive ethical theory. Points of disagreement and conflict exist between these theories, as is true of most areas of human knowledge. Different theories about human nature, about health and illness, or about religion offer us alternative ways of constructing our lives. We may learn from all of them, despite their conflicts and disagreements.

Rule ethics, virtue ethics, and feminist ethics each frame the issues of ethics differently and propose divergent processes for resolving moral issues. Nonetheless, there are some elements of ethical analysis that are relevant regardless of the particular ethical theory that is being applied. Box 1–3, Framework for Ethical Analysis, summarizes these common elements, which will be applied throughout this text. Each of the framework's five elements is described below.

➤ Identify the Problem

Describe the problem: What is going on, who are the parties or stakeholders involved, what are the value issues in this case/issue? Stakeholders are all persons who will be affected by this problem and its resolution.

➤ Analyze the Context

Identify contextual factors of this case/issue that are critical to understanding and resolving this problem. These may include political, economic, organizational, legal, or cultural aspects. Cultural aspects are those characteristic beliefs, attitudes, and practices that define a social group such as views of illness and death, family, sexuality, tradition, gender roles, education, and religion. Consider how these shape and impact values relevant to this case/issue. Consider also how these affect your ability to implement a desired solution.

Box 1–3   Framework for Ethical Analysis

1. Identify the problem or issue.
2. Analyze context.
3. Explore options.
4. Apply the decision process.
5. Implement the plan and evaluate results.

➤ Explore Options

Identify possible choices and/or solutions relevant to this case/issue, a preliminary consideration of options that seem to offer viable solutions. Application of the ethical decision process in the next step may reveal better options, but it is helpful to envision what sort of choices seem possible. It is always possible to imagine all kinds of options, but many are so unrealistic that they can be promptly ruled out. Focus only on those genuinely worthy of consideration—the best two or three possibilities.

➤ Apply the Relevant Ethical Decision Process

This text will present ethical decision processes for three different ethical theories: rule ethics (including rule utilitarianism and Kantian ethics), virtue ethics, and feminist ethics. A decision process will be outlined for each of these ethical theories. In practice, nurses will find that one of these approaches will sometimes be more appropriate than the others. In other cases, the application of more than one approach will be useful in resolving a particular ethical case/issue. Application of these decision processes lead to recommendations for action.

➤ Implement the Plan and Evaluate the Results

Once a plan is implemented, it should be evaluated to determine whether, in practice, the plan promoted the desired values, treated persons with respect, and enhanced a sense of community. This evaluation is essential to the ongoing dialogue of ethics, which requires communities to reflect continually on how well their values and principles promote community living that is as fulfilling as possible. As moral judgments are made and recommendations are implemented, communities may find that individual rules and practices need to be revised. In some cases, feedback may be so momentous that communities must consider revising fundamental values or principles.

Box 1–4   Communities in Dialogue:

Cultural Conflict and Informed Consent

The Roma are an ancient people whose original homeland is in and around Delhi in northern India. There are some 15 million Roms across the world, and roughly 1 million Roms living in the United States. While frequently referred to as "gypsies" and portrayed as romantic nomads, persecution and discrimination has often been the cause of their frequent movement. Half a million Roms were killed in the Holocaust. As a result of this history, Roms may be reluctant to disclose their ethnic heritage and reluctant to trust authorities, including health care providers.

    Contrary to the stereotype, many Roms are not nomadic. They hold various jobs, including many professional positions. The Roma culture is rich in music,

---

Box 1–4   Communities in Dialogue:

Cultural Conflict and Informed Consent

dance, art, literature, and religious beliefs. Dispersed across the world, the Roma are a nation in spirit; they are proud of their heritage and actively seek to preserve and revive their culture. Traditionally, this culture has been male- and age-dominated. As a result, decision making among Roma will be governed by different culture norms than in mainstream Western culture. Conflicts such as those in the following case may occur as a consequence.

Racing toward the goal, 10-year-old Lianne Rozelle was hit hard in the shin with a soccer ball. Shrieking in pain, she collapsed and was carried off the field. Three days after admission to Evergreen Community Hospital for tests that revealed a diagnosis of bone cancer, Lianne has not been informed of her status. The nursing staff are disturbed that her parents, 29-year-old Michael and 21-year-old Marie, have also not been told. In addition to withholding this information from Lianne and her parents, Michael's family has not allowed him or his wife to see Lianne since she was admitted. The paternal grandparents have insisted that the physician speak only with them, after which they huddle with the various aunts and uncles to discuss the situation. Lianne's nurses learn that the Rozelles are Romani people. Family members frequently ask the staff for information about Lianne's condition and prognosis. When the staff call a care conference to discuss Lianne's treatment, the paternal grandparents and two aunts attend, excluding the parents.

The absence of Lianne's parents and their lack of involvement in their daughter's care disturbs the staff. When they express concern, the family explains that the parents are "just babies" and thus much too young to make decisions about Lianne's treatment. Astonished by this statement, the physician informs the family that the parents are legally responsible for Lianne and will need to sign consent forms for the surgery and therapy that she will need. The paternal grandfather explains that in Roma culture marriages are arranged when couples are in their teens. Young married couples usually live with the husband's parents for many years after marriage. Although married, they do not assume full adult responsibilities and decision making for some time. They are still considered children and major decisions are made by the husband's parents, especially the father.

Lianne's nurses express respect for Roma culture and note that Michael and Marie are fortunate to have the support and counsel of their elders. Nonetheless, they believe her parents should participate in care conferences, and they reiterate that one of them must sign the consent forms. The paternal grandfather assures the staff that he will have Michael sign the necessary forms, but that he himself will make the decisions regarding his granddaughter's care.

continues

Box 1–4   Communities in Dialogue:

Cultural Conflict and Informed Consent (concluded)

Questions

1. Would Michael Rozelle's signature on a surgical consent form constitute a genuinely informed consent, legally and morally, for his daughter's surgery?
2. Should the physician and nursing staff insist on speaking directly with Michael and Marie Rozelle about their daughter's condition and care? Why or why not?
3. Are there other patient care situations in which information is withheld from patients because of cultural and/or family dynamics? How can nurses demonstrate respect for both the moral principle of informed consent and cultural/family dynamics in these situations?

KEY POINTS

- Ethics is a dynamic discipline in which members of a community critically assess their values and principles.

- Nursing ethics refers to the ideal norms and actual moral beliefs that guide and define nursing, as well as to the discipline that analyzes these norms and moral beliefs.

- Nursing codes are public statements of the goals, values, and responsibilities of the nursing profession. They provide moral guidance to nurses, which serves as a foundation for professional practice. Nurses will benefit from adding knowledge of ethical theories and the process of ethical decision making to this foundation.

- While ethical relativism seeks to promote tolerance for diverse cultural moral beliefs, it fails to provide guidance for resolving moral conflicts. Ethical objectivism recognizes the necessity of cross-cultural moral judgments and the need to stand up against egregious moral wrongdoing, but it depends on an unjustified assumption of transcendent moral values.

- Ethical pluralism respects cultural diversity and the existence of multiple moral standards. At the same time, it requires moral standards to be justified and recognizes that some moral standards are not justifiable and should therefore be resisted.

REFLECT AND DISCUSS

1. What moral values motivated you to become a nurse? Have some of these values changed or have others been added that sustain your professional work?
2. How do nursing codes of ethics inform your professional practice? Are these codes sufficient to guide the resolution of ethical issues in nursing practice?
3. Describe one or two instances in which you have observed an effect on patient care of different cultural beliefs about health or illness. Have you also experienced situations in which conflicting cultural beliefs and values led to different moral judgments regarding patient care? Were these conflicts adequately resolved? How does the perspective of cultural pluralism illuminate these conflicts?
4. Ethical pluralism is sometimes confused with ethical relativism. How is pluralism distinguished from relativism? What objections would an ethical objectivist have to pluralism? Does ethical pluralism avoid the relativist problem of reducing moral judgments to simply a matter of personal or cultural opinions?
5. How would an ethical relativist, ethical objectivist, and ethical pluralist assess the decisions made about Lia's care by the Lees and by Drs. Ernst and Philp?

REFERENCES

American Nurses Association. (1985). *Code for nurses with interpretive statements.* Washington, DC: American Nurses Publishing.

American Nurses Association. (1992). *Registered nurse utilization of unlicensed assistive personnel.* Available: http://www.ana.org/readroom/position/uap/uapusae.htm [2000, November 27].

American Nurses Association. (2000). *Code of ethics for nurses* (working draft #9). Available: http://www.ana.org/ethics/code9.htm [2000, November 17].

Canadian Nurses Association. (1997). *Code of ethics for registered nurses.* Ottawa: Author.

Crow, K., Matheson, L., and Steed, A. (2000). Informed consent and truth-telling: Cultural directions for healthcare providers. *Journal of Nursing Administration, 30*(3), 148–152.

Fadiman, A. (1997). *The spirit catches you and you fall down.* New York: Noonday Press.

Fowler, M. (1997). Nursing's ethics. In A. Davis, M. A. Aroskar, J. Liaschenko, & T. S. Drought. *Ethical dilemmas & nursing practice* (pp. 17–34). Stamford, CT: Appleton & Lange.

Hinman, L. M. (1998). *Ethics: A pluralistic approach to moral theory* (2nd ed.). Fort Worth, TX: Harcourt Brace.

International Council of Nurses. (1973/2000). *Code for nurses: Ethical concepts applied to nursing.* Geneva: Author.

Kekes, J. (1993). Pluralism and conflict in morality. *Journal of Value Inquiry, 26,* 37–50.

MacIntyre, A. (1984). *After virtue* (2nd ed.). Notre Dame, IN: Notre Dame Press.

Newman, D. M. (1995). *Sociology: Exploring the architecture of everyday life.* Thousand Oaks, CA: Pine Forge Press.

Sherwin, S. (1992). *No longer patient: Feminist ethics and health care.* Philadelphia, PA: Temple University Press.

Solomon, R. C. (1993). *Ethics: A short introduction.* Dubuque, IA: Brown & Benchmark.

Spector, R. E. (2000). *Cultural diversity in health & illness.* Upper Saddle River, NJ: Prentice Hall.

Wallace, J. D. (1988). *Moral relevance and moral conflict.* Ithaca, NY: Cornell University Press.

Walker, M. U. (1998). *Moral understandings: A feminist study in ethics.* New York: Routledge.

Wolf, S. M. (1992). Two levels of pluralism. *Ethics, 102*(4), 785–798.

2

Rule Ethics: Reason and Impartiality

EXPERIENTIAL ACCOUNT: Interpreting Advanced Directives

Hospitalized for complications, 64-year-old Mr. Aiken has been treated for chronic obstructive pulmonary disease (COPD) for over 20 years. A responsible patient, he has sought timely treatment for complications of COPD. He has also worked hard to maintain a reasonable exercise program. From time to time he has struggled to overcome severe depression related to his chronic illness.

    Mr. Aiken has made it clear for some time that he never wants to be placed on a ventilator. After completing an advanced directive that clearly states this decision, Mr. Aiken discussed his decision with his primary physician, Dr. Long, and his daughter, Johanna, who lives nearby. Johanna has been especially helpful in assisting him to manage his disease and activities of daily living since the death of her mother five years earlier.

During a current hospitalization for bronchitis and pneumonia, Mr. Aiken becomes weak and confused. It is determined that he needs the support of a ventilator to breathe. Johanna insists that to honor her father's wishes no ventilator should be used. The staff tries to make Mr. Aiken comfortable. Soon Alice, Mr. Aiken's younger daughter whom he has not seen in 12 years, arrives at the hospital. Alice insists that her father be placed on the ventilator. Johanna tries to persuade her sister to change her mind, explaining that their father absolutely did not want this. She also appeals to her father's nurse, Melissa Kimball, RN, to talk to Alice. Melissa tries to discuss the situation with Alice, but Alice keeps repeating that they cannot simply let their father die. Dr. Long warns Alice that her father will likely never come off of the ventilator, but he eventually acquiesces and begins the respiratory therapy.

Rule Ethics in Contemporary Health Care

Rule ethics has dominated moral philosophy since its development in the eighteenth and nineteenth centuries. The goal of this ethical model is to capture our moral duties and obligations within a manageable set of rules. Thus, applied ethics, such as nursing ethics, involves the application of abstract, universal rules to particular situations or cases. This attempt to distill ethical decision making into a list of rules reflects both the strength and weakness of this theory's roots in the Western European Enlightenment period.

Since its emergence as a discipline in the 1960s and 1970s, contemporary health care ethics has tended to rely on a simplified or abbreviated form of rule ethics. The analysis of cases has focused primarily on a short list of rules. The most common list has included four rules or principles: nonmaleficence, beneficence, respect for autonomy, and justice. From these principles more particular rules of conduct are derived that address issues such as truth-telling, confidentiality, promise-keeping, and negligence. Beauchamp and Childress in their influential *Principles of Biomedical Ethics* codified this four-principle summary of ethical rules early on in the health care ethics movement (1979). The Preamble of the American Nurses Association (ANA) *Code for Nurses with Interpretive Statements* (ANA, 1985) includes these four among those basic moral principles that "prescribe and justify nursing actions" (p. i). These principles appear directly or indirectly throughout interpretative statements that illuminate the guidelines of the 1985 code and the recently revised code (ANA, 2000). To understand more about these four ethical principles, let's apply them to the opening scenario.

Case Analysis

The first responsibility of all health care professionals is a duty of *nonmaleficence:* a duty not to intentionally inflict harm on patients. Although Mr. Aiken's physician,

Dr. Long, warns Alice that her father will probably become ventilator dependent, the ventilator will help Mr. Aiken breathe more comfortably. The treatment, intended to help and not to harm Mr. Aiken, does not, therefore, violate the duty of nonmaleficence. This duty is implied in Interpretive Statement 3.5 of the *Code of Ethics for Nurses* (ANA, 2000) when it states that the nurse's primary commitment is to the health, welfare, and safety of the client.

The second consideration in this case is the duty of ***beneficence:*** a duty to promote the well-being of others and oneself. The *Code of Ethics for Nurses* (ANA, 2000) opens with the recognition that concern for the health and well-being of the sick, injured, and vulnerable is the very foundation of nursing. Clearly, each of his daughters and his physician want to help Mr. Aiken. Alice sees her father's labored breathing and believes that using a ventilator to assist his breathing will promote her father's well-being. Johanna and Dr. Long, however, who have conversed extensively with Mr. Aiken about this very subject, know that Mr. Aiken believed that becoming ventilator dependent would significantly diminish his quality of life. Although he knew it would likely provide relief in the short run, Mr. Aiken understood that the ventilator would impose further burdens and only postpone his respiratory failure. Considering his advanced COPD, the ventilator offered no genuine hope of recovery. Beneficence does not, therefore, appear to require ventilator use for Mr. Aiken. Clearly, however, the decision makers in this case disagree about how to fulfill the duty of beneficence.

The duty to ***respect patient autonomy,*** a critical consideration in this case, requires that health care providers and families respect the ability of competent patients to hold views, make choices, and take actions based on their personal values and beliefs. In light of his confused state, Mr. Aiken is probably no longer competent to make his own treatment decisions. Mr. Aiken, however, was clear about his values and choices when he communicated to Dr. Long and Johanna his desire not to be ventilated. He completed an advanced directive that explicitly stated this desire.

Patients are identified, in the *Code of Ethics for Nurses,* as the primary decision makers with regard to their own health, treatment, and well-being. Their moral right to refuse treatment and to receive emotional support for their informed choices is further outlined in Interpretive Statements 1.3 and 1.4. Had Mr. Aiken remained competent after his hospitalization, Nurse Kimball would have been responsible to advocate vigorously in support of his refusal of the ventilator. The *Code of Ethics for Nurses* notes that a surrogate decision maker should be designated in situations like this one in which the patient lacks decision-making capacity. Unfortunately, Mr. Aiken did not appoint a legal surrogate for health care decisions. Presumably, he would have designated Johanna for this role, but without a legal designation, Johanna and Alice share decision-making authority.

Although advance directives, when properly witnessed, are legally valid, physicians and hospitals are reluctant to enforce them when they conflict with the decisions of family members. Some have suggested that although patients may make competent decisions when they prepare advanced directives, no one can be certain that they would make the same choices when critical situations arise. As a result, in the absence of a legally appointed surrogate, consensus among competent family members is desirable. Nonetheless, it is appropriate for Mr. Aiken's nurse and doctor to educate Alice about the negative consequences of respiratory therapy in this case and to advise her that use of a ventilator contradicts her father's wishes. It is unlikely that Mr. Aiken, who has lived with this disease for a long time and was well informed about its progression and the relative futility of the ventilator at this stage in COPD, would have changed his mind.

It is understandable that Alice might initially find it difficult to accept her father's decision not to be ventilated. Unlike her sister, she has not observed her father's decline in health. The significant changes in her father's condition may be difficult for her to assimilate. Because she has apparently been estranged from her father for some time, it may be difficult to accept her father's imminent death without further opportunity for reconciliation or closure. Alice needs some time to grieve and to accept her father's condition. Beneficence toward Alice might justify a decision to place Mr. Aiken temporarily on a ventilator to give Alice some time to come to terms with the situation. The decision to withdraw the ventilator could then be revisited in a few days. At that time, Dr. Long, Nurse Kimball, and Johanna should again insist that the ventilator be removed to honor Mr. Aiken's autonomous choice.

The issue of justice also emerges in this scenario. The duty of *justice* requires us to distribute benefits, resources, and burdens fairly. This is a social justice issue—it is primarily a responsibility of society, though nurses have a special role. The *Code of Ethics for Nurses* (Interpretive Statement 8.1) describes this as the responsibility of nurses to collaborate with other health professionals and citizens in promoting community, national, and international efforts to meet the health needs of all people. Nurses are also responsible to work collaboratively with others to ensure a just distribution of nursing and health care resources.

Scientific and technological developments have greatly enhanced the ability of health care professionals to prolong human lives. The ability of individuals and society to pay for these advanced treatments is not unlimited, however. Choices must be made about what research to support and what treatments to include in both government-financed and privately financed health plans. With an increasing number of elderly patients dependent on government-financed health care, decisions about how to fairly distribute societal resources (for health care and other needs) must be made. Presently, 30 percent of all Medicare dollars are spent during the last year of a person's life—most of this is spent in the last month (Hooyman and Gonyea, 1995). Had Mr. Aiken chosen to be placed on a ventilator, many would not regard this as a waste of health care resources. Nonetheless, the ethical issues of how health care dollars will be distributed, who will make these decisions, and through what process must be addressed.

In spite of the tremendous impact and dominance of this four-principle model, we should recognize that it represents merely one possible summary of moral rules relevant to health care. The four principles are general categories that provide a helpful approach to grouping moral rules. Other groupings with different categories are possible. Beauchamp and Childress's (1979/2001) four-principle model has been attractive for a number of reasons, including the ease with which it can be taught to health care professionals. A more important reason is that it has provided a common language for public discussion of health care ethics issues in an increasingly pluralistic culture. An understanding of the early history of health care ethics in America helps to explain the strong attraction of this simplified version of rule ethics.

Emergence of Health Care Ethics

Health care ethics developed as a discipline in the 1960s and 1970s in ~ States, at least a decade earlier than elsewhere. Much like the Enlightenmen~ in Western Europe where rule ethics was born, this was a turbulent time in Ame~ culture. Virtually all institutions and authorities were being questioned. Watergate, the Vietnam War, the civil rights movement, and the women's movement exerted a marked influence on society. Secularism crested as a social movement, shaking the traditions and foundations of religious communities. This was a period of dissension and shifting social consensus about basic values and conceptions of what constitutes a good life.

During this turbulent era, health care institutions were the subject of social criticism as well. In particular, the traditional paternalism and presumed authority of medicine was called into question. Americans who questioned whether governmental authorities should be trusted to serve the best interests of their citizens also questioned whether their health interests should remain in the hands of their health care providers. Widely publicized instances of unethical conduct in medical research fueled public interest in ethical standards in medicine.

At the same time, new technologies dramatically expanded the ability of medicine to intervene, to extend life, and to assist in the reproduction of new life. Dialysis machines, organ transplant techniques, mechanical organ support systems, intensive care units, lifesaving surgeries, and in vitro fertilization created new opportunities and new ethical problems. From the beginning there were socioeconomic issues of access and distribution of these scarce resources. Concerns about the intrusiveness of these interventions quickly followed as the media focused on cases like Karen Quinlan's. With this case Karen's parents, the health care community, and the American legal system struggled to understand the implications of prolonging life for an unconscious brain-injured patient (made possible by new but crude feeding tubes) and to define the rights of patients or their families to make decisions in cases about death and dying. Many ordinary Americans shared in this struggle as a result of unprecedented months of media coverage of the case.

Several factors account for the dominant role of rule ethics in the new field of health care ethics. First, the fragmentation and social upheaval of this period produced an increased pluralism of values. Second, discussion of these ethical issues was multidisciplinary, involving people from medicine, nursing, philosophy, theology, law, sociology, and economics. As a result of these two factors, both public discussions and academic/professional discussions of these emerging ethical issues involved a wide variety of people with diverse backgrounds and values. A third factor was the presidential and congressional appointment of task forces to address these issues. Political pressure led to the need to show the public that something was being done. As a result, those who were charged with developing guidelines and solutions perceived the need for a single, common language and process for resolving moral problems (Fox, 1994; Drane, 2000). Consensus appeared possible by sticking with a rather short list of broad moral rules. Adopting such a list allowed people from a wide variety of philosophical, theological, and cultural backgrounds to discuss moral issues without assuming a shared theoretical foundation.

There is a need for shared language and values in public discussion about health care ethics. The abbreviated rule models like the Beauchamp and Childress model have played a critical role in enabling broad participation of professionals, academics, citizens, patients, and policy makers in ethics discussions. Nonetheless, it is essential for dialogue participants to understand the theoretical foundations of the ethical concepts and language they use. Beauchamp and Childress provide thoughtful and insightful analysis of cases and policies using their model. Their analyses depend on underlying ethical theories, especially utilitarianism and Kantianism, two important rule ethics theories. Frequently, however, their model and other similar models often are employed rather mechanically with little understanding of their theoretical foundations. Nursing codes of ethics may be invoked with a similar lack of understanding. These codes are important statements of professional values and standards. But nurses need to be able to articulate reasons for why they subscribe to these particular rules and standards rather than others.

Disagreements about cases or issues will be impossible to resolve without the ability of dialogue participants to articulate their reasons for how and why they apply rules to specific cases. Similarly, modification or development of rules to address new situations requires an understanding of the theoretical foundations of moral rules. Given the constantly changing nature of the health care environment, this understanding is essential for everyone who makes decisions in this context.

Utilitarianism and Kantianism are the most influential theories of rule ethics in modern moral philosophy and in contemporary health care ethics. This chapter will consider how moral rules are justified and how particular rules are derived from these theoretical foundations. Furthermore, it will explore the social context that gave rise to rule ethics—and promoted the shift from virtue ethics.

Utilitarian and Kantian theories of ethics each begin with a basic, fundamental principle that states the essence of ethics from its theoretical perspective. From this principle, these theories derive action-guiding rules of ethical behavior. These rules are then applied to specific cases in order to make judgments about the right action to take in particular situations. Although there are significant differences in utilitarianism and Kantianism, both theories derive similar sets of moral rules. These rules are grounded in ethical theories that we will now explore, focusing on the four categories of nonmaleficence, beneficence, autonomy, and justice.

The Enlightenment Context

Like all ethical theorists, the authors of utilitarianism and Kantian ethics were thinking, discussing, and writing within a particular historical, cultural context. These two theories of rule ethics clearly reflect their origin in the modern Enlightenment period. This does not make them irrelevant for our contexts; it does mean that we must be aware of their context in order to understand the concepts and principles that they highlight. We must then ask how these are relevant to our contexts and whether any modifications of them are needed in light of our different experiences.

The Enlightenment period was an intellectual movement that celebrated the power and value of individual human reason. Philosophers, politicians, and scientists claimed the right of individuals to think for themselves, to work for themselves, and to govern themselves. Within this historical context, these rights generally applied only to white men. All men were declared equal in virtue of their capacity to reason, to deliberate, and to choose. The Enlightenment was a heady time in which the "common man" threw off the shackles of the religious and intellectual authority of the Church, the political authority of royalty, and the economic authority of feudal lords. Modern science with its emphasis on empirical and quantitative evidence asserted the right of men to explore questions such as why the physical world behaves as it does, what it is made of, and how our world came to be. Individual reason rather than religious institutional authority was celebrated as the arbiter of truth. The rise of nation states and republican forms of government asserted the right of individual men to have their interests represented in the process of governing. Finally, the collapse of feudalism and the rise of capitalism elevated the value of individual effort and ingenuity over social positions due to birth.

Rule-based theories that emerged from this context reflect this rejection of authority due to accidents of birth, inheritance of wealth, or social position. These theories vested moral authority not in kings, feudal lords, or bishops, but in the power of individuals to rationally discover universal truths. The virtue ethics tradition, dominant prior to the emergence of rule ethics, had emphasized the indispensability of a good upbringing, good education, and good mentors in the development of moral judgment and character. To Enlightenment thinkers, this emphasis on education and experience smacked of social privilege and special advantages available only to upper classes. Box 2–1 summarizes the key movements of the Enlightenment context.

Box 2–1   The Enlightenment Context

Themes

1. Challenged authority based on birth, social, or institutional status
2. Celebrated the power of individual human reason

Three Influential Movements

Transition		Result
From	*To*	
Religious authority	Modern science	Emphasis on empirical and quantitative evidence
Feudalism	Capitalism	Individual effort and integrity valued over social status due to birth
Monarchies	Nation states and republican forms of government	Belief that all free men should be able to shape the rules and organizations that govern their lives

In contrast to the virtue ethics tradition, rule ethics emphasized the importance of rational analysis and the logical deduction of conclusions from universal principles. All moral agents begin on an equal footing with regard to moral judgment in rule ethics. The uneven advantages of being born into a respectable family, of having access to a good education, or even of having a generous or courageous disposition were to be mitigated by the distillation of moral judgment into a list of rules. The reasonableness of these rules could be affirmed by all reflective persons, and every rational person could be taught how to apply these rules to concrete situations. Although they differ in other respects, utilitarianism and Kantian ethics share this common vision of a universal ethic based on a common set of moral rules.

Utilitarianism

Utilitarianism begins with the basic insight that acting morally should make our world a better place by increasing human happiness. The classical utilitarians, Jeremy Bentham and John Stuart Mill, believed that the one thing that has value in itself—the one thing that we desire for itself and not as a means to something else—is pleasure. Therefore, they believed that increasing happiness meant maximizing pleasure and minimizing pain. Utilitarianism begins with the *principle of utility:* Actions are right in proportion to their tendency to promote the greatest good for the greatest number of persons affected by these actions.

Thus, for the utilitarians, *consequences* alone are what is important. It is the utility of actions—their likely ability to produce good consequences (pleasure/happiness) and not bad ones (pain/unhappiness)—that is morally relevant for utilitarians. Box 2–2 illustrates this key utilitarian principle.

It is easy to see how utilitarianism supports the rules related to beneficence and nonmaleficence. Beneficence involves acting in ways that benefit others, including both acting to prevent some harm as well as producing positive benefits for others. Clearly, beneficence is a primary obligation of nursing and other health professions. Nurses are committed to acting for the benefit of patients, families, and communities by addressing health needs. Nonmaleficence is a corollary to beneficence: It directs us to refrain from actions that cause harm. This includes not merely avoiding malicious actions that intend to harm, but also exercising due care and caution to avoid causing harm while working to benefit someone. For the utilitarian, it is the consequences that count: A careless disclosure of patient information can be equally as harmful as an intentional disclosure.

Box 2–2   Principle of Utility

Actions are right in proportion to their tendency to promote the greatest good for the greatest number of persons affected by the action.

Beneficence as an ideal in nursing is uncontroversial. In practice, nurses face difficult decisions when conflicts occur. A decision to choose or refuse treatments may appear to be contrary to well-being. Or actions that support patient well-being may conflict with family or community needs. These conflicts will raise important issues about patient autonomy and justice or fairness. Utilitarianism places the rules of autonomy and justice as secondary to and derived from the primary obligation to maximize pleasure and minimize pain.

Bentham as Legal Reformer

Jeremy Bentham (1748–1832) was a social reformer who wanted to remodel the British legal system at a time when the well-established industrial revolution had produced highly stratified social classes. The new industrialists were becoming enormously wealthy at the expense of the working class who worked long hours with dangerous machinery for wages that barely kept their families alive. Workers included children who shared with their parents long days in poorly ventilated, poorly heated, and unsafe workspaces. The risk of loss of fingers, hands, and arms was a daily reality. As a jurist, Bentham saw the consequences of this social hierarchy in the courts. The legal system, accurately and vividly portrayed in Charles Dickens's novels, was corrupt—only those who could afford to buy their legal rights had any legal rights. Those who owed money were kept in debtors' prison until their debts could be paid. Bentham wanted to reform this corrupt system by developing a simple rule and a concrete decision-making procedure that would apply to everyone equally, rich or poor. He outlined a blueprint for reform in his *Introduction to the Principles of Morals and Legislation* (1789/1970).

MAXIMIZING PLEASURE

Bentham wanted a procedure that would be objective. By this he meant that it would be public, measurable, and quantifiable. This ideal inspired Bentham's ***hedonistic calculus,*** a mathematical process for choosing the right actions. All actions were to be evaluated in terms of their ***utility***—how useful they would be in maximizing pleasure. Bentham was not interested in people's motives for acting; he was concerned only with the results or consequences of actions. People's motives are not public: We cannot observe them or measure them. The consequences of actions are public, and, therefore, measurable and quantifiable. If what we ultimately desire is pleasure, then we should measure and quantify the consequences of our actions by measuring the amount of pleasure that our actions produce.

Pleasure, Bentham argued, is the only thing that has intrinsic value and, thus, whatever promotes pleasure has utility—it is useful. Each person's pleasure counts equally; no more weight is given to the pleasure of the rich man who can buy legal favors than to the pleasure of the poor factory worker. Bentham advocated taking the position of impartial, objective observers in making moral decisions. This means that we should consider all the consequences of our actions without regard for whose pleasure is increased or decreased. Every unit of pleasure counts equally whether it is your pleasure, your mother's pleasure, your employer's pleasure, or the mayor's pleasure. Focusing on the objective and measurable consequences of actions defeats attempts by the wealthy to use their money and influence to promote their interests over the equally valid interests of others and exposes any such attempts for all to see. If the anticipated consequences do not support their case, then giving preference to these opportunists will simply be wrong.

Contrary to what is often supposed, utilitarianism is not merely an ethic of self-interest. The utilitarian reformers of nineteenth-century England campaigned for numerous social changes, ranging from the elimination of debtors' prisons and the use of capital punishment for petty thefts to advocacy of public hospitals and proper sewage disposal. The intent was to give weight to every person's pleasure and pain and then to maximize the group welfare. The pleasure and pain of everyone affected by an action must be considered in utilitarianism. It is a demanding ethical theory that not only forbids preferential consideration of special interests, but also requires us to sacrifice our own pleasure for the sake of the greater pleasure of others if necessary to maximize happiness.

Hedonistic Calculus

The hedonistic calculus provided a democratic procedure for determining which of several possible actions would produce the best consequences. For each viable alternative, we must calculate the good and bad consequences of the action for those directly and indirectly affected, including an estimate of the likelihood of their occurring. We then choose the action that is likely to produce the greatest amount of pleasure for the greatest number of persons affected. The procedure sounds simple, but Bentham showed considerable sensitivity for the subtleties of calculating pleasure. He recognized that there are several variables of pleasurable consequences that need quantification. Besides the intensity of pleasure, we must also calculate how long the pleasure will last (duration), the relative immediacy in experiencing pleasure (immediacy), the tendency of an action to continue to produce similarly good or bad consequences (fecundity), the ratio of good to bad results produced by an action (purity), and how widely the effects will be felt (extent). Finally, he instructs us to consider and weigh the relative importance of these factors in a particular situation. We may sometimes prefer deferred pleasure of long duration and high fecundity over an immediate and intense experience of pleasure. But certainly, a life of only delayed gratification would seem to lack a needed balance of spontaneity and playfulness.

Victorian Influences and Mill

Bentham's hedonistic calculus is thoroughly democratic: Not only does each person's pleasure and pain count equally, but each person is allowed to decide what counts as pleasure for him- or herself. One person's preference for Agatha Christie counts equally with another's preference for Shakespeare's *Hamlet*. Bentham's theory is admirably inclusive. Every human being has the right to pursue pleasure and avoid pain, regardless of social standing. In fact, Bentham included in the moral universe all beings, human and nonhuman, who can suffer. This was a remarkably enlightened ethical theory for its time. In the Enlightenment "Age of Reason," Bentham no doubt simply regarded his view as logically consistent. If pleasure is what has intrinsic value, then everyone's experience of pleasure should be equally valued.

The inclusive impulse of utilitarianism is again reflected in the work of Bentham's godson, philosopher and economist John Stuart Mill (1806–1873). Mill's influential book *The Subjection of Women* (1869/1988) was an exposé of the profound inequality in Victorian Britain between men's and women's lives. Mill was the first influential male writer in the modern Western world to advocate for political equality between men and women. Yet, although Mill shared with Bentham a deep commitment to social and political equality, his utilitarianism reflects a cultural elitism. In his book, *Utilitarianism* (1861/1957), Mill introduced a qualitative distinction between types of pleasures. Some pleasures, he claimed, are more valuable or "higher" than others are.

HIGHER AND LOWER PLEASURES

Early critics of Bentham's utilitarianism dismissed it as "the pig's philosophy" because they identified it as mere gratification of physical pleasures. Although Bentham never limited pleasure to the satisfaction of physical desires, Mill seemed anxious nonetheless to reassure his readers that utilitarianism was not merely physical hedonism. He argued that utility should be defined in terms of happiness rather than pleasure. Mill's anxiety probably reflected the fact that his England was moving into the Victorian Era, which frowned on any displayed interest in or enjoyment of physical pleasures.

But Mill's distinction between higher and lower pleasures was more than simply a reflection of his respect for Victorian sensitivities. It also reflected a deep-seated confidence in the value of education. Mill argued that more cultured pleasures, such as those derived from an appreciation of classical music and literature or from solving an intricate logical puzzle, are better than the simple gratification of eating, drinking, or engaging in sex. Bentham would not object if Mill's claims were based on empirical evidence that these cultured pleasures do, in fact, provide quantitatively more pleasure.

Mill's argument, however, seems to be more complex than the simple notion that certain cultural activities produce more pleasure than physical experiences. His famous line, *"It is better to be a human dissatisfied than a pig satisfied, better to be Socrates dissatisfied than a fool satisfied,"* suggests that there is something especially gratifying about the process of engaging in distinctly human activities even if we are not always successful in them. Mill seemed to believe that the very process of striving for truly human experiences is fulfilling. The experiences of learning, of developing an appreciation for finer things, and of achieving something that takes effort and concentration are themselves highly pleasure intensive.

EDUCATING DESIRES

Social equality was as much Mill's goal as it was Bentham's, but Mill believed that it could not be achieved without education of the masses. We should not simply take a vote of people's present preferences. Rather, we should provide everyone with the opportunity to learn to appreciate a wider range of pleasures and to experience the joy of successful efforts. This observation is an important one that probably most would accept. We give similar arguments for mandatory public education.

Nonetheless, if Mill is a consistent utilitarian, he should be willing to allow those who have experienced both higher and lower pleasures to choose which ones are ultimately more pleasure intensive. If you are sufficiently educated to appreciate a wide range of cultural events, but prefer to stay at home and watch televised wrestling matches, then your preference should be valid.

Mill's distinction between higher and lower pleasures can be maintained, while remaining true to the fundamental utilitarian insight that only pleasure has intrinsic value, only if the distinction is, in the end, a matter of intensity. If pleasure is our only measure, then if some pleasures are better than others, it must mean that they are overall quantitatively more pleasure intensive. Furthermore, if education will maximize pleasure overall by expanding our opportunities and capacities for pleasurable experiences, then there are some utilitarian moral grounds for requiring education for all. But once education is attained, Bentham's democratic principle of one person, one vote is the only consistent utilitarian position.

Case Study: The Placebo Effect

We turn now to consider the following case from a utilitarian perspective.

Ms. Reed, a 33-year-old patient with irritable bowel syndrome (IBS), for the last six months has been treated in the outpatient clinic for episodes of abdominal cramping, pain, bloating, and diarrhea, followed by episodes of constipation. She visits the clinic two to six times a month and is well known by the clinic staff. She is considered "difficult" because she is usually upset and hard to please. She has been placed on standard treatment protocols for IBS with little success in treatment. Because she does not improve, she is considered noncompliant about her diet and medication. Drugs utilized in her care are associated with side effects that she does not tolerate and she often asks to be taken off these medications. She is usually anxious, and her anxiety appears to be readily transferred to those around her. She has been treated with high doses of a benzodiazepine, typically a highly addictive anxiolytic medication. Many patients on long-term anxiolytics develop tolerance, needing more of the drug to obtain an effect.

Everyone at the clinic is tired of handling the phone calls from Ms. Reed for her anxiolytic refills. The physician becomes irritated with these requests and often then takes it out on the staff. It was decided that Ms. Reed's anxiety disorder requires a more long-term treatment and that short-acting anxiolytics, like benzodiazepines, were inappropriate. The patient needed to be weaned from the benzodiazepine, however, in order to make the medication change. Every time this was tried with her knowledge, she had a relapse, resulting in her return for her typical dosage. Repetition of this process further increased Ms. Reed's anxiety. The physician and the clinic staff decided that they would tell the patient that they were providing the regular dosage of the medication, but actually they would be reducing the milligrams available. The pharmacist was instructed to leave the dosage off the medication label. The dosage was slowly decreased over time until she was taking only a placebo. When the patient asked why the pills were different, the staff told her that the generic medications differed in shape, color, and size.

During the six years that Terry Devlin, RN, has worked in the clinic, he has provided care for Ms. Reed on several occasions. Although he shares the staff's frustrations in this case, he is uncomfortable with deceiving Ms. Reed. Furthermore, he thinks that it is wrong to charge a patient money for inert pills. He voices his concerns, but other staff feel that Ms. Reed is harmed by her current addiction and that this plan offers a good chance of helping her.

ANTICIPATED CONSEQUENCES

The action to be evaluated in this case is the act of weaning an addicted patient from a prescription drug through the use of a placebo without the patient's knowledge or consent. From a utilitarian perspective, no actions are in themselves right or wrong. Deceiving patients, for instance, is not intrinsically wrong, and telling patients the truth is not intrinsically right. Obtaining the patient's informed consent for the gradual withdrawal of the medication will be the right action only if it is the action that most maximizes happiness in this particular situation.

As we will see, this case has the potential to affect a number of people, even those beyond Ms. Reed and those who care for her. The anticipated good consequences of this action are that Ms. Reed is weaned from an increasingly ineffective and addictive drug, making it possible to try potentially more effective medications for her anxiety disorder. Decreasing her anxiety will have positive benefits for her in managing her IBS as well. Whether the alternative medications will be effective is uncertain, but it is clear that if she remains on the benzodiazepine, Ms. Reed will need increasing doses to get the same effect. Long-term use of anxiolytics will result in serious, negative health effects. The likelihood of successfully weaning Ms. Reed from the medication with her informed consent is very low. The likelihood of successfully weaning her without her knowledge is high. In addition, it is likely that the physician and nursing staff stress level will be reduced as a result of successfully transferring Ms. Reed to the new medication.

One bad consequence of the proposed action is the discomfort of Terry Devlin. Other potential bad consequences are the feelings of betrayal and the resulting undermining of trust that would likely occur if Ms. Reed found out about the deception. It is possible that she would feel relieved if she learned of it after the weaning process was completed, but feelings of betrayal and lost trust seem much more likely. Anger is also a likely response if Ms. Reed discovers the deception. If it is, she is likely to publicize the incident and the clinic would suffer a loss of reputation. Other patients at the clinic might also lose their trust in their health care providers as a result of the publicity. If the weaning process is accomplished gradually, there is little risk that she will experience any withdrawal symptoms and, thus, there is no reason to think that Ms. Reed will discover the deception, making these secondary bad consequences very unlikely.

WEIGHING THE CONSEQUENCES

For simplicity's sake, we will use a 1 to 10 rating system for measuring the good consequences and a -1 to -10 for measuring the bad consequences. The results are summarized in Box 2–3; readers are encouraged to refer to the box as we go along.

Box 2–3   Consequences of Gradual Withdrawal of Ms. Reed from a Benzodiazepine Without Her Knowledge or Consent

Good Consequences	Intensity	Duration	Immediacy	Fecundity	Likelihood	Total
1. Ms. Reed is weaned from ineffective and addictive medication; necessary for transition to more effective medication.	6	6	6	6	× .90 =	21.6
2. Eliminate harmful side health effects of long-term use of anxiolytics.	6	6	6	6	× .90 =	21.6
3. Decrease stress for physician and nursing staff.	5	3	6	5	× .90 =	17.1

Extent: *small*   60.3

Bad Consequences

	Intensity	Duration	Immediacy	Fecundity	Likelihood	Total
1. Discomfort of Terry Devlin	−5	−6	−10	−1	× 1.00 =	−22.0
2. Feelings of betrayal and loss of trust by Ms. Reed if she learns of the deception.	−9	−9	−6	−9	× .01 =	−.33
3. Anger leading to Ms. Reed's publicizing the incident; this would damage reputation of the clinic and undermine trust of other patients.	−9	−9	−6	−9	× .01 =	−.33

Extent of potential consequences: *large*   −22.7
Extent of actual consequences: *small*

Purity of the action: *9*

➤ *Summary of consequences: Good consequences significantly outweigh the bad consequences.*

Intensity: How Strongly the Effect Will Be Felt or Experienced

There are three good consequences to consider. Withdrawal from the benzodiazepine is an essential first step in controlling Ms. Reed's anxiety. Weaning her from this medication also will allow her to avoid harmful side health effects of long-term use of anxiolytics. These two consequences are neither trivial nor the most significant events in Ms. Reed's life. Ms. Reed is likely to experience these effects as having a medium intensity, so we will rate them each as +6. The transition to an alternative medication is likely to produce the third good consequence, the decrease in stress experienced by the physician and nursing staff in interacting with Ms. Reed. This seems a bit less intense than the first two, so we will give it a +5 rating. On the side of bad consequences, Terry Devlin feels mental and emotional discomfort about this action, again at a medium level of intensity. Give it a −5 rating. The potential bad consequences of anger and loss of trust by Ms. Reed would be quite intense, though presumably not the most intense negative experience she might have. The intensity of the effects on other patients and the clinic that would result from publicizing the deception if it is discovered would be similarly high in intensity (imagine a front-page story in the local newspaper). We will rate both of these consequences as −9.

Duration: How Long the Effects Will Be Felt or Experienced

The duration of being weaned and of avoiding further harmful effects of the anxiolytic is rated as medium duration. Each is given a +6 rating. The duration of the effects of reduced stress for the staff may be less enduring since new difficulties with this patient may arise. We will assign a +3 rating. The duration of Terry Devlin's discomfort probably is also medium or −6, while the duration of the potential undermining of trust in Ms. Reed and in other patients is high in duration because recovery from lost trust is a long process. Give each of these a −9 rating.

Immediacy: How Soon the Effects Will Be Felt or Experienced

The good consequences will be experienced within weeks, making the immediacy of each of the good consequences medium or +6. Terry Devlin will feel the discomfort immediately, making this effect a −10, while the immediacy of potential discovery is −6 since it is likely to occur within weeks if it occurs at all.

Fecundity: The Tendency of an Action to Continue to Produce Similar Effects

The importance of fecundity is reflected in the old proverb that "it is better to teach a man how to fish than to feed him." Generally, we prefer actions that will continue to produce further positive effects over one whose effect is limited to its immediate impact. Similarly, we try to avoid negative effects that continue to have a negative rippling effect. Withdrawal from the benzodiazepine will facilitate the further positive effect of using potentially more effective medications to moderate Ms. Reed's anxiety and this in turn would have positive benefits for her IBS. Fecundity for the weaning is thus +6. In addition, continued long-term use of the benzodiazepine will produce harmful side effects. Thus, withdrawal from this drug will avoid the medium fecundity, +6, of these bad effects. Decreasing stress for the physician and nursing staff will have some rippling effect in terms of better focus and increased efficiency, which will promote better patient care. Let's rate this as +5.

On the other side, the undermining of trust that would occur if the deception were discovered would likely spread to other health care relationships for Ms. Reed and other patients who learn of the incident. Fecundity for this bad effect is high; we assign a −9 for Ms. Reed and −9 for other patients. There does not seem to be any significant ripple effect from Terry Devlin's discomfort, so the fecundity for this effect is low or −1.

At this point, we can add up the numbers for each consequence to determine our estimate of total pleasure units and pain units. For the good consequences, we have 24, 24, and 19 units. For the bad consequences, we have −22, −33, and −33 units.

Likelihood: How Likely It Is That These Consequences Will Occur

Now we need to consider the likelihood of each consequence. If the benzodiazepine is withdrawn slowly, it is very likely that Ms. Reed will be weaned successfully and that she will avoid the further harmful effects of long-term use of this drug. Let us say that there is a 90 percent (or .90) chance of each of these consequences occurring. The likelihood of reduced physician and staff stress levels is also very high. If Ms. Reed is successfully transferred to a more effective medication, the staff stress is nearly certain to go down. Because this consequence depends on the first two, we will assign a 90 percent chance of occurrence to this third consequence as well. Thus, for each good consequence, we multiply the total pleasure units of that consequence by its chance of occurring. Box 2–3 shows that the total result for the good consequences is a total of 60.3 pleasure units.

The same process is applied to the bad consequences. It is certain that Terry Devlin will experience discomfort if the placebo is used without Ms. Reed's knowledge, so likelihood here is a 100 percent (or 1.00) chance of occurrence. On the other hand, since there is such a small chance that the deception will be discovered, the feelings of betrayal, loss of trust, and anger resulting in negative publicity are very unlikely to occur. Likelihood here is a 1 percent (or .01) chance of occurrence. This is a critical point since these latter effects would be high in intensity, duration, and fecundity for Ms. Reed and other patients. But because their likelihood is so low, these potential consequences will have little weight in our assessment of this action. Box 2–3 shows that the total units for this action are −22.7.

Extent: How Many People Will Be Affected by This Action

Our estimate so far is that the action of withdrawing Ms. Reed from the benzodiazepine without her knowledge will produce 60.3 pleasure units and −22.7 pleasure units (or 22.7 pain units). Now we must consider the extent of this action: how widely these pleasure and pain units will be distributed. This action will positively affect only Ms. Reed, her physician, and the clinic nurses. The effects on each of these persons are already included in our calculations of the good consequences. On the negative side, we have calculated the intensity, duration, and so on of the loss of trust and the negative publicity if the deception is discovered. But if the deception is discovered, the extent of these feelings would be large. The clinic may serve several thousand people, and other patients who do not use this clinic may be distressed when they read about this news as well. Clinic staff may suffer also from the damage done to the clinic's reputation. Thus, the −22.7 units would be multiplied by this large number of affected people. If 5,000 patients experienced a loss of trust as a result of this deception, the negative units would quickly increase to −113,500, demonstrating the significance of the extent of the effects. But because, in this case, the chances of discovery seem very slim, the *actual* extent of the pain being experienced will likely be limited to the one nurse who experiences mental and emotional discomfort.

Purity: The Ratio of Good to Bad Effects Produced by This Action

Many actions will produce mixed results—some good consequences and some bad ones. Bentham's point here is that we may care not only about whether an action produces more good than bad consequences overall, but we may also wish to consider how mixed the results are. We might prefer an action with fewer net good consequences but a high purity rating, than one that produces more net good consequences but has many undesirable, bad side effects. The messiness of an action that produces considerable "collateral damage" is itself a negative consequence. We may have won the battle, so to speak, but we made a lot of enemies in the process. The use of the placebo without Ms. Reed's knowledge is not pure because there are both good and bad consequences. But since most of the bad consequences are unlikely to occur, we will give this action a high rating, +9, on purity. The purity rating is not directly added on to the total pleasure and pain units. When the projected results of alternative actions are considered, the purity ratings of each action will be compared to each other. If the total amount of net pleasure produced is roughly the same, we will prefer the action with the highest purity rating.

SUMMARY OF CONSEQUENCES

As Box 2–3 summarizes, the good consequences outweigh the bad ones. The decisive factor is the relatively low risk that Ms. Reed or other patients will discover the deception. The consequences of discovery would be significant, and if the risk were high, these combined with the known negative feelings of Terry Devlin would outweigh the positive benefits. But because the risk is low, the known positive benefits of weaning Ms. Reed from the benzodiazepine and the likely improvement in managing her anxiety clearly outweigh the known bad consequence and the low risk of other consequences.

We need to repeat this analysis for other actions that would be realistic alternatives. It is not enough to determine that one alternative action will produce more good than bad consequences. The principle of utility requires us to *maximize* utility: to choose that action that will produce the *most* good (or the least bad, if none produces more good than bad) among those available. Since previous attempts to wean Ms. Reed with her permission have failed, there are few good alternatives in this case. One alternative might be to develop a plan with Ms. Reed that would encourage her to permit the staff at some point to begin the withdrawal process. Ms. Reed would not know when this would begin—only that the medication would be gradually decreased at some point in the future. Given the level of Ms. Reed's anxiety, this plan may have little hope of success, but it would allow the patient to be a collaborator in her care plan.

You may be uncomfortable with this justification of the deliberate deception of a patient. Perhaps you feel that something still seems missing in this utilitarian assessment of this action. Let us consider some of the problems with the analysis.

PROBLEM: MEASURING CONSEQUENCES

This case analysis reveals some problems with the hedonistic calculus. First, you may challenge the numerical ratings. You may have wanted to assign different ratings in some cases. How, after all, do we quantify pleasure and pain? This is an important concern, especially in light of the fact that Bentham and Mill were both committed to developing a public decision-making procedure that would guide social reform. They wanted a procedure by which communities could determine public policies. The pleasures and pains of all citizens would be given equal weight. It was not that difficult to assign values in the case above since what was important was the *relative* value of the ratings—is this pleasure more, less, or about the same as the pain in each category? However, it would be difficult to tabulate these relative rankings for large groups of decision makers.

We need a common yardstick to apply to our measurement of consequences. But no such yardstick of pleasure units exists. This realization should not lead us to immediately dismiss the utilitarian approach. As difficult as it is to assign values to pleasure and pain, we do it in practice all the time. We personally weigh the pros and cons of alternative choices of action on a daily basis. Nurses prioritize their patients' needs in order to allocate their time among several needy patients. They regularly make similar calculations about their personal and professional time and resources. Groups who cooperate and share resources similarly make frequent utilitarian assessments of benefits and burdens. Work assignments, budgets, and policy making all reflect these kinds of calculations. We must conclude that we do assign values to benefits and burdens on a regular basis. This process of decision making, however, is almost certainly not as objective as Bentham and Mill envisioned.

PROBLEM: PREDICTING CONSEQUENCES

Another difficulty with the utilitarian calculus is our ability to predict consequences. The morally right thing to do for a utilitarian is that action that will maximize happiness. Often, however, we cannot imagine all of the consequences of our actions. Also, as in the case above, we can imagine that Ms. Reed may become suspicious about the changes in her medication and that she might uncover the deception, but it is difficult to estimate accurately the likelihood of this occurring. It is also difficult to predict what will happen once she is removed from the benzodiazepine, whether she will tolerate and respond well to alternative medications. But utilitarianism asks for no more than any other ethical theory—make your best judgment. We are responsible only for the reasonably foreseeable consequences of our actions and not for the unforeseeable ones.

One further problem should be noted. This is the difficulty of determining another person's pleasure or happiness. Your values, what is pleasurable to you, will bias your ability to assess the effects of possible actions on others. This will again be a significant problem when people try to choose actions that will affect many other persons, especially if they are not personally known by the decision makers. Once again, we see that the utilitarian calculus is not as objective as Bentham and Mill's ideal.

Accounting for Obligation: Act Versus Rule Utilitarianism

Bentham and Mill may adequately handle the problems of measurement and prediction. But some see a deeper problem in the placebo case above. In spite of the fact that the good consequences in this case clearly outweighed the bad consequences, some may be left feeling that Bentham's calculus lacks some essential moral consideration. Some suggest that a sense of obligation is missing. In the placebo case, the nurse who feels that an implicit obligation to informed consent was being violated expresses this. Even if it turns out that Ms. Reed makes a successful transition to new medication and her anxiety improves as a result, Terry Devlin would probably still feel that an implicit promise to this patient was broken. Most people believe that keeping one's obligations is an essential element of what we mean by being moral.

Utilitarian theorists in the twentieth century have responded to this concern through a major modification of classical utilitarianism. The classical formulation of Bentham and Mill, which require us to evaluate each singular action, was revised to require evaluation of rules governing types of actions. This formulation is called *rule utilitarianism* because it evaluates a rule for types of situations considering the consequences if everyone lived in accordance with this rule. Instead of evaluating the consequences of the act of lying in a specific situation, for example, a rule utilitarian evaluates the consequences of everyone's following a particular rule about lying. Nearly all twentieth-century utilitarians have advocated rule utilitarianism over what is now referred to as *act utilitarianism*. Rule utilitarianism modifies the principle of utility to reflect the shift from evaluating individual actions to evaluating rules. Box 2–4 illustrates this revised principle. Note again that it is not enough to demonstrate that a rule will produce a positive ratio of pleasure to pain. The rule we adopt should be the rule predicted to produce the *greatest* such ratio of pleasure to pain.

One might think that rule utilitarianism is preferable merely on timesaving grounds. However, rule utilitarianism is motivated by a much more profound intuition about morality than mere time efficiency. Bentham acknowledged that over time we observe that one type of action generally promotes utility more effectively than alternatives. And he recognized that most daily actions would be guided by past experiences. Thus, only situations that are unusual or complex require a detailed analysis

Box 2–4   Revised Principle of Utility

Rules of action are right in proportion to their tendency to promote the greatest good for the greatest number of persons affected by these rules.

of consequences. Rule utilitarianism is primarily motivated by the need to account for our sense of moral obligation. The following admittedly contrived example will illustrate this point.

Suppose that you are stranded on a deserted island with one other person. This person develops pneumonia and is dying. In her last hours, she describes to you her passion for bird-watching and asks you to promise that if you are rescued, you will see that her $2 million estate is given to the Audubon Society. You promise to fulfill her request, and soon thereafter you are rescued. When back in your familiar environment, however, you begin to reconsider your promise to the dying woman. After careful consideration, you conclude that deserted island deathbed promises are for the birds and $2 million could provide prenatal care for a lot of pregnant women. You ignore your promise and instead use the money to endow such a program. Surely, an act utilitarian cannot argue with this decision. The dead woman cannot feel harm. No one else will know that the promise was broken, so there are no negative consequences. You will maximize happiness in this particular case by breaking your promise. But many may feel that something important is lost in the act utilitarian analysis because it attributes no value to promise keeping or the sense of being obligated by a promise.

THE UTILITY OF RULES

The rule utilitarian would argue that although in this case breaking a promise increases overall happiness, generally, the practice of keeping promises does promote happiness. Instead of evaluating each individual action, the rule utilitarian evaluates a rule that will guide a *type* of action—in this case, promise keeping. We must ask whether a society in which everyone followed the rule "Keep uncoerced promises" would maximize happiness more than one in which people followed the rule "Keep uncoerced promises only when it maximizes happiness in a particular case." A society in which keeping promises is contingent on changing circumstances would be a chaotic, unpredictable place to live and not one in which happiness is maximized. An absolute rule that required promise keeping no matter what, however, probably would not maximize happiness either. We can readily imagine a situation in which a promise should be broken in order to produce a greater good. For instance, a nurse stops to provide emergency care, which results in breaking a promise to meet a friend for dinner. Our rule can be revised to require us to "Keep uncoerced promises except to avoid great disaster such as loss of life."

REASSESSING THE PLACEBO CASE

Let us reconsider the placebo case from a rule utilitarian perspective. The rule utilitarian will not consider the positive and negative consequences of this *individual action* as we did previously. Instead, the rule utilitarian will note that this is a case about providing patients with relevant information about possible treatments and fostering adequate decision making. The ethical issue is then to determine what rule(s) concerning informed consent will maximize happiness if everyone follows this rule. Ethical rules will be public rules: They are derived from a communal conversation of rational persons, and they are publicized as the ethical rules that have been agreed on by this community. This is a critical factor in the placebo case in which withdrawal from the medication is done secretly without patient consent. A rule utilitarian considers what rule regarding informed consent would be adopted by rational persons who understand that everyone will know this rule.

Certainly, a rule such as "Treat a patient without consent whenever it will benefit the patient" will not maximize utility. This rule would breed patient insecurity and undermine trust between patients and health care providers. These consequences would have disastrous long-term effects on patient care. Effective patient care critically depends on patients' confidence that they will be kept informed and allowed to make decisions about their own care. The days of medical paternalism are not far behind us. Patient trust is fragile and must be nurtured through reliable actions.

Rule utilitarians will adopt a rather strict rule regarding informed consent, such as: "It is impermissible to treat competent patients without their adequately informed consent." This rule is generally believed to be exceptionless. In some other cases, exceptions are considered justified to maximize happiness. For instance, society's interest in prosecuting criminals justifies the sacrifice of patient confidentiality in order to report gunshot wounds. This exception is built into the rule (see Box 2–7); it is not an exception that will be determined by individual practitioners.

A rule utilitarian may sympathize with the staff's desire to help Ms. Reed, but would oppose the use of the gradual withdrawal of the medication without her consent. Even though treatment without the patient's consent in this particular case would maximize pleasure, the rule utilitarian argues that adhering to the strict rule of informed patient consent will maximize greater pleasure overall in the long run.

The Problem of Justice

We have stressed Bentham and Mill's commitment to a democratic decision procedure in which each pleasure unit counts regardless of whose pleasure it is. As admirable as this is, many critics of utilitarianism believe that it does not go far enough, that both act and rule utilitarianism lack an adequate account of justice. *Justice* requires us to give each person his or her due; it requires the fair distribution of a community's resources and burdens. Utilitarianism allows us to maximize pleasure or happiness for a community by treating some people very badly. Because individuals have no intrinsic value (only pleasure does) and no rights that guarantee fundamental freedoms or minimum welfare, the pain of some individuals may be traded off for the greater total pleasure of others. No individual's interests are excluded from the decision process, but the collective interests of others may simply outweigh his or her well-being. Such an approach clearly fails to provide for the fair and equitable treatment of all persons that justice requires since some individuals will bear a disproportionate share of burdens.

INJUSTICE IN HEALTH CARE

The history of health care ethics includes several instances wherein the health of a few was deliberately sacrificed to benefit a greater number of others. One famous example occurred in the 1950s and 1960s at the Willowbrook Institution in New York State.

Mentally retarded children at this institution were isolated in a special medical unit and injected with hepatitis cells to enable researchers to study the disease in a controlled environment. The goal was to develop a vaccine. Immunity-boosting gamma globulin was regularly administered to the staff, but withheld from these children. The U.S. Army, with its own special interest in controlling hepatitis, was a major funder of this research. The research proposal was reviewed and approved by a prestigious group of medical schools and state medical agencies (Krugman and Giles, 1983).

If the Willowbrook study was well designed and if there was a reasonable chance of developing a new vaccine, then it is difficult to see how utilitarianism could do anything but support and, in fact, require us to perform the study. The researchers and the Willowbrook administrators justified their support for the project by arguing that the children would inevitably contract hepatitis in the institution anyway since it was rampant there, that by participating in the study the children would receive better medical care through the course of their illness, and that the children's parents gave consent (Edsall, 1983). This self-serving justification ignores the facts that systematic cleaning and sanitation throughout the institution combined with gamma globulin could have significantly reduced the incidence of hepatitis. Also, the parents had few or no alternatives for their children. The interests of a vulnerable population, entrusted to the state's care, were considered expendable in the Willowbrook study.

MILL'S SOLUTION

Aware of the utilitarian problem of justice, Mill discussed it in *Utilitarianism* in a section called "On the Connection Between Justice and Utility." He recognized that a society in which a majority abuses a minority is not a good society, arguing that in the long run abusive practices would undermine overall happiness in society. Mill advocated treating people as if they have intrinsic value and individual rights because this would maximize happiness in the society. This argument encourages rules such as "Individuals should not participate in nontherapeutic research unless they give informed and voluntary consent." Justification for these rules is like that for all rule utilitarian rules: If everyone follows these rules, they will maximize happiness in this society.

In many cases, Mill's empirical claim seems not to be true. There do seem to be many instances in which sacrificing the interests of a minority does benefit many others. For instance, the money spent on research for some rare diseases, which affect only a small percentage of the population and are expensive to treat, could instead fund a lot of basic health care for many. Or the money spent on education for children with significant learning disabilities could buy resources for many other children. Thus, a rule such as "Every person should receive a fair share of health care resources" does not seem to produce the greatest overall happiness in society.

But Mill's argument is subtler. He argued that a society that treats all individuals as if they have intrinsic value and basic rights provides a level of security that is itself very pleasure intensive. A society that guarantees that your basic individual needs and interests will not be traded off for the greater benefit of a group of other persons frees you from being constantly on guard to protect your safety and well-being. This frees you to pursue those more pleasure-intensive cultural activities that Mill so valued. In short, a society in which citizens participate in education, science, the arts, politics, and religion will be a much happier, more fruitful society than one in which citizens invest the bulk of their energies in simply protecting themselves from harm.

FATAL FLAW?

This argument goes a long way toward solving the utilitarian problem of justice. As insightful and powerful as it is, however, we must note that the claim made is still merely an empirical one. In many parts of the world today, basic civil rights have been suspended by ruling elites on the grounds that it is essential for the government to enforce political stability so that these countries can attract needed multinational investments in their economies. Political dissent and freedom of speech and of assembly are regarded as luxuries that these countries cannot afford given their economic conditions. Even the use of intimidation and torture is justified on these utilitarian grounds. Whether these claims are empirically true or not is beside the point, because when individual rights rest solely on empirical claims of utility, individuals are vulnerable to the calculations of those in power. Many theorists regard utilitarianism's lack of an adequate account of justice as a fatal flaw in the theory. Other advocates of utilitarianism acknowledge that its theory of justice is inadequate, but believe that utilitarianism is nonetheless overall the best account of ethics.

Individual Autonomy

Mill used similar arguments to defend the importance of *autonomy* or, as he called it, individual liberty. The issue is what freedom individuals should have to make choices based on their own personal values and beliefs. It is surprising that the same theorist, who denies that individuals have any individual rights or intrinsic value, also offers one of the strongest defenses of individual liberty. Mill, in his essay *On Liberty* (1859/1973), defended what he called the "harm principle." This principle states that others, especially governments, may interfere with the actions of an individual only to prevent harm to others. Interference with the actions of competent adults by others cannot be justified by claims that such interference is for the individual's own good, either physical or moral. Others may reason with, persuade, remonstrate, or entreat the individual to change his or her behavior, but unless the conduct will harm others, interference is unjustified. Others sometimes must attempt to dissuade an individual when his or her views are false or ill conceived. A nurse, for instance, would be obligated to reason with a competent patient who refuses surgery for the amputation of a gangrenous leg, believing that he cannot live in this world as a man with one leg. The nurse can provide accurate information, provide emotional support for the patient's fears, and offer resources that may help to imaginatively expand this patient's vision. But, in the end, the nurse must respect the patient's own assessment of his well-being and his treatment choice.

Mill supports his position on individual liberty with two claims: (1) that individuals are in the best position to assess their interests, and (2) that the process of shaping their lives and developing according to their own convictions is itself extremely pleasure intensive. A society that strictly observes the harm principle, therefore, will maximize utility. Like his arguments regarding justice, Mill's position depends on empirical claims that are at least sometimes questionable.

While recognizing the vulnerabilities of utilitarianism, we may draw from this theory a regard for the importance of consequences and the intuition that being moral should make us better off. Utilitarianism continues to be used widely in contemporary society, especially at the level of public policy making.

Kantian Ethics

Kantian ethics, like utilitarianism, begins with a basic principle and derives rules from it that guide actions. Immanuel Kant (1724–1804) was the most influential modern deontologist. His ethics is referred to as ***deontological*** because it emphasizes what we are supposed to *do* (from the Greek, *deon*, meaning *duty*). While utilitarianism advances the belief that only the utility of actions has intrinsic value, Kant believed that some actions are in themselves right or wrong and not simply because of their consequences. In fact, Kant took the rather extreme view that some ethical rules should never be broken regardless of the consequences. Most contemporary deontologists argue that since ethical rules are intended to protect and benefit human beings, even the most basic ethical rules may need to be broken in unusual circumstances to avert major human catastrophes. In all but very extreme cases, however, deontologists regard respect for individual human beings as taking priority over maximizing happiness.

Kant's ethical theory reflected the optimistic confidence in the objectivity of human reason and the value of individual autonomy, which was characteristic of the Enlightenment. His basic principle, summarized in Box 2–5, is one of universal respect for all persons.

From this principle, duties not to harm and duties to help all human beings can be derived. It is difficult to overestimate the influence of Kant's ethics in Western cultures. Recognizing persons as autonomous beings, capable of deliberation and choice, rationally demands that we treat them as worthwhile in themselves. Kant described this as treating persons as "ends-in-themselves," rather than as mere means to other persons' ends as the children at Willowbrook were. This core Kantian insight has had a profound impact on Western moral, political, and legal traditions. Furthermore, it has been absolutely central in modern health care ethics.

Box 2–5   *Principle of Universalized Respect*

Act always so that you respect every human being, yourself and others, as a *rational* being (Donagan, 1977).

Kant's Categorical Imperative

Unlike utilitarianism, wherein one's motives are irrelevant and only consequences matter, in Kant's ethics, motives are everything. An action is morally good and praiseworthy only if it is done from a sense of duty, or what Kant calls a "good will." It is not enough to do the right thing; it must be done because the one who acts believes that this action is morally right and that it is, therefore, his or her duty. Kant proposes a test for determining whether our will is good or whether an action is our duty. The test that he outlines, called the *Categorical Imperative,* has two requirements that he discussed in his book *Groundwork of Metaphysics of Morals* (1785/1964).

UNIVERSALIZATION

The first requirement is that when we are considering an action we must ask whether we can imagine our intentions for an action as a general rule for everyone. This is the requirement of *universalization:* Could my intention be stated as a principle—or maxim, as Kant called it—that could be generalized to apply to all cases of the same kind? Kant's examples of universalization emphasize the need for logical consistency. For instance, Kant argues that you could not will that you be allowed to lie when it serves your interests while, at the same time, willing that all other people tell the truth even when it is to their disadvantage to do so.

Kant's argument here is not the utilitarian one that a lie will be effective only if people can generally assume that others are telling the truth. Utilitarians note that if we all agree to lie when it suits us and we all know that this is going to happen, then we will stop trusting each other and our attempts to get away with a lie will not work. But Kant's argument is not about the bad consequences of universalizing our intention to lie. Rather, his argument is that it is logically inconsistent to apply one rule to yourself and a different rule to other persons. Logical consistency is a requirement that rational people impose on their own actions. Kant concluded that the universalization of our moral maxims is also then a requirement that we impose on ourselves simply because we are rational beings.

How exactly we should understand and apply Kant's Categorical Imperative is controversial among Kant scholars. But it is clear that one of the basic insights behind the Categorical Imperative is the claim that we cannot make arbitrary exceptions for our own actions. This is consistent with one of our first moral lessons about fairness. Parents encourage their children to think about fairness when they ask a child to stop and consider "How would you feel if your brother or sister did that to you?". This simple lesson encourages children to universalize their actions—to imagine that their actions are open to assessment by any rational person. Would that person see the action as one that says "what's fair for me is fair for you"? Or would that person see an action that says "my interests and preferences count more than yours"? Fairness is a consistency requirement that is embodied in Kant's requirement of universalization.

Of course, some exceptions to rules are legitimate. Ambulances should be allowed to run red lights, surgeons should be allowed to cut into abdomens with a knife to remove inflamed appendices, and nurses should be allowed to spend more time with a patient in critical condition than with one whose condition is stable. However, these are all exceptions that we expect *any* rational person to recognize as legitimate. The ambulance rushing to the hospital is in a different situation than the driver who is merely anxious to get to work. Their different situations deserve different considerations. We can still say that drivers generally should not run red lights, while allowing exceptions that are of the same kind as the ambulance, that is, a life-saving kind. Our maxim would then be that "Drivers should not run red lights unless it is necessary to save a life." This maxim can be universalized and, thus, passes this first requirement of Kant's Categorical Imperative test.

RESPECT FOR PERSONS AND AUTONOMY

The second requirement of the Categorical Imperative is one of *respect for persons.* To be morally praiseworthy, the maxim of your action must not only be universalizable to all persons in the same type of situation, but it must also contain the intention to show respect for all persons as rational beings.

The Moral Value of Rationality

Without doubt, Kant was an Enlightenment man who reveled in the power and potential of human reason. But why did he think that our rationality is morally relevant? Why does the fact that beings have the capacity for reasoning make them valuable and deserving of respect? Is it simply that reasoning ability is what makes human beings unique? If so, this may seem rather self-serving. (Today, we are beginning to appreciate that dolphins and whales may have similarly complex reasoning capacities.) Does the fact that other living beings have unique characteristics make them objects of respect as well? Kant tells us to respect others and ourselves *as rational beings.* Should we then respect horses and lions as swift and graceful beings or bats as echo-locating beings? Do their unique characteristics endow these animals with a morally relevant value? What *moral* value does human rationality have? We can see how Kant answered this by looking at what he thought it meant to treat rational beings with respect.

One formulation of the Categorical Imperative, which Kant provides in *Groundwork of Metaphysics of Morals* (1964, p. 96), is the following:

> Act in such a way that you always treat humanity, whether in your own person or in the person of any other, never simply as a means but always at the same time as an end.

This formulation suggests that treating rational persons with respect means that we treat them as "ends" and never as mere "means." An end is a goal or something that is valued for itself rather than valued only as a means to another goal or value that motivates a person's action. Kant thought that human rationality had moral value precisely because their capacity for rationality makes human beings capable of being goal setters. Rationality enables human beings to deliberate about what actions to take and about what ends or goals are worth pursuing. Our behavior is not simply the result of instincts, biological conditioning, or learned responses to environmental stimuli. We are capable of choosing our goals and not merely following ones that are imposed on us by nature or environmental conditioning. If we are capable of deliberating, choosing our ends, and determining actions consistent with these ends, then it is also appropriate for us to be held accountable for these choices and actions.

Persons As Mere Means

This is exactly what it means to be a moral agent. Ethics is the process of reflecting and deliberating about what has value, what end is worth pursuing and how it should be pursued. A moral agent is someone who is capable of entering into this process of reflection and deliberation and, then, of being held accountable for his or her actions. This is why Kant thinks that rationality is morally relevant. It is what makes human beings capable of moral reflection and action. This is what gives us value and makes us "ends" deserving of respect. When we treat people simply as "means," we deny them the respect that they deserve as deliberators, goal setters, or moral agents. In fact, it means that we act as if they have no goals or values of their own, but instead that their value is merely their usefulness in helping truly autonomous beings to achieve their own goals.

We have all likely experienced both being "used" and using others as mere means. Service roles especially lend themselves to this treatment. It is not wrong, of course, for others to expect those in service jobs to do their jobs. But bosses, customers, and patients can sometimes forget that secretaries, clerks, and nurses are more than just providers of service. When they do forget, they treat these people as mere means to their own ends. If we treat our secretaries as mere means, we treat them like Xerox machines that exist solely to serve our production needs. We fail to remember that they are also agents who are capable of deliberation and goal choosing. This is, in fact, why many employees feel alienated from their daily work when they are not invited to be part of the process of choosing goals and the effective means to achieve them. They are simply assigned tasks and expected to carry them out. Kant regards treating people this way as demeaning and immoral.

Human beings have an absolute value, according to Kant, because of their ability to reason and, on the basis of this, their ability to choose actions. This, Kant suggests, is the basis of human dignity. Each human being is unique and is, therefore, irreplaceable. One human being cannot be substituted for another or traded off for another. The unique, intrinsic value of each human being imposes limits on the means that we may choose to pursue our goals. We may never violate the autonomy of any rational human being as a means to achieving other goals, even if these goals are themselves for the benefit of other human beings. On the other hand, we must also recognize that there are limits on individual autonomy: Individuals may not exercise their autonomy in ways that cause significant harm to others.

Sadly, the history of medicine, is filled with examples of exactly this. In the Willowbrook case, the mentally retarded children were deliberately harmed in order to benefit other, "less expendable" human beings. Before the institutionalization of informed consent, the autonomy of many patients was violated in the interests of training health care personnel or advancing medical knowledge. Medical interns routinely performed multiple pelvic exams on women anesthetized for surgery, without their knowledge or consent. Indigent patients were frequently used to test new drugs or procedures that had no therapeutic value for these patients, again without their consent and, sometimes, without their knowledge. The case study of the deceptive use of a placebo with Ms. Reed suggests that all such violations of patient autonomy have not disappeared today.

Obligations Related to Autonomy

For Kant, respect is a feeling, but it is most of all a way of acting required by the Categorical Imperative. An action will be moral if it satisfies the tests of universalization and respect for persons. Most importantly, respect for persons *as rational beings* requires that we do not take away the conditions of their moral agency or autonomy. Autonomy is the ability to choose one's own actions based on relevant information. It is easy to see why lying, deception, withholding relevant information, and paternalistic treatment of autonomous patients are all fundamentally wrong from this perspective. It should also be clear why informed consent and the right of patients to refuse treatment have been recognized in contemporary health care as basic patient rights. Ensuring privacy and confidentiality are two other moral obligations that respect for autonomy prescribes. Respecting patients (and colleagues) as autonomous decision makers includes respecting the decisions these persons make about what information they wish to provide about themselves, for whom, and for what purposes.

PRINCIPLES OF UNIVERSALIZED RESPECT

Kant did not attempt to summarize his ethical theory into the four principles of autonomy, nonmaleficence, beneficence, and justice, which are ubiquitous in contemporary rule-based bioethics. But, as noted earlier, the rules derived from Kant's principle of universalized respect can be grouped into these four categories. We have already seen that respect for autonomy is inherent in Kant's basic principle of universalized respect for persons. We will briefly discuss the other three categories and note the distinction that Kant makes between "perfect" and "imperfect" duties.

Nonmaleficence

The injunction to "do no harm" has been the most basic principle in the history of health care ethics. It is easily derived from Kant's basic principle of universalized respect. Because human beings have intrinsic value and dignity, we demonstrate respect for this value by taking care not to harm these persons. The category of nonmaleficence will include rules that prohibit killing, physical and emotional harm, negligence, stealing, sexual exploitation, and breaking promises or contracts.

Beneficence

The provision of health care is as fundamentally tied to beneficence as it is to nonmaleficence. Health care professionals commit themselves to the care of the sick and to the promotion of health. Our duty of universalized respect for persons implies that we all have duties to promote the well-being of others as well as our own well-being. This duty follows both from our recognition that each human being has intrinsic value and from our recognition that physical and mental health is a necessary foundation to our autonomy. Healthy bodies and minds enable us to pursue our chosen goals.

Patients do not have an unlimited obligation to promote their own well-being. Neither is the obligation of health care providers to promote their patients' well-being unlimited. Kant distinguished two kinds of duties, perfect and imperfect (1964, p. 91; 1797/1964, pp. 48–53). *Perfect duties* must be observed at every opportunity. These are duties not to harm. Every time that we have the opportunity to murder, rape, steal, deceive, and so on, we have an obligation not to do so. On the other hand, *imperfect duties* are duties that we are obligated to perform, but the time and manner are more open. These are duties of benevolence and self-development. For example, as you leave a department store during the holidays, the Salvation Army bell ringer may not grab your scarf and bark "Fulfill your duty of benevolence. Put some money in the kettle." You do have an ongoing duty of benevolence, but you are not obligated to be benevolent at every opportunity. Some choice about how and when is permitted. Benevolence is a duty as long as there are others who need help, but you are permitted to make choices about where you will invest your time, effort, and money. A rational, responsible person will not overlook grave and urgent needs for trivial ones. In some cases, you will be obligated to help a person, here and now. If the need is urgent, if you have the ability to help and no other help is available, and if the cost of helping would not be too great, then you are obligated in a particular situation to give help.

Respect for persons requires that we do our part to give aid to others and to ourselves, but there are some limitations. The first is that we may not violate a perfect duty in order to fulfill an imperfect one. Consequently, it is impermissible to intentionally lie, deceive, exploit, or physically or emotionally harm an innocent person (one not threatening any other person) in order to give help to that person or other persons. The researchers at the Willowbrook Institution clearly violated their perfect duty not to harm its residents when they intentionally infected children with hepatitis as a means to potentially benefit others. Less dramatic but equally significant violations of perfect duties may occur as a result of misguided attempts by health care professionals and families to protect patients. Consider the following case:

> Mr. Gahn, 79, is in your care following an episode of angina. He is alert and talks of being discouraged because he feels so tired recently. He lives with his son and daughter-in-law, Jeb and Stacie. Dr. Bender has told them that Mr. Gahn's angina is well managed, but that recent tests she reviewed revealed untreatable pancreatic cancer. Jeb informs the physician that his father is planning to leave with a friend of his on a Caribbean cruise in two weeks. It is a trip that his father has dreamed of taking for many years. Mr. Gahn and his friend have been planning this trip for two years. Jeb and Stacie ask the physician if Mr. Gahn is strong enough to make the trip. Dr. Bender states that he is. The couple begs the physician not to tell Mr. Gahn about the cancer until he returns from the trip, saying that it would be a huge disappointment if he could not go, and receiving the news about his cancer will certainly ruin the trip for him. Dr. Bender thinks that Mr. Gahn should have an accurate diagnosis of his condition and be free to make his own decisions about how he will spend his remaining time. But Jeb and Stacie persist in their request that he not be told. The physician reluctantly agrees to abide by the family's wishes and instructs the nurse to do so as well. She agrees not to reveal the cancer diagnosis to Mr. Gahn.

Jeb and Stacie clearly believe that withholding the truth about Mr. Gahn's condition is in his best interests. Although the physician is not so sure that it is, she goes along with the family's request and the nurse follows suit. For Kant, this is a violation of Mr. Gahn's autonomy. Jeb and Stacie presume to substitute their judgments for Mr. Gahn's. In doing so, they deny him both the respect that he is due as a competent adult and also the opportunity to use his remaining time as he judges most appropriate. For their part, the physician and nurse respect the family's autonomous choice at the expense of their patient's autonomy. Consequently, although Jeb and Stacie are motivated by genuine concern for Mr. Gahn, the means used is unacceptable. Furthermore, although the physician and nurse may believe that their actions are necessary in order to respect Jeb and Stacie's autonomy, this is false. Jeb and Stacie's autonomous choice in this instance violates their perfect duty not to violate Mr. Gahn's autonomy by withholding critical information about his health status. Consequently, their action is unjustified, and Mr. Gahn's health care provider should not cooperate with this deception.

Finally, although Kant argued that no violation of perfect duties is ever justified, most contemporary Kantians believe that catastrophic (not merely serious) costs to others may sometimes justify violation of a perfect duty.

Disproportionate Care

Imperfect duties are limited not only by perfect duties, but also by the costs of fulfilling them. We are obligated to help only up to the point at which the costs would be disproportionate to the benefits. Kant's insight here seems consistent with ordinary moral intuition. We expect greater efforts and sacrifice as the needs for assistance increase. But we do not believe that individuals are obligated to risk everything even to save another human life. For instance, although a person who does not know how to swim would surely be obligated to help a drowning swimmer by throwing out a life preserver, this person would not be obligated to jump in over his or her head to attempt a rescue. Kant provides us with no specific criterion or guidelines for determining when the costs are too high. In the context of health care, however, the concept of an imperfect duty of benevolence is reflected in the long tradition of the proportionate and disproportionate care distinction. This distinction evolved in Catholic moral theology (McCartney, 1980), but a look at this distinction can help us understand why Kant refers to benevolence as an imperfect duty. Consider the case of Mara Jones.

> In the late stages of lung cancer, Mara Jones, 48, has been hospitalized due to excessive fluid in her lungs. She has endured three days of frequent suctioning to clear the fluid. The procedure is now performed every 15 to 20 minutes. Although his wife is heavily medicated and sleep deprived, Mara's husband is convinced that Mara understands the consequence of her decision when she insists that the nurses discontinue the suctioning. He informs Mara's nurse that "while I dread the moment when she will drown in her own fluid, I do not want to continue to torture her."

Mara Jones has a duty of benevolence to preserve her life and to promote her health. Her husband and her nurses also have a duty of benevolence to promote Mara's health. Is Mara obligated to continue with the suctioning? We are not asking whether Mara has a *right* to refuse this treatment: As a competent individual, she has the right to control what is done to her body. If she refuses further suctioning, continued suctioning would violate her autonomy. The question in this case is about Mara's obligation to herself: She must ask whether the burdens of continued suctioning are disproportionate to the reasonably anticipated benefits of this treatment. The burdens include the pain, effort, and cost of the treatment. The costs that patients are obligated to consider are primarily the costs to themselves. The costs to family or other primary caregivers, however, are also relevant. Obviously, different individuals may weigh the burdens and benefits of treatments differently, but for nearly all patients, there will come a point when the burdens will seem disproportionate relative to the benefits of treatment.

In Mara's case, the burdens of further suctioning include the significant discomfort of the suctioning process itself and the feeling of suffocation associated with the repeated buildup of the fluid in her lungs. These burdens are significant, while the brief minutes of clearer breathing are a small benefit that will continue to rapidly decrease. It is reasonable to conclude that the burdens are disproportionate to the benefits in this case. Consequently, Mara is no longer obligated to continue with the suctioning.

The distinction between proportionate and disproportionate care was traditionally known as the ordinary/extraordinary means distinction. Over time, health care practitioners tended to label certain treatments or procedures as in themselves *ordinary* or *extraordinary*, meaning usually done or not usually done. Antibiotics, for instance, were often considered ordinary means, while bone marrow transplants were typically considered extraordinary. This use of the terms *ordinary* and *extraordinary* obscures the fact that the moral distinction requires an evaluation of treatments *relative* to the burdens and the benefits *in a particular case*. Suctioning a patient briefly after major surgery could well be a treatment whose burdens are proportionate to the benefits (an "ordinary means"), while in Mara's case the burdens are disproportionate to the benefits (an "extraordinary means"). The language of proportionate and disproportionate care reminds us that these judgments are always contextual because they imply the question of proportionate or disproportionate to what? Box 2–6 summarizes guidelines for discontinuing treatment.

Box 2–6   *Guidelines for Discontinuing Treatment*

- Every competent patient has the right to refuse medical treatment, based on the right of individuals to decide what happens to their bodies and to be protected from unwanted interference from others.
- Life is valuable. We have an obligation to maintain our health and to preserve our lives, but this obligation is *not unlimited*.
- We are not obligated to preserve our lives when the burdens of treatment become *disproportionate* to the benefits of the treatment.
- *Disproportionate care* exists when the burdens of treatment in terms of pain, effort, or other costs, primarily from the patient's perspective, are disproportionate *relative to* the anticipated benefits of the treatment.

It is clear now why Kant described the duty of benevolence as an imperfect duty. Although we always have the duty to give aid to others as well as to ourselves, the rule of benevolence is imperfect because it does not instruct us precisely about how, when, or how much help to give. There are no specific guidelines that can lead us to definitive judgments about when a treatment imposes a disproportionate burden relative to its benefits. The proportionate/disproportionate distinction, however, does provide us with a conceptual framework that can help patients to assess their obligations of benevolence to themselves and help surrogate decision makers assess their obligations to others. As medicine's technical abilities to intervene in the dying process have dramatically increased, along with the burdens frequently imposed on the dying, it is critically important that both patients and care providers recognize that respect for life does not ethically require that every treatment available must be pursued as long as a patient is still breathing. Nurses sometimes feel that what they are required to do to patients in critical care units is closer to torturing their patients than to caring for them. Education and thoughtful application of the guidelines for disproportionate care can help to avoid such soul-depleting treatment of patients.

Of course, health care workers assume a special responsibility for promoting the well-being of others. By assuming these social roles, these professionals accept a responsibility to risk their safety to a greater degree than others do and to invest more of their time and skills in alleviating human suffering. Even so, there will still be points at which the costs are too great. In the early years of acquired immune deficiency syndrome (AIDS) treatment, some health care workers wondered whether the personal costs of caring for persons with AIDS are so great that health care providers are not obligated to provide this care. The widespread conclusion of health care professionals has been that risk of infection under prescribed infection control measures is currently so low, that such care does not impose disproportionate burdens, and that it is therefore obligatory. As the degree of risk rises in treating persons with life-threatening diseases, at some point the costs may become too burdensome, and treatment would be heroic rather than obligatory. The care that some nurses provided during the 1918 influenza epidemic seems to fall into this category.

Principle of Justice

Also a critical responsibility in health care, justice requires that we give each person his or her due. This includes an obligation to distribute the benefits, risks, and costs that belong to a community and to allocate health care resources fairly. Universalized respect for persons demands that we give each person his or her fair share. Since individuals have intrinsic and equal value, individuals in similar circumstances will require similar treatment. Kant did not offer any particular model for how shared resources should be fairly allocated. Contemporary deontologists, however, have offered a variety of models, which vary depending on which "similar circumstances" are considered most relevant. Is it similar needs, similar talents, similar efforts, similar promises by others, or similar achievements that should be given priority? Does it make a difference what is being allocated so that we might emphasize need in the case of health care, but emphasize talent in the case of education? These are critical questions for our communities faced with growing needs and limited resources. Ultimately, they can be answered only in the context of careful community dialogue.

Box 2–7 summarizes rules that are relevant to nursing practice. All of these rules can be derived from both the utilitarian principle of utility and from the Kantian principle of universalized respect for persons. The lists are illustrative and do not necessarily include all the moral rules that could be derived. It is important to note that rule utilitarians and Kantians produce similar lists of rules, but also to keep in mind that their justifications for these rules are quite different.

Box 2–7   Summary of Moral Rules Relevant to Nursing Practice

Requirement of Nonmaleficence: **Do not intentionally inflict harm.**

- Do not kill or physically harm others without justified cause (e.g., self-defense or the use of physically harmful treatment as a necessary and consented means to promoting patient welfare).
- Do not impose unreasonable risks of harm. Negligence is conduct that falls below a standard of due care.
- Do not harm others by slander, insult, or ridicule.
- Do not break a freely made promise or contract to do something in itself morally permissible.
- Do not engage in sexual acts that are exploitative or life diminishing. This includes all sex with patients.
- Do not steal the legitimately obtained property of others, including their intellectual property (e.g., published ideas, research data, and computer programs).

Respect for Autonomy: **Respect the ability of competent patients to hold views, make choices, and take actions based on personal values and beliefs.**

- Respect the choice of competent patients to refuse medical treatment and/or nursing care.
- It is impermissible to lie to patients or to withhold information necessary for an adequate understanding of their conditions.
- It is impermissible to treat competent patients without their adequately informed consent. Such consent requires disclosure of relevant information, probing for and ensuring understanding and voluntariness, and fostering adequate decision making.
- Establish a clear process for the identification of surrogate decision makers in the case of incompetent patients.
- Respect and protect patient privacy and confidentiality, providing confidential information to others only as required by law or to prevent grave harm to others.

continues

Box 2–7　Summary of Moral Rules
Relevant to Nursing Practice (cont.)

Requirement of Beneficence: **Promote the well-being of others and oneself, using morally permissible means, insofar as one can do so without disproportionate cost.**

♦ Maintain one's competence in nursing; participate in efforts to maintain and improve standards of nursing; participate in efforts to maintain working conditions that support quality nursing care; support the development of nursing's body of knowledge.
♦ Make reasonable efforts to protect patients and the public from harm due to incompetent or unethical practice by other health care professionals.
♦ Participate in efforts to promote the health needs of one's communities.
♦ Promote one's own mental, physical, emotional, and spiritual development.

Requirement of Justice: **Distribute benefits, resources, and burdens fairly.**

♦ Nursing resources should be allocated fairly among patients served.
♦ Communities should develop processes for the fair access and allocation of health care to all members of the community.
♦ Workplaces should ensure that all health care providers receive fair compensation for their work and that appropriate appeal processes are in place to ensure fair distribution of wages, compensation, and workloads.

Rationality and Competence

The rationality of human beings is fundamental in Kantian ethics and utilitarianism. For Kant, rationality is the basis for the fundamental duty of respect for persons. Utilitarianism requires rational observers capable of calculating the utility of their actions. We have already noted that it is possible that some living beings other than humans may satisfy Kant's requirement of rationality. If so, logic would demand that we extend universalized respect to these nonhuman persons as well. A more pressing issue for nursing ethics is whether all human beings qualify as persons worthy of respect or as utilitarian rational calculators. Clearly, there are human beings who do not have the capacity for rational deliberation. Fetuses and young children, severely brain damaged and severely senile human beings, and those who are in persistent vegetative states all lack the ability to deliberate, reflect, and choose ends. Writing before the technological possibilities of late-twentieth-century medicine, neither Kant nor the classical utilitarian thinkers addressed this issue.

Contemporary ethicists have discussed this issue at length. A few have taken the extreme position that only those who presently possess the ability to rationally deliberate are persons whose interests require full moral consideration (Tooley, 1983; Warren, 1994). Most conclude, however, that all living human beings do have the status of moral persons deserving universalized respect or whose pleasure and pain must be given full weight. This conclusion is often supported by recognition of the potential rational capacity in the case of fetuses, children, or the temporarily comatose (Noonan, 1994). Others note that as members of the species whose members characteristically exhibit the rational capacity to deliberate, even human beings who lack either present or future reasoning capacity have the status of full moral persons (Devine, 1982).

Assessing Decisional Capacity

Even human beings that presently appear to have rational capacity may sometimes make decisions that call into question their competence. We are inclined to call some choices "irrational." But do "irrational" choices necessarily demonstrate that a person is incompetent?

First, we must distinguish decisional capacity from "competence." *Competence* refers to a person's overall or general ability to act responsibly and to care for self. Incompetence is frequently determined by a mental health professional. A person who is determined to be legally incompetent may still be *decisionally capable* of particular choices about medical treatment. The capacity to make such a decision requires three abilities: (1) to understand information relevant to the decision, (2) to consider the alternatives and make a choice, and (3) to communicate with others about the decision. There are, of course, degrees of abilities to understand, to deliberate, and to communicate. Someone who possesses these three capabilities is entitled to be the primary decision maker for his or her own health care.

Judgments regarding minimum capacity will need to be made, but nurses take care to protect patient autonomy. Individual choices that most people would regard as irrational do not alone demonstrate a lack of decisional capacity. For instance, a person may refuse an amputation of a gangrenous limb saying that he "cannot go through life as a one-legged man." Or a woman may refuse to try any chemotherapy even when her breast cancer has been diagnosed at an early stage, citing the horrific experience of her aunt 20 years ago.

But apparently irrational choices do not necessarily show that these individuals lack, in general, the capacity for the deliberative, purposeful behavior which characterizes either Kant's or Mill's concept of "rational beings." After all, many of us make choices about our diets and our exercise that may undermine our health. Some persons choose to smoke and others choose not to wear seatbelts. Aren't these irrational choices? But do we cease to be rational beings when we make these choices? No, we do not. Individual irrational choices, even repeated ones, do not necessarily demonstrate the loss of the underlying rational capacity, nor the loss of decisional capacity regarding one's health care. Of course, some extreme choices may call this into question. It will be necessary at times to intervene temporarily in order to assess the person's decisional capacity.

The Enlightenment Context Today

Rule ethics emerged from the heady, optimistic period of the Western European Enlightenment. The events and concerns of this period significantly influenced this approach to ethics. Utilitarianism and Kantianism share three characteristics that reflect their Enlightenment context. They both emphasize the rationality and individuality of the moral agent, the impartiality of the moral point of view, and the confidence that moral judgments can be summarized in a set of universal rules.

The classical utilitarians and Kant shared a confidence in the ability of rational thinkers to derive a common set of moral rules. The utilitarian method reflects the influence of the emerging fields of modern mathematics and science. The process of ethical decision making is mathematical and scientific: Pleasure and pain are objectively and impartially observed, measured, and quantified. Ethical rules are perceived as being much like scientific rules or laws of nature. These rules are universal and discoverable by objective, reflective observers. Kant shares this perspective speaking about the moral law as universal principles that rational beings naturally impose on themselves once they recognize the logic of these principles. Scientists expect their research results to be replicable by any other researchers who apply the same rational principles of the scientific method. The Enlightenment ethicists shared a similar expectation regarding ethics: Careful, rational thinkers would eventually derive essentially the same set of moral rules.

The model of ethics as the logical application of moral rules to concrete cases reflects the democratic impulse of the Enlightenment thinkers to level the playing field for all rational thinkers. They celebrated the intellectual and political authority that rationality conferred on each (free and male) human being. This understandable "bias," however, led them to discount or simply ignore any need for moral judgment beyond a logical application of moral rules.

Although we may acknowledge inadequacies in rule ethics, it is essential that we do not lose sight of the tremendous contributions of this tradition to ethical theory in general and to health care ethics in particular. We tend to take for granted the value of human reason and the rights of all to participate in shaping their society. The radical nature of these ideas in Enlightenment Europe is clear, however, when we recall Galileo's censure by the Church and the several bloody attempts of French peasants to overthrow their monarchy (including the 1830 Paris Revolution portrayed in Victor Hugo's *Les Miserables*). Box 2–8 highlights key points of rule ethics.

Critiques of Rule Ethics

Rule ethics has been the subject of serious criticisms during the last two decades. Some of the recent developments in virtue ethics and feminist ethics can be seen as attempts to develop more adequate ethical theories in light of these critiques. Recent criticisms of rule ethics in the nursing literature suggest that it alone does not provide an adequate account of nursing ethics. Critics argue that rule ethics neglects or

Primary Questions

♦ What actions are right or wrong?
♦ How can moral obligations be summarized into moral rules?

Key Features

♦ The ability of individual human beings to deliberate and choose purposeful actions sets them apart and makes them moral agents.
♦ All human beings are equal in virtue of their capacity to reason and to choose actions.
♦ Moral duties can be summarized in a set of universal moral rules; moral decisions require the logical application of moral rules to particular cases.
♦ Looking at situations from a moral point of view requires an impartial viewpoint in which the interests of all rational persons are given similar consideration.

---

excludes important aspects of the moral experience of nurses. These include the contextual nature of moral judgments, the significance of emotions and experience, and the relational nature of nursing practice. As Chapters 4 and 6 will show, these are aspects that are emphasized in both virtue and feminist ethics.

Contextual Nature of Moral Judgments

Modern moral philosophy, and especially health care ethics, has focused on resolving moral dilemmas. Short, abstract cases are presented for resolution, and discussion ensues about the proper application of ethical principles to these cases. The moral life, therefore, appears to be episodic, involving the resolution of a series of discrete cases: whether to tell the patient with cancer that his case is terminal, whether to abort the child with Down's syndrome, whether to terminate artificial nutrition for a person in a persistent vegetative state, and so on. Furthermore, it is assumed that all ethical decision making can be reduced to the logical application of rules. Yet, some moral aspects of nursing care are not adequately described through a set of rules (Parker, 1990). Being morally sensitive and responsive to one's relational responsibilities is one area that does not lend itself to rule making. There is a need in nursing for contextual judgments such as how to embody compassionate care and how to be genuinely responsive to the needs, hopes, and fears of patients, their families, and their communities.

Being sensitive and responsive in this way, Parker notes, is a dynamic process that requires engaged listening, keen attention to context and detail, openness to being emotionally touched and changed, negotiation, and mediation. Each of these responses must be appropriately balanced, timed, and integrated with the technical aspects of nursing care. And all must be done in the context of multiple nursing responsibilities that arise in a typical day. In addition, nurses operate from the center of a web of interconnected relationships of patients, families, colleagues, physicians, other care providers, and administrators (Parker, 1990). As a result, they must balance their responsibilities for their patients' needs and for coordinating patient care within these other relationships. What is needed here is something more than the will to do the right thing and the analytic skills to apply rules to cases. One needs the capacity to make contextual moral judgments, that is, to discern the morally appropriate response to particular situations.

Even if all ethical decision making could be summarized in a set of rules, the process of developing moral rules itself requires complex moral judgments. Many moral rules attempt to build in legitimate exceptions. Determining the exact nature and extent of these exceptions requires a sustained communal conversation and reflection on the community's experience. This process relies on more contextualized judgments than those suggested by the Enlightenment emphasis on abstract, logical, and deductive thinking. The North American community's understanding of legitimate exceptions to patient confidentiality, for instance, has evolved over time in the light of new experience. The famous *Tarasoff* v. *Regents of the University of California* case crystallized the struggle to balance patient confidentiality with the need to protect third parties from harm (Torbriner, 2000). The courts ruled that therapists have an obligation to warn others who they believe, based on confidential patient disclosures, may be in imminent danger of harm.

Today, there is considerable discussion about the responsibilities of health care professionals to warn sexual partners when one partner tests positive for the human immunodeficiency virus (HIV). Our rule regarding confidentiality (Box 2–7) states that confidentiality may be violated only when required by law and in order to avoid grave harm to others. Some argue that contact tracing and case reporting laws should be no different for HIV than for other sexually transmitted diseases (Gostin et al., 1997; Richardson, 1998), while others believe that in our homophobic societies HIV exceptions to these practices are justified (Colfax & Bindman, 1998; Hecht et al., 1997). The discussion clearly reflects the fact that the development of moral rules is an ongoing process that requires communal reflection and contextual moral judgment to determine and interpret legitimate exceptions to these rules.

Integration of Affective and Intellectual Responses

Kant distrusted feelings, believing that they were too unstable and easily biased to be reliable sources of moral judgment. His ethics, and rule ethics in general, emphasize the need for objective, detached judgments based only on an impartial application of abstract principles. The devaluing of their emotional responses, however, frequently contributes to nurses' burnout and decisions to leave the profession (Parker, 1990). When our emotional responses to situations are repeatedly devalued, Parker notes that "detachment, numbness, and apathy begin to filter our perception of reality" (1990, p. 36) Over time, this suppression of emotions may produce technically competent nurses who neither perceive nor care about the moral dimensions of nursing care. Benner (1991) also criticizes the emotional detachment prescribed by rule ethics and argues that nurses need ethical comportment, which is an embodied knowledge in which thoughts and feelings are fused with physical presence and action. Cooper (1991) suggests such an integration of emotional and intellectual responses provides for a more holistic understanding of the moral practice of nursing.

Relationships and Community

Ray (1994) notes the neglect of relationships and community in rule ethics. Rule-based theories emphasize the necessity of taking an impartial point of view detached from all particular relationships and the value of individual autonomy. Communities are groups of people who are bound together by a common purpose or goal. Moral communities are bound together by values that transcend their personal interests or gain. Ray argues that the themes of moral community and nursing care within relational contexts are emerging in nursing as a critical element of ethics research (1994). Chinn (1990), Benner (1984, 1991), and Aroskar (1995) also emphasize the importance of community as the context in which values and virtues are collectively shaped and where practical moral reasoning is exercised. We will see that community and relationships are central themes in both virtue ethics and feminist ethics.

Masculine Bias of Rule Ethics

Another criticism of rule ethics that appears in recent nursing literature is the claim that it has a masculine bias. This critique has largely been motivated by the work of Carol Gilligan (1982) and Nel Noddings (1984). Both of these authors articulate a feminine ethic that they contrast with the more masculine ethic of mainstream ethics. They note that conventional rule ethics reflect typically masculine characteristics of autonomy, rationality, and independence of the moral subject. In contrast, they articulate an ethic of care that reflects more typically feminine characteristics of responsiveness to relational responsibilities, emotional connectedness, and contextuality.

It is not surprising that nursing theorists have found Nodding's and Gilligan's voices helpful in rearticulating the goals and virtues of the female-dominated profession of nursing. An ethic of care and responsibility has emerged as the dominant model in nursing ethics today through the work of Benner (1991), Bishop and Scudder (1991), Leininger (1984), Ray (1994), Schultz and Schultz (1990), and Watson (1985). We will return to this discussion of gender bias and the ethic of care in Chapter 6.

Conclusion

The emphasis on rational human reason and the codification of moral judgment reflect the Enlightenment belief in the power of every rational individual to discover universal moral truths. This democratic stance has had enormous and lasting influence on Western ethics. Kant's insistence on the evenhandedness of morality has had a similarly important impact on Western ethics. Although Kant uniquely articulates this in the requirement of universalization, his ethics shares with utilitarianism a modern emphasis on impartiality. The Enlightenment advocacy of this position has been so persuasive that many contemporary ethicists suggest that to take the moral point of view is to take an impartial point of view (Baier, 1965; Donagan, 1977; Rawls, 1971).

Decision processes for rule utilitarian and Kantian ethics are outlined in Chapter 3. The rules in Box 2–7 are derived from these decision processes and may be directly applied to particular cases. No set of ethical rules will anticipate and cover every possible ethical problem. Nurses will encounter situations that are not covered by these rules. Understanding the underlying foundation for these rules will enable nurses to return to these decision processes in order to develop new rules relevant to emerging situations.

KEY POINTS

- The goal of rule ethics is to capture our moral duties and obligations within a manageable set of rules.
- Nursing ethics, then, involves the application of abstract, universal rules to particular situations or cases. Understanding the theoretical foundations for these rules is essential.
- Enlightenment philosophers rejected the view that moral authority is vested in kings, feudal lords, and bishops, emphasizing instead the power of individuals to rationally discover universal truths and to derive moral rules.
- Utilitarians evaluate moral rules based on their tendency to produce desired consequences; moral rules that maximize happiness in society are valid.
- Kantians evaluate moral rules based on the criteria of unversalized respect for persons; some actions are morally wrong in themselves because they violate these criteria.
- Individual "irrational" choices do not necessarily demonstrate the loss of a person's capacity to make informed choices regarding health care.
- Even if, as critics charge, rule ethics neglects important aspects of nurses' moral experience, it provides a critical piece of ethical theory and concrete tools for moral decision making.

REFLECT AND DISCUSS

1. How did the social, political, and economic climate influence Bentham's and Mill's ideas? Note the contextual parallels with the emergence of Beauchamp and Childress's four-principle model of rule ethics in twentieth-century health care ethics.
2. What are the most serious objections to Bentham's hedonistic calculus? How did these problems contribute to the twentieth-century shift to rule utilitarianism?
3. The strongest criticism of the utilitarian theory of ethics is that it requires us to sacrifice the interests of a minority to maximize happiness in society. How is this problem illustrated in the Willowbrook study? How might Mill have argued that a utilitarian should oppose the use of the Willowbrook children in this hepatitis study? Is his solution to the problem of justice adequate?

4. Describe two or three instances in nursing practice in which patients are treated as "mere means" to other persons' ends. Give some examples of possible policies or practices in a nursing work context that would violate Kant's requirement of universalizability.

5. Kant's fundamental principle requires us to respect every being as a rational being. Why does he think that our rationality is morally relevant? Are there other aspects of human beings that you believe are morally relevant? Why? Are there other aspects of animals that you think are morally relevant? Why or why not?

6. Outline a case in which the use of antibiotics could be considered disproportionate care. Outline another case in which you think that reasonable people might disagree about whether the burdens of a particular treatment will be disproportionate to the anticipated benefits of that treatment.

7. Describe two instances from nursing practice, particularly from your own nursing experience, where rules from the categories of autonomy, beneficence, nonmaleficence, and justice conflict. How would you resolve the conflicts as a utilitarian and as a Kantian?

8. In spite of the contrasts between Kantianism and utilitarianism, how do both theories reflect their roots in the Enlightenment? What do you see as the main strengths and weaknesses of rule ethics? What do you think makes rule ethics so attractive to those working in health care?

REFERENCES

American Nurses Association. (1985). *Code for nurses with interpretative statements.* Washington, DC: American Nurses Publishing.

American Nurses Association. (2000). *Code of ethics for nurses* (working draft #9). Available: http://www.ana.org/ethics/code9.htm [2000, November 17].

Aroskar, M. A. (1995). Envisioning nursing as a moral community. *Nursing Outlook, 43,* 201–209.

Baier, K. (1965). *The moral point of view.* New York: Random House.

Beauchamp, T., and Childress, J. (1979/2001). *Principles of biomedical ethics.* New York: Oxford University Press.

Benner, P. (1984). *From novice to expert: Excellence and power in clinical nursing practice.* Menlo Park, CA: Addison-Wesley

Benner, P. (1991). The role of experience, narrative, and community in skilled ethical comportment. *Advances in Nursing Science, 14*(2), 1–21.

Bentham, J. (1970). *Introduction to the principles of morals and legislation.* New York: Free Press (original work published 1789).

Bishop, A. H., and Scudder, J. R. (1991). *Nursing: The practice of caring.* New York: National League for Nursing.

Chinn, P. L. (1990). Toward the 21st century: Nursing theory, research, and practice. Paper presented at the 1990 23rd Annual Communicating Nursing Research Conference, Western Institute of Nursing, Boulder, CO.

Colfax, G. N., and Bindman, A. B. (1998). Commentary: Health benefits and risks of reporting HIV-infected individuals by name. *American Journal of Public Health, 88*(6); 876–879.

Cooper, M. C. (1991). Principle-oriented ethics and the ethic of care: A creative tension. *Advances in Nursing Science, 14*(2), 22–31.

Devine, P. (1982). Abortion. In T. Beauchamp and L. Walters (Eds.), *Contemporary issues in bioethics* (pp. 260–266). Belmont, CA: Wadsworth Publishing.

Donagan, A. (1977). *The theory of morality.* Chicago: University of Chicago Press.

Drane, J. F. (2000). Bioethics: How the discipline came to be in the U.S. Available: http://www.vchile.cl/bioetica/drane4.htm [2000, June 23]

Edsall, G. (1983). Letter from *The Lancet,* July 10, 1971. In S. Gorovitz, R. Macklin, A. L. Jameton, J. M. O'Connor, and S. Sherwin (Eds.), *Moral problems in medicine* (pp. 606–607). Englewood Cliffs, NJ: Prentice Hall.

Fox, R. (1994). The entry of U.S. bioethics into the 1990s: A sociological analysis. In E. R. DuBose, R. P. Hamel, and L. J. O'Connell (Eds.), *A matter of principles.* Valley Forge, PA: Trinity Press.

Gilligan, C. (1982). *In a different voice.* Cambridge, MA: Harvard University Press.

Gostin, L., et al. (1997). National HIV case reporting for the United States: A defining moment in the history of the epidemic. *New England Journal of Medicine, 337*(16), 1162–1167.

Hecht, F. M., et al. (1997). Name reporting of HIV: Attitudes and knowledge of those at risk. *Journal General Internal Medicine, 12*(Suppl. 1), 108.

Hooyman, N. R., and Gonyea, J. (1995). *Feminist perspectives on family care: Policies for gender justice.* Thousand Oaks, CA: Sage Publications.

Kant, I. (1964). *Groundwork of a metaphysics of morals* (H. J. Paton, Trans.). New York: Harper & Row (original work published 1785).

_____. (1964). *The metaphysical principles of virtue* (J. Ellington, Trans.). Indianapolis: Bobbs-Merrill (original work published 1797).

Krugman, S., and Giles, J. P. (1983). Letter from *The Lancet,* May 8, 1971. In S. Gorovitz, R. Macklin, A. L. Jameton, J. M. O'Connor, and S. Sherwin (Eds.), *Moral problems in medicine* (pp. 603–604). Englewood Cliffs, NJ: Prentice Hall.

Leininger, M. (1984). *Care: The essence of nursing and health.* Thorofare, NJ: Charles B. Slack (reprint 1988 by Wayne State University Press).

McCartney, J. J. (1980). The development of the doctrine of ordinary and extraordinary means of preserving life in Catholic moral theology before the Karen Quinlan case. *Linacre Quarterly, 47,* 215–224.

Mill, J. S. (1982). *On liberty.* New York: Viking Penguin (original work published 1859).

_____. (1988). *The subjection of women.* Indianapolis: Hackett Publishing (original published 1869).

_____. (1957). *Utilitarianism* (E. O. Piest, Ed.). Indianapolis: Bobbs-Merrill (original work published 1861).

Noddings, N. (1984). *Caring: A feminine approach to ethics and moral education.* Berkeley: University of California.

Noonan, J. T. (1994). An almost absolute value in history. In T. Beauchamp and L. Walters (Eds.), *Contemporary issues in bioethics* (pp. 279–282). Belmont, CA: Wadsworth Publishing.

Parker, R. S. (1990). Nurses' stories: The search for a relational ethic of care. *Advances in Nursing Science, 13*(1), 31–40.

Ray, M. A. (1994). Communal moral experience as the starting point for research in health care ethics. *Nursing Outlook, 42,* 104–109.

Rawls, J. (1971). *Theory of justice.* Cambridge: Harvard University Press.

Richardson, J. L. (1998). HIV infection. In E. A. Bechman (Ed.), *Behavioral medicine and women: A comprehensive handbook.* New York: Guilford Press.

Schultz, P. R. and Schultz, R. C. (1990). Nodding's caring and public policy: A linkage and its nursing implications. In M. Leininger (Ed.), *Ethical and moral dimensions of care* (pp. 81–87). Detroit: Wayne State University Press.

Tooley, M. (1983). Abortion and infanticide. In R. Munson (Ed.), *Intervention and reflection: Basic issues in medical ethics* (pp. 61–76). Belmont, CA: Wadsworth Publishing.

Torbriner, M. O. (2000). Majority opinion in *Tarasoff* v. *Regents of the University of California.* In R. Munson (Ed.), *Intervention and reflection* (6th ed., pp. 446–449). New York: McGraw-Hill.

Warren, M. A. (1994). On the moral and legal status of abortion. In T. Beauchamp and L. Waters (Eds.), *Contemporary issues in bioethics* (pp. 302–311). Belmont, CA: Wadsworth.

Watson, J. (1985). *Nursing: Human science and human care: A theory of nursing.* Norwalk, CT: Appleton-Century-Crofts.

3

Applying Rule Ethics

Chapter 2 outlined a set of rules relevant to nursing (see Box 2–7). These rules were derived from utilitarian and Kantian ethics. Health care, however, is a complex and constantly changing context. As new issues arise, some ethical questions can be answered by directly applying the rules in Box 2–7. But some issues will require a more in-depth analysis. This chapter considers the issue of whether recovering alcoholics should receive transplanted livers. This issue is covered by the second rule under the category of justice: "Communities should develop processes for the fair access and allocation of health care to all members of the community." But, of course, the critical question is what is "fair" in the allocation of scarce livers for transplant. To answer this, we need to go back to the foundational ethical theories and consider what rule about allocating livers these theories would support.

    This chapter will demonstrate the application of the framework for ethical analysis introduced in Chapter 1 and presented in Box 3–1. In step 4, we will demonstrate

Box 3–1 Framework for Ethical Analysis

1. Identify the problem or issue.
2. Analyze context.
3. Explore options.
4. Apply the decision process.
5. Implement the plan and evaluate results.

the application of the rule ethics decision process. Step 4 appears twice, however, so that we may consider this process from both the Kantian and utilitarian rule ethics decision processes. The chapter concludes with suggestions of additional issues in nursing that would benefit from the application of rule ethics.

Liver Transplants for Recovering Alcoholics

Step 1. Identify the Problem or Issue

According to the United Network for Organ Sharing (UNOS), which maintains a registry of transplant candidates and recipients, in the United States 14,709 people were waiting for a liver transplant at year end in 1999. In 1999, 4,697 livers were transplanted, while 1,753 persons on the list died while waiting (UNOS, 2001). Alcoholism is the leading cause of liver disease; roughly 50 percent of resulting deaths are alcohol related. Yet, in spite of these statistics, fewer than 10 percent of liver transplants were performed on alcoholics in 1989 (Office of Health Technology Assessment, 1990) and a mere 14 percent in 1993 (American Liver Foundation, 1996).

These statistics raise important ethical questions about the selection criteria for liver transplants. It appears that patients with alcohol-related end-stage liver disease (ARESLD) are given a lower priority or, in some cases, excluded altogether from consideration for transplant. Given the scarcity of these precious organs, we need as a community to address the question of *whether persons with ARESLD should be considered equally with other end-stage liver disease (ESLD) patients when liver organs are distributed for transplant.*

As concerns about the costs of health care continue to grow, the issue of patients' responsibility for their health status will need to be addressed. Should patients whose behavior has significantly contributed to their illnesses be denied health care? Should they be given a lower priority for treatment than others who are ill through no fault of their own? These are critical value questions that are raised as we consider whether persons with ARESLD should be given equal consideration for liver transplants.

While nurses may not work with patients who are candidates for liver transplant, all nurses care for patients who engage in unhealthy or unsafe behaviors that cause or exacerbate their illnesses. Health care resources are finite, and allocation decisions must be made. Consequently, the issue of patients' responsibility for their health status arises in all contexts of patient care.

Step 2. Analyze the Context

Cohen and Benjamin (2000) propose that the unwillingness to transplant livers into alcoholics is tied to two common but unsupported beliefs that are held by many persons both within and outside of health care. First, many believe that alcoholism is the result of individual misconduct and a reflection of poor character. Second, there is a common belief that even alcoholics who are in recovery when they receive transplants will have poor survival rates after transplantation. We could add to these a third common belief that persons with ARESLD will return to excessive drinking after transplant and, as a result, destroy a second liver. These beliefs reflect social stigmas and bias more than medical facts. The most significant contextual factors that must be considered then are social and medical factors. We will consider the medical factors first.

SURVIVAL RATES

There is considerable research data that contradicts the last two medical beliefs about survival rates and recidivism. Virtually all recent studies conclude that there is no significant difference in the survival rate among ARESLD patients and patients who received transplants following non–alcohol-related liver failure. The American Liver Foundation reports a 70 percent to 80 percent one-year survival rate for alcoholics who receive new livers. The same range of survival rates is reported for nonalcoholics. Kelso (1994) summarizes the results of four studies whose results were published between 1990 and 1993. All four studies (three in the United States and the fourth in France) found no statistical differences in one-year survival rates for the ARESLD group and the non-ARESLD group.

RECIDIVISM RATES

Concerns about recidivism among ARESLD transplant patients are of two sorts. First is the straightforward concern that these patients may return to previous drinking patterns and, as a result, damage or destroy their new livers. The second concern is that a relapse into heavy drinking will dramatically undermine the ability of these patients to follow through on the demanding post-transplant regimen of multiple medications for immunosuppression and survival. Since heavy drinking generally results in a chaotic or disorderly lifestyle, this is a significant concern.

Current guidelines for liver transplantation candidacy, established by the National Institutes of Mental Health in 1983, require that candidates exhibit progressive liver failure despite medical treatment *and abstinence from alcohol.* Although research studies do not suggest a clear guideline for the period of pretransplant abstinence, a remarkably low rate of recidivism has been documented. Studies by Knechtle, Kumar, Osorio, and Pageaux reported recidivism rates of 13 percent, 11.5 percent, 19 percent, and 9 percent, respectively (Kelso, 1994). Similar results are reported in a Mayo Clinic study that found "moderate to large" consumption of alcohol among 12.5 percent of alcoholics who survived surgery for more than one year (American Liver Foundation, 1996). It is also noteworthy that Knechtle, Kumar, and Osorio found similar post-transplant rates of alcohol consumption among non-ARESLD patients (Kelso, 1994). (Pageaux and associates did not report data for the non-ARESLD patients.) Although these non-ARESLD patients presumably did not have the sort of history of alcohol abuse and/or dependence that the ARESLD patients had, the alcohol they consume has the same physiological effects on their livers as it does on the ARESLD patients.

Some studies report a significantly higher rate of postoperative drinking for patients who were abstinent for less than six months prior to transplant, compared to those who were abstinent for more than six months. Kumar and colleagues reported a 43 percent recidivism rate in the first group and only 6.7 percent for the latter group. Similar results were reported in the Osorio study, but Pageaux's study found no statistical difference in the recidivism rate among those abstinent fewer than six months prior to surgery and those abstinent for greater than six months (Kelso, 1994). In 1995, an international conference on liver transplantation could not agree on how long an alcoholic cirrhotic patient should be sober prior to transplant (American Liver Foundation, 1996). Clearly, further research is needed to determine whether a reliable correlation between length of preoperative abstinence and postoperative abstinence exists.

STIGMA AND BIAS

Thomas (1993) notes that alcoholism is not only an unhealthy lifestyle like smoking or a high-cholesterol diet. It also carries a heavy social stigma. In spite of the fact that alcohol is widely and conspicuously consumed by many in the United States, there is widespread condemnation of alcoholics in our society. Alcohol consumption is glamorized and vigorously promoted throughout our media, but there is a striking lack of sympathy for alcoholics by many. Alcoholism has been recognized as a disease for more than 35 years. It is identified as such by the American Medical Association, American Psychiatric Association, World Health Organization, National Council on Alcoholism, various government agencies, and insurance companies (Killeen, 1993). Nonetheless, many people perceive alcoholics as a group of societal freeloaders responsible for societal devastation including auto accidents and deaths, domestic violence, lower productivity and safety in the workplace, and a disproportionate use of health care resources and government assistance (Cohen & Benjamin, 2000; Thomas, 1993). For many persons, alcoholism is perceived as a moral failing. It is important to be aware that this social stigma may influence some people's arguments concerning whether patients with ARESLD should be considered for liver transplants.

ECONOMIC FACTORS

We cannot ignore the fact that liver transplants are expensive. The average cost is $145,000. The cost for continuous maintenance on cyclosporine is about $6,000 per year. Even when covered by health insurance policies, these costs are shared by the public through increased premiums. There was a public outcry when Oregon's Medicaid system announced in 1987 that heart, liver, and bone marrow transplants for leukemia would be excluded from its health plan. Yet, it is reasonable to ask whether these transplants are a responsible use of limited health care dollars in either publicly funded programs such as Medicaid or in privately insured health programs. This issue of fair allocation of health care dollars is a complex and increasingly urgent issue in North America. We will focus our discussion here on the question of whether patients should be given equal consideration for transplant regardless of the cause of their liver disease.

Step 3. Explore Options

There are three likely policy positions that could be adopted on this issue. We could adopt a policy that excludes all patients with ARESLD from being considered for a liver transplant. Alternately, we could require that ARESLD patients who meet other criteria for transplant, including other medical criteria, should be given equal consideration for a liver transplant. The third policy would allow patients with ARESLD to be considered for a liver transplant but require that they be given a lower priority than patients with other forms of ESLD are. We should recognize, however, that given the long waiting lists for livers, it is unlikely that an ARESLD patient would ever actually receive a liver for transplant under this third policy. Considerations, therefore, will focus on the first two policy positions.

Step 4. Apply the Rule Ethics Decision Process: Kantian Ethics

Reasonable arguments can be offered from Kantian and utilitarian perspectives both in favor of equal access of ARESLD patients to liver transplants as well as opposing such equal access. This fact does not mean that it makes no difference what one thinks about this issue. Rather, it means that members of a community must be prepared to give thoughtful reasons for their positions on this issue. Only through thoughtful, responsible dialogue can a community reach a justifiable position. We will present arguments that apply both the Kantian and utilitarian decision processes. The Kantian decision process is summarized in Box 3–2.

✓ *Accurately state the rule to be considered.*

The heart of the Kantian perspective is the recognition that all human beings have intrinsic value and that they all, therefore, deserve equal respect. This is Kant's basic principle of universalized respect for persons. It would seem then that the most critical point in this case, from a Kantian perspective, is that all ESLD patients are human beings with intrinsic value. The presumption, consequently, is that a Kantian would support the action of providing equal opportunity for a liver transplant to all patients who satisfy the basic medical criteria. The intention behind this action is to recognize the intrinsic value of all of these persons and to treat them with equal respect by providing them all with an equal opportunity for transplant. We may discover that there are other morally relevant factors that will override this presumption, but we will begin by examining this proposed action.

Box 3–2   Rule Ethics Decision Process: Kantian Ethics

4. Apply the Rule Ethics Decision Process: Kantian Ethics

Basic Principle: **Act always so that you respect every human being, yourself and others as a rational being.**

♦ Accurately state the rule of action to be evaluated.
♦ Consider whether the action considered can be universalized: Could one consistently desire that everyone in similar circumstances should intend the same action? If not, then this is not a morally permissible action. If it can be universalized, then go on to the next step.
♦ This action must also treat all affected persons with respect: All persons must be treated as ends and never merely as a means to serve the interests of others.
♦ If a perfect duty conflicts with an imperfect duty, the perfect duty will override in all but extremely exceptional circumstances.

All of the patients being considered must satisfy the medical criteria for transplant. These criteria include a period of abstinence from alcohol prior to transplant. As noted earlier, there is no consensus at this point on what the length of this period should be. Some research suggests that patients who were abstinent for six months or longer had significantly lower recidivism rates than those who were abstinent for a shorter period. Further research on this issue is needed.

In addition to an evaluation of their basic physical health, all potential transplant candidates are evaluated in terms of their likely ability to follow through on the demanding post-transplant regimen. This may include an assessment of the patient's mental well-being, support system, and social/familial stability. Although they go beyond strictly medical criteria, these factors may significantly affect a patient's ability to comply with the prescribed medical regimen essential to post-transplant survival. For recovering alcoholics, the likelihood of a return to heavy drinking is an important element in assessing ability to follow the prescribed post-transplant plan of care and, therefore, to survive. If further research confirms that there is a significantly lower rate of recidivism after a six-month or longer period of pretransplant abstinence, then we would be justified in limiting transplants to those ARESLD patients who have achieved this level of recovery. This would simply be one criterion among others that would be used to predict a patient's likelihood of survival and benefit from the transplant.

Although further research is needed, for purposes of this discussion we will assume that patients with ARESLD who have been abstinent for six months or longer will have a significantly lower rate of recidivism. Our proposed rule, therefore, is that *patients with ARESLD who have been abstinent six months or more and who meet other medical criteria should be given equal consideration for a liver transplant as other ESLD patients who satisfy basic medical criteria.* It is important to note that many patients with ARESLD will not qualify for transplant consideration either because they have not achieved six months of sobriety or because their overall physical condition does not make them reasonable transplant candidates. The policy proposed here does not imply any obligation to provide a liver transplant to an alcoholic who continues to drink. The overall physical health of such a person is likely to be poor; the ability of this person to follow through on the post-transplant regimen is extremely low; and continued drinking, of course, will destroy the new liver as well. This person clearly would not meet the minimum medical transplant criteria. A transplant under these conditions would simply waste a valuable and scarce resource.

Equal consideration for transplant can be assured by means of a formal lottery system or through the informal lottery system of "first come, first served." Allowances must be made for the fact that livers must be used within hours of being harvested. As a result, these organs will be transplanted in patients who are reasonably accessible. This may not always be the next person in the queue. The important point in our discussion, however, is that a recovering alcoholic's history of alcoholism should not count against this person's qualification for a transplant.

✓ CONSIDER WHETHER THIS ACTION CAN BE UNIVERSALIZED

We must test our proposed action by asking whether we could universalize the intention behind it. The intention in this case is to provide equal opportunity for a liver transplant to all persons who have a reasonable chance to significantly benefit from one. Could this intention be universalized to apply to all similar cases? Kant would direct us to think about what basic principle is underlying our action. The basic principle here is not simply one about liver transplants, but is more general. When considering whether we would apply this principle to similar cases, what would count as a similar case? The crucial facts of this case are that although we have two sets of patients who would benefit equally from a proposed treatment, the behavior of recovering alcoholics significantly contributed to their liver disease. We are proposing that the morally relevant factor here is that the allocation decision should be based on whether the patient meets the medical criteria for treatment and not on the cause of the disease. The underlying basic principle is then a principle about access to health care: Patients should not be denied equal access to medical treatment simply because their behaviors have significantly contributed to their illness.

Consider what it would mean to universalize the principle to deny equal access to those whose behaviors significantly contribute to their illness. The treatment of chronic smokers who develop lung cancer or emphysema would clearly be affected. Many communities increasingly are attempting to discourage smoking and to make smokers bear some of the costs of their habit. Smoking is forbidden in many public spaces, smokers are charged a higher premium for health and car insurance, and significant taxes are assessed on tobacco products. Some antismoking activists demand that smokers either be required to pay all the costs of their health care or be denied all but the most basic palliative care for smoking-induced illnesses. After all, the effects of smoking are well documented and well publicized. Smokers knowingly continue behavior that contributes to their illness and, as a result, they have no right to expect society to utilize limited, expensive resources to assuage their self-induced suffering.

As maddening as the self-destructive behavior of smokers may be for many in health care and in the larger community, some may object that the smoking issue is not sufficiently similar to the case of providing liver transplants for ARESLD patients. In the latter case, the resource is absolutely scarce. That is, there is an absolute number of livers available—a number that is drastically short of the demand for them. Moss and Siegler (1991) make this argument, stating that generally health care providers should treat patients based on their actual medical needs and not on the factors that cause the problem. In the case of chronic smokers, obese people with type 2 diabetes, or motorcyclists who ride without helmets and sustain severe injuries, they argue that the resources needed to treat these and similar self-induced conditions are only relatively or moderately scarce. Each person with these conditions can be allocated a share of resources necessary to meet their need. But the fact that there are not sufficient livers to meet the needs of all patients with ESLD, Moss and Siegler argue, justifies some discrimination in choosing the recipients of this absolutely scarce resource (1991).

Consider the case of the diabetic who does not follow prescribed diet restrictions, who fails to carefully monitor his blood sugar level, and who has been repeatedly hospitalized for diabetic shock. Eventually, this person requires extensive dialysis treatment and, finally, is in dire need of a kidney transplant. If the diabetic had responsibly cared for his condition, he might have avoided the need for a transplant. At the least, the need for a transplant could have been postponed for a significant amount of time. Although not as scarce as livers, the shortage of kidneys needed for transplant is still significant. Would we as a society deny this person an equal chance for the kidney that he needs? It is doubtful that many would argue for this conclusion. Are we more likely as a society to deny the recovering alcoholic a needed liver than we are to deny the noncompliant diabetic a kidney? If so, it appears that the social stigma attached to alcoholism biases our judgments, making us inconsistent in our policy.

If we accept Moss and Siegler's argument, we would be justified in giving both recovering alcoholics and noncompliant diabetics a lower priority for the organs that they need. Their distinction between absolutely scarce and relatively scarce resources requires closer examination. It is true that transplantable organs are a nonrenewable and scarce resource. Nonetheless, all of our health care resources are limited. The dollars that pay for chemotherapy for the smoker with lung cancer, or the dollars that pay for expensive intensive care for the patient with severe head injury resulting from failure to wear a seat belt come from limited sources. If allocated for these purposes, these dollars will not be available for prenatal care for indigent women, public education, or to increase the number of police officers who serve our community. Because we do not have unlimited resources to meet the needs of our society, we must always make choices. These limits are just as real as the limits imposed by the number of organs donated for transplant. In all of these cases, we must decide whether a patient's culpability for an illness should be grounds for denying equal opportunity for treatment.

The requirement of universalization alone cannot answer this question. Kant's requirement of universalization simply insists that if we claim that patient responsibility should count, we must be certain that it does so in all cases—and not simply in those, like alcoholism, that carry a social stigma. We must consider respect for persons—the second requirement of Kant's Categorical Imperative—to determine whether all patients with self-induced illnesses should be denied equal opportunity for treatment or whether none of them should.

✓ Treat All Affected Persons with Respect

Respect for all persons is central to Kantian ethics. All human beings have intrinsic value and, therefore, deserve respect because of the kind of beings that they are. It is their rational, autonomous nature that endows human beings with intrinsic value. Notably, this respect is not contingent on one's social utility or one's achievements. It also does not depend on consistently acting in a rational manner. Simply *being* an autonomous kind of being warrants respect.

All patients with ESLD share the same basic nature as rational beings and deserve equal respect. This respect requires that they not be harmed and that each patient be given an equal chance for help. The help they each need is a liver transplant. It does not matter whether this need is the result of a genetic liver disease or if it is the result of a long history of alcohol abuse. For a Kantian, the relevant consideration in allocating the scarce organs is not what one has contributed to society or what one may potentially contribute. Nor is it a matter of one's character. All human beings have the same intrinsic value and deserve equal respect. If not all persons who need a liver transplant (and who meet the minimum medical requirements) can receive one, then the recipients should be selected through a random process in which each person has an equal chance of being selected. Universalizing this action results in the principle that all persons should have an equal opportunity for those treatments for which they medically qualify, regardless of whether their illness or injury was self-induced.

This position is consistent with the long tradition in health care of treating patients' diseases or injuries regardless of their cause. This nonjudgmental stance has been a cornerstone of health care ethics for centuries. Health care providers give care because of a person's medical need and not because of his or her character. Public policy that would require health care providers to monitor and evaluate patient behavior to determine who deserves medical care would constitute a radical shift in this health care tradition. Such a shift would clearly be inconsistent with a Kantian ethics perspective.

✓ Prioritize Perfect Duties

When a perfect duty and an imperfect duty conflict, the perfect duty overrides in all but the most extreme circumstances. Violating a perfect duty in order to fulfill an imperfect duty would mean intentionally harming one person in order to produce good consequences for another person(s). Kant believed that this would always be wrong no matter what the consequences would be. One the other hand, nearly all contemporary deontologists believe that if the consequences of not performing the imperfect duty to give aid to others would be truly catastrophic, then it is permissible to violate the perfect duty.

The present case does not involve such a conflict of duties. The ethical issue in this case is one of deciding who should be helped when not all can be helped. The conflict that exists is one between helping some rather than others—a conflict between imperfect duties to provide help. From a Kantian perspective, the only fair way to resolve this conflict is through a random process of selection, such as a lottery.

CONSIDERING OBJECTIONS

Our application of the Kantian decision process has led us to conclude that ARESLD patients who meet the medical criteria for transplant should be equally eligible to receive a liver transplant as those whose ESLD is the result of other causes. The application of ethical principles, however, always requires some judgments about how the principles apply in a particular case. As a result, different opinions may emerge about how to apply Kantian principles to this issue. We will consider two objections that some might make to the application of Kantian principles to the issue of liver transplants.

Objection on the Grounds of Fairness

One objection to the position advanced above is the cry, "It isn't fair!" That someone who is dying through no fault of his or her own should forfeit a chance of survival because an available organ goes to someone else who has destroyed his or her liver through many years of alcohol abuse is unfair. After all, the effects of alcohol abuse are well known and treatment is available. Even if we acknowledge that alcoholism is itself a disease and not a weakness of character, it is essential to note that it is a treatable disease. They could have sought help much sooner instead of waiting until death was imminent to do so. Furthermore, if some did try treatment but failed, then they should have tried again. Those with congenital biliary cirrhosis have no opportunities to prevent their disease, nor do most with chronic liver diseases. They are innocent of blame for their condition.

Of course, no patients should be completely abandoned—all are human beings with intrinsic value. Those with ARESLD should receive palliative care, but they should not compete equally for the scarce organs. It is simply unfair to treat those who could not prevent their disease the same as those who destroyed their liver function through a long process of irresponsible behavior. Kant requires that we treat similar cases alike. But these are not similar cases and to treat them as if they are is unfair.

We can empathize with patients and their families who make this argument. The objection cannot easily be dismissed as the mere railing of those frustrated by their helplessness in the face of tragedy. The demand for fairness strikes at the core of Kantian ethics. Universalization is fundamentally a requirement of fairness and thus, the essential question again is whether the case of patients with ARESLD is significantly different than those of other ESLD patients.

Although this objection acknowledges that alcoholism is a disease, the implications of this fact are not sufficiently recognized. Waiting many years to seek treatment for alcoholism suggests grossly irresponsible behavior. Yet, though successful treatment of alcoholism is available, the treatment is an arduous process. Many alcoholics begin treatment, but do not complete it. This may not necessarily indicate a lack of will power. Rather, it may be, at least partly, an indication of the intractability of this disease. It is also notable that even when alcoholics do complete a treatment program, they may not find the treatment helpful. Moss and Siegler cite a comprehensive review of alcohol treatment programs that concluded that more than two thirds of patients were helped by their treatment. They cite this fact to support their argument that alcoholism is a treatable disease. But even this encouraging statistic reveals that somewhat less than one third did not improve with treatment. Thus, the fact that a person drank significantly for many years does not necessarily demonstrate that efforts were not made to control this disease. The fact is that alcoholics often make repeated efforts at recovery before they have significant success.

Another critical aspect of alcoholism is that denial is one of its primary symptoms. For some, there are obvious public indications of their problem. Others are able to maintain an acceptable public persona, restricting their behavior to the privacy of their home and family. In either case, alcoholics have an amazing ability to deny the obvious symptoms of an underlying disease. Often, it is only after the loss of primary relationships, jobs, social status, and/or economic security that alcoholics break through their denial to begin facing their illness. Denial is not part of a pattern of an irresponsible joyride—it is an insidious component of the disease itself.

The objection based on considerations of fairness presents a stark contrast between blameless individuals who were powerless to prevent their desperate condition and prodigal individuals who threw away precious years and ignored opportunities to halt the deterioration of their livers. These facts about alcoholism suggest, however, that this contrast may itself be unfair. Recovery from alcoholism is extremely difficult. We cannot assume that a person with ARESLD made no efforts or even only one failed attempt to control the disease until faced with imminent death. Many may have made repeated efforts and suffered numerous humiliating failures before gaining sufficient control of the disease.

Suppose that some of the people with ARESLD did not make genuine efforts to control their alcoholism until it became clear that their liver function was severely damaged. Is it unfair for these persons to receive equal consideration for a liver transplant? The critical facts are that these patients have demonstrated their commitment and ability to follow through with the rigorous post-transplant regimen by remaining abstinent for at least six months. As a result, they have a chance of survival equal to that of other liver transplant patients. In short, they meet the established medical criteria. Furthermore, they are human beings with as great a need as other candidates and with equal intrinsic value. It is these facts that are relevant in Kantian ethics.

Finally, the Kantian would remind us that the action that we take in this case must be one that we could universalize to other similar cases. Do we believe that it is appropriate for health care practitioners to judge who has made sufficient efforts to control their illnesses and who, therefore, deserves treatment and who does not? Or do we believe that their duty is to respect the equal dignity of all human beings and limit their assessments to medically relevant factors?

Objection About Accountability

Our rationality and capacity to make autonomous decisions is what gives us intrinsic value and grounds Kant's basic principle of respect for persons. Respect for the autonomy of persons requires that others do not take away the conditions of personal moral agency or autonomy. Holding people accountable for the choices they make is also a requirement of respect for autonomy. As a result, a Kantian may argue that we must hold people accountable when their alcohol abuse causes end-stage liver disease.

Earlier efforts to control the alcoholism should be credited, but those who fail to seek treatment until their liver disease is well advanced should be denied candidacy for a liver transplant. To hold people with ARESLD to any lower standard implies that we do not regard them as genuinely autonomous persons.

The fact that a person with ARESLD has achieved sobriety for six months or more is significant, but it is not the only relevant fact from this perspective. This person's whole history of behavior is relevant. Autonomous persons are responsible for all of their choices and are accountable for them. The only justifiable reason for not holding those with ARESLD accountable for their alcohol abuse would be if we do not believe that these persons are competent and autonomous, that is, if we believe that they cannot choose to stop their alcohol abuse. Presumably, we do not consider alcoholics incompetent or incapable of making responsible choices about their alcohol consumption. If we did, we would be justified in committing them to treatment centers without their consent to protect them and the safety of others.

Certainly, accountability is a fundamental aspect of moral agency. Society does hold alcoholics accountable for their behavior in many ways. A significant number of people involved in vehicular accidents, homicides, and domestic violence have been drinking alcohol. Society holds these people responsible for their actions in spite of their alcohol consumption. Parents who neglect or harm their children as a result of their alcoholism may have their children removed from their homes. Alcoholics also are held accountable when their drinking behavior leads to failure to perform their jobs adequately. On the other hand, many employers provide and pay for treatment if employees voluntarily seek treatment for their alcohol addiction.

Alcoholics are thus held responsible for harm that they do to others in multiple ways. Shouldn't they also be held responsible for the harm that they do to society through their high use of limited health care resources, especially livers? This question returns us to the complex issues of addictions and autonomy. Alcoholism is an addiction that clearly undermines autonomy. It is generally believed that alcoholics are capable of choosing to seek treatment in all but very advanced cases. In fact, the choice to seek treatment is an essential component of treatment. Respect for persons requires that we acknowledge that alcoholics suffer from an addiction and that this addiction undermines their autonomy. It also requires that we encourage the efforts of alcoholics to overcome their addiction. Excluding recovering alcoholics from being candidates for liver transplants seems to discount the mitigating effects of alcohol addiction on these persons' autonomy. These persons have taken responsibility for their health and have overcome significant obstacles to achieve their sobriety. This hard work should be encouraged rather than dismissed.

The claim that accountability requires us to deny transplant candidacy to recovering alcoholics is linked to the issue of universalization. We could not fairly deny treatment in this case unless we are prepared similarly to deny all but palliative care to others with allegedly self-induced illnesses. Cohen and Benjamin (2000) caution against such an attempt noting the difficulty involved in developing a "detailed calculus of just deserts for health care based on good conduct" (p. 792). Such a calculus would involve complex analyses of the multiple contributing factors to disease, deciding what percentage of patient contribution is necessary to warrant denial of treatment, and nightmarish dilemmas related to monitoring patient behaviors. Such a calculus is almost certainly impossible to develop and to apply fairly. A Kantian would conclude that although individuals should be held accountable for their behavior out of respect for their rational autonomy, society has a duty not to apply a policy unjustly, as this policy would necessarily be.

CONCLUSION OF KANTIAN DECISION PROCESS

Our conclusion is that a Kantian would support the proposal for giving equal consideration for liver transplants to recovering alcoholics who have been abstinent for six months along with other ESLD patients. This proposal satisfies both Kant's requirement of universalization and respect for persons.

Step 4. Apply the Rule Ethics Decision Process: Utilitarian Ethics

We turn next to apply the utilitarian decision process, which is summarized in Box 3–3. Utilitarians are concerned also about the personal responsibility of ARESLD patients. The issue for them, however, is not one of fairness but of social utility. A utilitarian must consider what policy would promote the greatest good for the greatest number of persons. Working with patients whose behaviors significantly contribute to their illnesses can be frustrating for nurses. It is commonly assumed that society could save a great deal of money and precious health care resources by strictly limiting health care for those with alleged self-induced illnesses. Careful analysis of the utility of such policies does not support this assumption.

✓ ACCURATELY STATE THE RULE TO BE EVALUATED

Rule utilitarianism requires us to consider the best options or rules and to compare the cost–benefit analyses of these alternative rules. The best options to consider in this case are either a rule that excludes patients with ARESLD as transplant candidates or one that includes them as equal candidates. We will consider the rule to exclude first: *Patients with ARESLD who have been abstinent for 6 months or more and who meet other medical criteria should* not *be given equal consideration for a liver transplant as other ESLD patients who satisfy the basic medical criteria. They should be provided with basic palliative care for their illness.*

✓ IDENTIFY ALL THOSE WHO ARE DIRECTLY AND INDIRECTLY AFFECTED BY THE RULE

Those directly affected by this rule include both the ARESLD patients and other ESLD patients who qualify for consideration. Many people are indirectly affected by this rule. The most significant of these include the families and others who will provide support for patients after transplant, health care providers involved in choosing transplant candidates, families of organ donors, and insurers who fund transplants (including government health plans).

✓ SPECIFY CONSEQUENCES OF THE RULE AND THEIR LIKELIHOOD OF OCCURRING

Reduce Personal and Social Costs of Alcoholism

One of the potential positive consequences of this rule is that it may motivate alcoholics to seek early treatment and thus reduce the personal and social costs of alcoholism.

Framework for Ethical Analysis
1. Identify the problem or issue.
2. Analyze context.
3. Explore options.
4. Apply the Rule Ethics Decision Process
5. Implement the plan and evaluate results.

Box 3–3 Rule Ethics Decision Process: Rule Utilitarianism

4. Apply the Rule Ethics Decision Process: Rule Utilitarianism

Basic Principle: **Rules of action are right in proportion to their tendency to promote the greatest good for the greatest number of persons affected by these rules.**

- Accurately state the rule to be evaluated.
- Identify all those who are directly and indirectly affected by the rule.
- Specify all the pertinent good and bad consequences of the rule for those affected, as far into the future as appears appropriate, and imaginatively consider various possible outcomes and the likelihood of their occurring (multiply likelihood by the effects.) Effects on those directly affected will generally carry greater weight than the effects on those indirectly affected.
- Consider whether there is some dominant, obvious consideration that carries such importance as to outweigh other considerations.
- Sum up the total good results and the total bad results of this rule.
- Imaginatively consider other good options to your rule and carry out a similar analysis for each of these options.
- Compare the results of the various rules. The rule that produces the most good (or the least bad, if none produces more good than bad) among those available is the morally correct rule to adopt.

Approximately one in every 10 Americans is a heavy drinker. The costs of alcoholism are high. One hundred thousand American deaths per year are wholly or partially attributed to drinking. Nearly half of emergency room admissions for injuries are alcohol related. Alcohol plays a major role in greater than half of automobile fatalities, and it is implicated in 67 percent of all murders and 70 percent of instances of domestic violence. In addition, alcoholism is the primary diagnosis in 25 percent of all people who commit suicide. The health effects of heavy alcohol consumption are multiple and serious. Ten to 20 percent of heavy drinkers develop cirrhosis, and 10 to 35 percent develop alcohol hepatitis. Other health effects include gastrointestinal problems; increased carcinogenic effects of substances such as tobacco; suppressed immune system, making heavy drinkers more prone to infections; and serious complications for diabetics (Well-Connected, 1998).

If the proposed rule encouraged even a minority of heavy drinkers to seek early treatment, the savings in health, productivity, and resources would be significant. We will consider this a large effect. There are good reasons, however, to question the efficacy of denying livers to patients with ARESLD. Telling alcoholics that they will not be eligible for liver transplants 10 to 15 years in the future is unlikely to motivate them to seek treatment now. The threat of the loss of family, friends, self-esteem, and jobs is often an insufficient inducement for alcoholics to seek help or to continue with treatment. It seems unlikely that consequences far in the future would provide a stronger incentive than these more immediate losses. Thus, although the positive consequences of motivating early treatment are large, their likelihood of occurring seems to be very small. Multiplying a very small likelihood by a large effect leaves us with a small positive result.

It is also possible that a policy denying equal eligibility for transplant to ARESLD patients who have been in recovery for six months or more could be counterproductive. After all, these persons have persevered to achieve their sobriety. In some cases, they required several attempts to reach this milestone. What kind of message would society be sending to other alcoholics with ARESLD who are still struggling toward recovery if they are told that regardless of their efforts, they will not be considered for treatment? (We might also imagine the effect on all heavy drinkers of similar policies that would restrict health care for other alcohol-related health problems.) Alcoholism is a disease that is difficult to overcome. It is highly unlikely that a rule denying the possibility of a liver transplant to those with ARESLD will motivate many who abuse alcohol to seek early treatment. Those few that might be so motivated will be canceled out by the larger numbers of those who might be discouraged from trying for recovery as a result of this rule.

Increase Organ Donations

Another potential positive consequence of a rule denying transplants to those with ARESLD is that this rule might encourage more organ donations. For every organ transplanted in the United States, two more people enter the waiting list. Only about 37 to 57 percent of eligible donors become actual donors of organs in the United States (Munson, 2000). We clearly need to improve the number of organ donors.

In light of the strong stigma and social bias against alcoholics that exists in our society, some people will be outraged by a policy that permits recovering alcoholics to receive liver transplants. It is foreseeable that some people will not sign organ donor cards out of fear that alcoholics might receive their livers. It is even more likely that some family members will refuse to consent to organ donation if they are aware of this policy. One need only imagine the response of a family who has just learned that a drunk driver killed their daughter or son. This family might refuse consent to organ donation knowing that their child's liver could end up transplanted in a recovering alcoholic. Others who consider those with ARESLD irresponsible might also refuse donation. Consequently, it is possible and perhaps likely that publicizing a policy denying liver transplants to all patients with ARESLD would lead to a moderate increase in organ donations. We will count this as a medium positive effect of this rule.

Reactions of Family Members

Many family members and friends of those with non–alcohol-related ESLD would respond favorably to a policy to exclude those with ARESLD from the pool of candidates for liver transplants. This policy will obviously increase the chances of their loved ones receiving a transplant. Many of these family and friends may also share the belief that those who did not cause their disease should have preference over those whose disease was self-induced. On the other hand, we can expect an opposite reaction from many family and friends of those with ARESLD, especially from those who have supported their loved ones through the difficult process of alcohol recovery. Thus, we can presume that these two sides of positive and negative effects cancel each other out.

Costs of Monitoring Patient Behavior

An anticipated negative consequence of the proposed rule is the cost of monitoring patient behavior. Monitoring the heavy drinking behavior that causes ARESLD is not particularly difficult. ARESLD can be fairly accurately diagnosed. Carbohydrate-deficient transferrin is a fairly accurate indicator of heavy drinking that can be used to detect a history of alcohol abuse. It is highly likely, however, that if a policy to deny liver transplants to those with ARESLD were formally adopted, there would be pressure to generalize the policy to deny all but palliative care for all other alleged self-induced illnesses as well. Although utilitarianism does not value fairness for its own sake, discriminatory policies often create negative tensions and undermine social stability. One family in every three in the United States has at least one member at risk for alcoholic cirrhosis. Although family members are often deeply hurt by alcoholic behavior, many family members will resent social policies that deny lifesaving treatment for family members who have worked hard to achieve sobriety and who medically qualify for a transplant.

Furthermore, if the primary utilitarian argument for the proposed rule is to encourage self-care and responsible use of health care resources, then the same calculus of social utility would support a more general rule denying all but palliative care to any patient with a self-induced illness. And the costs and practical difficulties of monitoring this broader policy would be overwhelming. The causes of some injuries or illnesses, such as not wearing a motorcycle helmet or a seat belt, are easily determined. But in other cases, such as heart disease, there may be multiple contributing factors. It is impossible to determine how much diet, genetics, exercise, stress, and side effects of medications have each contributed in any individual instance.

Even if this could be determined, how would health care providers monitor a patient's diet, stress-related behaviors, or exercise? Or imagine the difficulties involved in monitoring unsafe sexual behaviors. Would the presence of a sexually transmitted disease (STD) always mean that the patient has behaved irresponsibly? The effect of turning health care providers into "behavior monitors" would surely lead many persons with STDs to avoid treatment with further detrimental effects on public health.

✓ CONSIDER WHETHER THERE IS A DOMINANT CONSIDERATION

These are only a few of the costs and practical obstacles associated with monitoring patient behaviors that contribute to illness. One further major effect of a general rule denying all but basic palliative care for all self-induced illnesses would be the overall chilling effect that it would have on the character of health care itself. The relation of patients to their health care providers would be radically transformed and inescapably permeated with distrust. This weight of this consequence is large and its degree of likelihood is also large. This fact and the burdensome monitoring costs would outweigh any anticipated positive effects of this rule.

✓ Sum up Total Good Results and Bad Results of This Rule

We found only a small positive effect from the rule to deny candidacy for liver transplants to recovering alcoholics. We did not attempt to calculate possible positive effects of the general rule to deny all but basic palliative care to all patients with self-induced illnesses. Such a policy could encourage some patients to take more responsibility for their health and, consequently, could reduce the demand for limited health care resources. Yet, the negative effects associated with such a policy seem to far outweigh any savings in resources and increased patient well-being.

✓ Consider Alternative Rules

The best alternative to the proposed rule is this rule: *Patients with ARESLD who have been abstinent for six months or more and who meet other medical criteria should be given equal consideration for a liver transplant as other ESLD patients who satisfy the medical criteria. In addition, incentives to encourage healthy behavior regarding alcohol use should be instituted.* This rule would affect the same persons listed for the previous rule.

Positive Consequences

This rule would recognize and encourage the efforts of recovering alcoholics. Health care providers under this rule would assess the patient's medical status and likely success as a transplant candidate, rather than focus on whether the patient pursued treatment in a sufficiently timely and persistent manner. As a result, health care providers' time and resources would be devoted to patient care rather than to monitoring patient behavior. This nonjudgmental stance would in turn promote patient trust in health care providers and encourage patient–provider collaboration to promote wellness. This set of interrelated consequences is large, and its degree of likelihood is also large.

Incentives that reward healthy behavior are included in this rule. These might include discounts on health and car insurance premiums for nondrinkers or moderate drinkers. Employee assistance programs (EAPs) that provide confidential treatment for alcoholic employees also offer significant incentives for recovery. EAPs benefit both employees and employers. They encourage employees to stay connected to jobs and colleagues who often provide a critical source of self-esteem and motivation for treatment. Employers benefit from increased productivity, decrease in work-related accidents, reduced health care costs, and significantly lower costs for recruiting and retraining replacement workers. The Gillette Company reported a 75 percent reduction in inpatient alcohol and other drug abuse treatment costs, while the City of Los Angeles Department of Water and Power reported savings of $350,000 over a five-year period in reduced sickness absenteeism for employees with alcohol problems (Montgomery General Hospital, 1999). There is a 5:1 return on investment for EAP costs, with 85 percent of the savings due to decreased medical claims (Employee

Assistance Program, 2000). The positive effects of incentive programs of this kind are large and their degree of likelihood is also large.

At present, only 31 percent of American workers work for companies with EAPs (U.S. Department of Labor, 1999). Consequently, there is a need for further development of similar programs in the remaining companies. Many businesses are recognizing the mutual benefits of corporate wellness programs and are developing similar incentives to encourage healthy behaviors in other areas such as diet, exercise, and stress reduction. Surveys of employee participants in EAPs report that employees are more highly motivated to change their behaviors out of concern for their health than out of fear of punitive measures (Cleaves, 1997). This provides further support for the social utility of a rule that encourages and rewards recovery rather than one that punishes unhealthy behavior.

Negative Consequences

If denying eligibility for liver transplants would motivate a significant number of heavy drinkers to seek and persist in treatment at an earlier point in their lives, the loss of this effect would be a significant consequence of this alternate rule. However, there seems to be little reason to expect such a result. The other possible negative consequence of this rule is that some may be discouraged from making organ donations if recovering alcoholics are candidates for liver transplants. It seems likely that some persons would make this decision though it is difficult to predict how many. This effect could probably be moderated through public education programs noting the post-transplant survival and recidivism rates of recovering alcoholics.

✓ COMPARE THE RESULTS OF ALTERNATE RULES

The alternate rule gives equal consideration to patients with ARESLD and those with other forms of ESLD, and it encourages incentive programs for healthy behaviors related to alcohol consumption. Our estimates of its effects lead us to expect large positive effects and small negative ones. Compared to the largely negative effects of the rule denying candidacy to patients with ARESLD, the alternate rule plainly promotes greater social utility.

CONCLUSION OF RULE ETHICS DECISION PROCESS

Our conclusion is that Kantian and rule utilitarians support equal consideration of recovering alcoholics for liver transplants as patients with other forms of ESLD. Nurses interact constantly with patients who choose not to follow medical advice, or who choose not to discontinue behaviors that contribute to illness or loss of function, or who choose not to adopt lifestyles and personal habits that could improve their health. These choices may disappoint or baffle health care providers. It is important to keep in mind that the reasons for individual choices are usually complex. Most patients do care about their health. But they may have to disagree with their health care providers about how to promote their health or they may prioritize their values differently than their providers do. In any case, the analysis here creates serious doubts about the ethical nature of punitive attempts to prevent the wasteful use of health care resources by patients with allegedly self-induced illnesses. It is likely that rules intended to achieve this goal would also fail to pass the tests of either Kant's universalized respect for persons or rule utilitarian's maximization of happiness. Positive incentives encouraging responsible patient behavior to promote health are much more promising.

Others may disagree with one or both of the applications of rule ethics decision processes outlined here. Advocates would need to offer their own arguments for their positions. Disagreements of this sort are quite common in ethics, leading some to conclude that ethical judgments are simply a matter of personal opinion. But the disagreements noted here are not merely opinions reflecting personal biases or emotive reactions. The differing positions on this issue are based on reasonable applications of ethical rules. Articulating the reasons for our positions on ethical issues allows us as a community to locate the particular points of disagreement. This is a first step toward respectful understanding and perhaps eventual consensus.

Step 5. Implement the Plan and Evaluate the Results

The recommended policy needs to be reviewed from time to time in light of any new research regarding transplant outcomes and recidivism rates for those with ARESLD. If further study demonstrates significantly lower survival rates or higher recidivism rates, we would need to reconsider the position taken here. Significant changes in these two rates would suggest that the condition of ARESLD patients and other patients with ESLD are not sufficiently similar to require similar treatment.

Further Connections

Rule ethics is applied frequently to ethical issues relevant to nursing. Several issues are highlighted here, noting how rule ethics is relevant. Emerging technology and changes in the context of care present nurses with new ethical issues. Many of these issues can be addressed through the application of traditional rules to new situations. Other issues may require major amendment of traditional rules or rethinking of fundamental ethical concepts that are central aspects of these rules. All of these issues highlight the ongoing dialogue within particular communities that is at the heart of ethics. Rule ethics provides a crucial framework for public debates regarding what principles and values are needed to promote civilized and fruitful life within our communities.

New Applications of Rules

As direct care providers and patient advocates, nurses encounter many situations in which patient autonomy is threatened. Threats to patient confidentiality are one such area. Protecting patient confidentiality has grown more complex as the number of parties with access to patient records has dramatically increased. The multidisciplinary nature of patient diagnosis and treatment in today's hospitals generates a "need-to-know" status for dozens of professionals. Beyond this direct scrutiny of patient charts, third parties such as insurance companies, employers, and government agencies through Medicare and Medicaid, may gain access to an individual's private medical information. Increased computerization and networking of computer systems creates additional opportunities for illegitimate access to patient files. Within another decade or so, individual health histories will likely include DNA profiles revealing actual and potential pathologies. A national DNA registry is likely. All of this heightens the obligation of health care practitioners and others to safeguard patient confidentiality.

The increasing shift from hospital-based care to home care and long-term care highlights daily conflicts between patient autonomy and nurses' duties of beneficence. Examples in home care include a paraplegic with pressure sores on his buttocks. While dependent on nurses to help him from his bed to his wheelchair, the patient refuses the bed rest, which his nurses insist is needed. The adamant refusal of restraints by an elderly Alzheimer's patient and her family is not uncommon in long-term care. Restrained patients may become fearful, humiliated, demoralized, or uncomfortable (Dawkins, 1998). They may also suffer from negative physical effects such as skin abrasions, urinary retention, and pressure sores (Quinn, 1996). Nurses, on the other hand, are responsible for protecting patients from harm and for providing the correct nursing interventions related to safety. Although evidence suggests that restraints are not effective when used to treat aggressive behavior or to prevent patient injury (Neufeld et al., 1999; Dodds, 1996), restraints are used every day throughout the United States. Chronic understaffing, particularly in long-term care facilities, exacerbates the pressures to employ restraints. Alternatives to restraints should be carefully explored.

Nurses face additional challenges related to their obligations of beneficence when patient safety and well-being are threatened by impaired, incompetent, or unethical behavior by health care practitioners. While nurses have clear obligations to report impaired or incompetent colleagues, difficult decisions must be made when nurses consider "blowing the whistle" on colleagues. Ideally, organizations will support nurses who act conscientiously to protect patients. In reality, organizations often do not provide this support. Misbehavior may be covered up, reports ignored or forgotten, and whistle-blowers may be reprimanded, shunned, or even fired. Nurses will need to weigh the risks and costs of whistle-blowing against their imperfect duties to protect their patients.

Amending Rules and Rethinking Ethical Concepts

Voluntary Active Euthanasia

Discussions about euthanasia exemplify ethics as an ongoing dialogue within particular communities. Active euthanasia involves interventions such as administering medication that has the intention of causing a patient's death. In a physician-assisted suicide, a physician assists a patient's death by providing a prescription and instructions for a lethal dose of medication. The demand to legalize euthanasia continues to grow louder in both the United States and Canada. Laws supporting assistance by physicians already exist in the Netherlands, Uruguay, Switzerland, Peru, Japan, and Germany.

Although the actions of physicians have been the focus of public debates and debates within health care ethics, nurses are directly involved in these practices. Nurses play an indispensable role in the delivery of appropriate care at the end of life. Because of their intimate interaction with dying patients, nurses are in a special position to understand the suffering and the wishes of patients and their surrogates. Asch (1996) reports on a study that attempts to determine the practices of critical care nurses with respect to assisted suicide and active euthanasia. Since the study relies on self-reporting, the data may not be entirely accurate. Nonetheless, the study indicates that critical care nurses receive significant numbers of requests from patients or family members to perform euthanasia or to assist in suicide and that some nurses sometimes engage in these practices. These practices are contrary to position statements of the American Nurses Association, endorsed by the American Association of Critical Care Nurses (Curtin, 1995). As the public demand for these interventions grows and if they are legalized more fully, nurses will, undoubtedly, be drawn more and more into these practices in critical care units and in home health care settings.

The euthanasia debate in the United States and Canada reflects the attempt by these communities to reevaluate their rules regarding morally justified killing. Traditionally, these communities have recognized only three instances of justified killing: self-defense, just war, and capital punishment. (Even the latter two of these have been hotly debated in the last few decades.) All three of these exceptions to the rule "Do not kill human beings" involve killing persons who are a threat to others' lives. In the case of euthanasia, these communities consider adding a fourth and very different exception: One that concerns killing persons who are no threat to others. This revision of moral rules has the potential to significantly reshape the health care professions. It is no wonder that this dialogue has been so passionate and difficult.

Advocates of euthanasia argue that it is supported by the values of individual autonomy and individual well-being (beneficence) in cases where competent patients request it (Brock, 2000). Some opponents of euthanasia object that the sanctity and dignity of human life makes it morally wrong to directly and intentionally kill these persons even if they themselves request this action (Callahan, 1992; Kass, 1991). Other authors raise equally important questions about the impact of cultural contexts on the euthanasia dialogue. Some analyze the way in which Western cultures conceptualize and institutionalize death. They shift the focus of ethical discussion from the question of whether euthanasia is morally permissible to questions about the obligations of society to support individuals in their last life stage (Byock, 1996). To what degree are people asking health care providers to end their lives because our health care system and our society fails to adequately assist them in living fully their last life stage (Scofield, 1995)? What role do financial pressures play in individual requests for physician-assisted suicide? These pressures come from two sources: (1) patients' concerns about becoming an economic burden on their families and (2) policies and incentives in some insurance companies that encourage physicians to undertreat seriously ill patients (Bilchik, 1996). These facts highlight the danger of creating a right to die before we create a right to treatment.

ACCESS TO HEALTH RESOURCES

The issue of euthanasia thus points to issues of access to care and the allocation of resources for health promotion and health care. These are pressing issues of justice. With increased concerns about cost-containment and efficiency, changes in the structure and delivery of health care are under way in the United States and Canada today. Unfortunately, there has been a huge gap between the abstract discussions of ethical theorists regarding what appropriate theories or models of distributive justice and actual health care reforms that are taking place. It seems unlikely that either the United

States or Canada will achieve consensus on an overall model of fair distribution of health care resources. Nonetheless, concrete changes in the management, delivery, and financing of health care contain implicit assumptions about fair distribution. Nurses are in positions to observe the effects of policy decisions and to monitor the quality and availability of care. Also, as members of the largest health care profession, nurses can and should be active participants in health care policy and planning decisions.

Related to the issues of fair access and allocation of health resources are questions about appropriate models of health care. In spite of significant changes, North American health care continues to be illness centered. Nursing must continue to challenge this model and to envision alternatives focused on wellness and health promotion. Such a shift could play a critical role in solving the challenges of cost-containment and fair allocation.

GENETICS

The number of nurses working in genetic counseling has rapidly increased in the past decade. More significant, however, is the fact that genetic knowledge will form the basis of medical science in the twenty-first century. The delivery of genetic services is shifting from specialized genetic clinics to primary care settings. As a result, nurses in all settings will care for patients facing genetic issues related to screening, testing, counseling, or treatment.

Genetic research offers hopeful possibilities for increased understanding of the causes of genetic disorders, followed by better treatments and/or the elimination of these disorders. But there are also increased opportunities for violations of patient privacy and discrimination against those who do not fit new definitions of "normal" or "healthy." Gene therapy may also produce unintended negative side effects, many of which may simply be unpredictable.

New diagnostic tests such as multiplex testing (performing multiple genetic texts on a single blood or tissue sample), preimplantation genetic testing, and fetal cell sorting (allows early prenatal genetic diagnosis) will require careful application of traditional moral rules regarding patient confidentiality, informed consent, and privacy (Scanlon and Fibison, 1995). Gene therapy, particularly alteration of the DNA in sperm or ova (germ-line therapy), will dramatically impact our conceptions of illness, health, disability, and health care. New rules or significant reconceptions of old ones may be needed to address these genetic issues. Nurses will have critical roles to play as these technologies are developed and applied.

"Genetics" is not a single practice, discipline, or social issue. Rather, it involves a series of choices made by parents, scientists, health care professionals, and government agencies. These choices reflect diverse interests and purposes. Many people are poorly educated about the basics of biological understandings of heredity as well as unreflective about the nature and goals of technology. As a result, much of public discussion about genetics careens back and forth between overly pessimistic views of the dangers of technology and overly optimistic promises to solve a multitude of individual and social problems (McGee, 1997). Consumers, patients, and parents, consequently, may face a panoply of products and options without the benefit of thoughtful public discussions concerning the goals of genetic technologies.

From the duties of nonmaleficence and beneficence we can deduce a nursing obligation to be informed and involved in ethical and political debates that will emerge. Nurses can play a crucial role in these discussions. Many lay people respect nurses as observant translators of technical medical information. Nurses will play this role in clinical settings as patient and parents struggle to make choices about genetic

---

Box 3–4   Communities in Dialogue:

Genetic Enhancements

Germ-line therapy in the future may make it possible not only to cure genetic diseases, but also to enhance or improve upon normal healthy lives. Consider the following futuristic scenario.

The AIDS pandemic has continued unabated into the third decade of the twenty-first century. Numerous countries in the developing world, particularly Africa, have been devastated by the enormous loss of lives, the societal burdens of orphaned and often infected children, and the stress on limited health care budgets. Promising treatments have failed to be effective in the long term. Those treatments that have significantly extended life for HIV-infected persons are expensive and, thus, entirely unrealistic as a global response to this disease.

New research in germ-line therapy has made it possible to insert gene coding for antibodies to AIDS. Extensive research with baboons has been overwhelmingly successful. More limited experimental therapy with human subjects in the last five years has revealed no undesirable effects thus far. No one can predict the long-term effects with 100 percent accuracy. But the continued effects of the AIDS pandemic are painfully clear.

Several African governments have approached the World Health Organization (WHO) with a proposal and request for assistance. They propose to make germ-line therapy to create AIDS immunity mandatory for all future children. They lack the technical and financial resources to implement this plan. They are seeking assistance from the WHO. The proposal is an expensive one, but the overwhelming global costs of the continued AIDS pandemic will be even greater.

Questions

1. Putting aside the cost issues for the moment, would you support this project? Why or why not?
2. If this form of germ-line therapy is morally acceptable, should it be made mandatory?
3. In a society in which this form of germ-line therapy is technically and medically possible, would we consider human beings who are not protected from AIDS in this way to be disabled?
4. What does it mean to be disabled, and is there an obligation for parents and/or society to prevent disability when it is feasible to do so?

information or therapy that will change their lives. They can play a similar role in public conversations as respected professionals with a knowledge of biology and as trusted patient advocates. Issues of justice will also emerge as questions of access to genetic counseling and therapy are discussed. In addition, justice demands that we consider whether an increasing allocation of limited health care dollars to genetic research is appropriate in light of our society's present failure to provide even basic needs for the poor, the disabled, uninsured workers, and the elderly. The scenario presented in Box 3–4 reflects the need for community dialogue about the use of genetic technologies and the allocation of funds for this use.

Conclusion

Health care is a complex and ever-changing context. Rule ethics provides clear processes to guide decision makers whether the issues require applications of established moral rules or development of new rules. In either case, Kantian and rule utilitarian theories provide reasons and justification for the rules and their applications.

KEY POINTS

- Mistaken beliefs about survival rates and recidivism for recovering alcoholics as well as social stigma and bias contribute to an unwillingness to transplant livers in those with ARESLD that meet medical criteria.
- Both Kantian and rule utilitarian decision processes support equal access to liver transplants for persons with ARESLD and other ESLD patients.
- The most important consideration for a Kantian in allocating all limited health care resources is whether a patient medically qualifies for a treatment. Whether the illness or injury was self-induced is not morally relevant.
- Rule utilitarian calculations do not support the intuition that a rule limiting liver transplants would maximize happiness in society by encouraging self-care and responsible use of health care resources.
- Kantians and rule utilitarians conclude that patient self-care and responsible use of health care resources are more fairly and effectively supported through positive incentives.
- Rule ethics provides nurses with clear guidelines for making ethical decisions. Understanding the theoretical foundations for Kantian and utilitarian rules enables us to develop and apply rules to new challenges in health care.

REFLECT AND DISCUSS

Consider the following case studies in light of the utilitarian and Kantian rules summarized in Box 2–7. For each case consider what rules are relevant to the case. If more than one rule is relevant, which rule will have priority and why?

Case 1   The Patient's Good

David Brooks, age 60, was admitted with a chief complaint of abdominal pain. Mr. Brooks was scheduled to have a common bile duct stone removed prior to this admission, but ended up in the emergency room with a suspected case of pancreatitis. An amylase of 4,200 confirmed this. His admission vital signs were 116/90, pulse 100, oxygen saturation 90 percent. The patient is admitted for pain control, intravenous hydration, and antibiotics.

History

The patient's history includes a left femoral bypass and a left to right femoral/femoral bypass graft. Although started on Coumadin, he developed a deep venous thrombosis and pulmonary embolus. Because of lack of therapeutic anticoagulation, the patient went on to further develop a left cerebrovascular accident (CVA) involving the right arm and leg. After recovery from the CVA, Mr. Brooks continued to have residual neurovascular deficits of his right leg that included weakness and vascular insufficiency. Additionally, he has some short-term memory loss and has become quite forgetful. A postrecovery workup revealed a left carotid lesion, which was treated with a left carotid endarterectomy.

Systems Review

Patient has a history of heart disease and previous coronary bypass 10 years ago. A recent chest x-ray and prostate-specific antigen were both normal. He smokes 2 packs/day and admits to drinking 6 to 8 beers/week. Patient is quite overweight, with body mass index at 32.

The morning following the current admission for abdominal pain, the nurse found that the patient had no pulses in his right lower leg and, after evaluation by his physician, he was transferred to the intensive care unit (ICU). An embolectomy was done, after which he became hypoxic and hypotensive. A Swan–Ganz was placed to monitor for cardiac output and possible sepsis. Bipap was used initially for hypoxia.

Two days after being admitted to ICU, patient had significant oxygen desaturation problems with sudden change in mental status, becoming agitated. He was intubated, placed on mechanical ventilation, and given medication for agitation. His wife was informed of his condition and of his poor prognosis.

Approximately five days later the patient appeared oriented and calm. He was still ventilated but needing only 10 cm of pressure support for mechanical ventilation. He continued to improve and was able to be extubated and advanced from total parenteral nutrition to jejunostomy feedings. He was moved to the surgical floor. Twenty-four hours later he developed acute pancreatitis with elevated amylase, severe abdominal pain, and nausea with hypotension. He was transferred back to ICU. Within a day he was reintubated and developed another arterial thromboembolism of the right leg. A second embolectomy had to be performed.

Mr. Brooks continued with abdominal distention and still needed common bile duct stone removal as well as medical support for his pancreatitis. Concurrently, his right foot continued to demonstrate ischemia and the surgeon recommended a below-knee amputation (BKA). About three weeks into this hospitalization, a conference was held with the attending physician, the consulting physician, nursing staff, and the patient's wife. Mrs. Brooks was willing to consent to the BKA surgery based on her belief that this was best for her husband; however, she did not want her husband to know about this. She felt that her husband would not agree to an amputation. The nursing staff from ICU felt that Mr. Brooks was alert and oriented enough to be included in the discussion of a pending BKA. Mrs. Brooks opposed this, saying that she not only feared that her husband would not agree to the surgery, but that with his current physical and medical status, he was in no condition to discuss his treatment options. The physician and surgeon agreed not to include Mr. Brooks in the decision, getting surgical consent from Mrs. Brooks.

Would Mrs. Brooks's consent for surgery be adequate? Is it permissible not to inform Mr. Brooks of the surgeon's recommendation? What should the ICU nursing staff do at this point? Explain your answers by applying the relevant rules.

Case 2 Baby Andy

Andy was born at home, the eighth child for Dan and Marsha. A prenatal exam had suggested potential complications, and a hospital delivery was strongly recommended. The baby presented in the breech position and suffered an anoxic event. Andy's 15-year-old brother did "mouth to mouth" while Dan drove to the closest hospital emergency room. Since this ER was not prepared to care for neonates, baby Andy was transported to another hospital. After weeks of care in the neonatal intensive care unit (NICU), Andy was sent home with 24-hour nursing care, funded through state Medicaid. Andy has constant seizures and he is on a ventilator. An electroencephalogram (EEG) shows minimal brain activity. He has been hospitalized six times since being discharged five months ago. Although Andy's parents do not seem to have any second thoughts about continuing Andy's intensive therapy, some of the nurses who have cared for him during his hospitalizations do have questions. They wonder if it would be morally wrong to remove Andy from the ventilator.

Would it be wrong to remove the ventilator? Are Andy's parents morally obligated to continue to do everything medically possible for their son? Explain your answers by applying the relevant rules to this case.

Case 3 Protecting the Elderly

Lilly, 78 years old and a vital member of her Pacific Northwest community, never had children and was widowed a decade ago. Her only living relative was a brother in Michigan whom she had not seen for nearly 20 years.

Betty, a friend and neighbor, checked on Lilly early each evening. Lilly has recently exhibited brief periods of confusion; sometimes, she cannot remember if she has paid a bill or taken a particular medication. Betty has been concerned about Lilly's diminished appetite and also for her safety. Lilly's house is terribly cluttered with what most people would consider junk, but to Lilly it is her life and all she owns. She often tells Betty how important it is for her to stay at home and how she fears long-term care (LTC) facilities.

One evening, Lilly casually mentioned that her brother was in town and had been to visit her. Betty asked Lilly to have her brother call her, thinking that it would be good to discuss her concerns about Lilly with him. The next evening, Lilly revealed that her brother took her to a lawyer that day and that she had given him power of attorney, "just in case something ever happens to me," Lilly quoted her brother.

The next evening, Betty as usual checked on Lilly. When she arrived, however, the house was dark. Betty let herself in and called Lilly's name. Lilly was nowhere to be found. Betty reasoned that one of Lilly's neighbors had taken her to dinner, as happened from time to time.

Early the next morning, Betty called Adult Protective Services, and a case-worker reported that they had just investigated Lilly's situation at the request of her brother. When Lilly wouldn't let them in, they obtained a warrant and, accompanied by police, took Lilly to a gero-psych hospital unit where she would remain for 14 days. Livid, Betty immediately went to the hospital to comfort her friend. Lilly demanded, "How could you do this to me?"

Lilly's levels of the cardiac medicine digoxin were found to be toxic, which contributed to her confusion. After her serum levels were normalized, she seemed much better. A legal hearing had already been held, however. Lilly was found to be incompetent, an independent guardian was appointed by the court to represent Lilly's interests, and Lilly was told that she could not return home. She asked Betty repeatedly, "Why is this happening to me?"

After 14 days, Lilly was moved into the first accepting LTC facility. Greeted by the admissions department, she appeared confused due to the change in environment and by all of the activity and questions. She was assigned a semiprivate room, and her clothes were unpacked and marked with permanent ink. Within two weeks, Lilly had lost the right to make choices about where she lives, when to get up or go to bed, when and if she bathes, and when, where, and what she eats. Even so simple a choice as what kind of toothpaste she uses had been taken from her.

What rules are relevant to this case? Assess the decisions and the processes in the case applying these rules. Do you think that Lilly was incompetent? Do you think that the process and the decisions in this case were appropriate? Did Betty do all she could to advocate for Lilly? Explain your answers.

REFERENCES

American Liver Foundation. (1996). Liver transplantation for alcoholic liver disease [Online]. Available: http://gi.ucsf.edu/ALF/pubs/progalc&tx.html [1998, September 2].

Asch, D. A. (1996). The role of critical care nurses in euthanasia and assisted suicide. *New England Journal of Medicine, 334*(21), 1374–1379.

Bilchik, G. S. (1996). Dollars & death: Money changes everything. *Hospitals & Health Networks, 70*(24), 18–22.

Brock, D. W. (2000). Voluntary active euthanasia. In R. Munson (Ed.), *Intervention and reflection: Basic issues in medical ethics* (6th ed., pp. 215–222). Belmont, CA: Wadsworth/Thomson Learning.

Byock, I. (1996). Beyond symptom management. *European Journal of Palliative Care, 3*(3), 125–130.

Callahan, D. (1992). When self-determination runs amok. *Hastings Center Report, 22,* 52–55.

Cleaves, E. (1997). The hidden benefits of employee assistance programs, part I. [Online]. Available: http://www.ccjmagazine.com/EAP.HTM [2000, June 13].

Cohen, C., and Benjamin, M. (2000). Alcoholics and liver transplantation. In R. Munson (Ed.), *Intervention and reflection: Basic issues in medical ethics* (6th ed., pp. 789–793). Belmont, CA: Wadsworth/Thomson Learning.

Curtin, L. L. (1995). Nurses take a stand on assisted suicide. *Nursing Management, 26*(5), 71, 73–74, 79.

Dawkins, V. H. (1998). Restraints and the elderly with mental illness: Ethical issues and moral reasoning. *Journal of Psychosocial Nursing and Mental Health Services, 36*(10), 22–27, 36–37.

Dodds, S. (1996). Exercising restraint: Autonomy, welfare, and elderly patients. *Journal of Medical Ethics, 22*(3), 160–163.

Employee Assistance Program. (2000). [Online]. Available: http://www.psychhealthnet.com/eap.htm. [2000, June 12].

Kass, L. (1991). Why doctors must not kill. *Commonweal, 118*(14, Suppl.), 472–476.

Kelso, L. A. (1994). Alcohol-related end-stage liver disease and transplantation: The debate continues. *Clinical Issues in Critical Care Nursing, 5*(4), 501–506.

Killeen, T. K. (1993). Alcoholism and liver transplantation: Ethical and nursing implications. *Perspectives in Psychiatric Care, 29*(1), 7–12.

McGee, G. (1997). *The perfect baby: A pragmatic approach to genetics.* Lanham, MD: Rowman & Littlefield.

Montgomery General Hospital. (1999). Employee assistance programs [Online]. Available: http://www.montgomerygeneral.com/bhs/eap.htm [2000, June 12].

Moss, A. H., and Siegler, M. (1991). Should alcoholics compete equally for liver transplants? *Journal of the American Medical Association, 265*(10), 1295–1298.

Munson, R. (Ed.). (2000). *Intervention and reflection: Basic issues in medical ethics* (6th ed.). Belmont, CA: Wadsworth/Thompson Learning.

Neufeld, R. R., Libow, L. S., Foley, W. J., et al. (1999). Restraint reduction reduces serious injuries among nursing home residents. *Journal of the American Geriatrics Society, 47*(10), 1202–1207.

Office of Health Technology Assessment, Agency for Health Care Policy Research. (1990). Assessment of liver transplantation. *U.S. Department of Health and Human Services, 1,* 3–32.

Quinn, C. A. (1996). The advanced practice nurse and changing perspectives on physical restraint. *Clinical Nurse Specialist, 10*(5), 220–227.

Scanlon, C., and Fibison, W. (1995). *Managing genetic information: Implications for nursing practice.* Washington, DC: American Nurses Publishing.

Scofield, G. R. (1995). Exposing myths about physician-assisted suicide. *Seattle University Law Review, 18*(3), 473–493.

Thomas, D. J. (1993). Organ transplantation in people with unhealthy lifestyles. *Clinical Issues in Critical Care Nursing, 4*(4), 665–668.

UNOS. (2001). Critical data [Online]. Available: http://www.UNOS.org [2001, March 12].

U.S. Department of Labor. (1999). Working partners for an alcohol-and-drug-free workplace [Online]. Available: http://www.dol.gov/dol/workingpartners.ktrn [2000, June 12].

Well-Connected. (1998). Alcoholism [Online]. Available: http://www.Well-Connected.com [2000, June 12].

4

Virtue Ethics: Character, Judgment, and Community

CHAPTER OUTLINE

EXPERIENTIAL ACCOUNT: Trust Between Nurse and Patient

The following excerpt from an interview with Elena D'Amico, RN, a home health nurse, illustrates how the issue of trust arose in connection with her patient, Kirsten, who developed pregnancy-induced hypertension:

As the nurse who cared for Kirsten during her third pregnancy, I had gotten to know her well. I discovered that Kirsten had experienced postpartum depression after her first two babies were born. Kirsten and I talked about that and, anticipating it might happen again, we tried to figure out ways to prevent it this time. After a successful delivery, Kirsten was discharged to home care, and the doctor said no visits were needed. I phoned and asked if she would like to continue with the in-home support program for mothers, First Steps. She agreed, so I phoned the doctor and got the okay for her to continue.

At first, it seemed Kirsten was doing okay. Then she began to feel depressed. I started seeing Kirsten a couple of times a week and was concerned about her depression. I consulted several social worker colleagues just to talk about where they might go with her. Soon after this, Kirsten began to sound like she might hurt herself. I became more concerned and called her doctor, who approved daily visits. So, we started making daily home visits, and sometimes these were nurses she knew. She wasn't very comfortable with strange nurses . . . she had a history of abuse in her childhood, and she is kind of guarded.

I could see that she was becoming more despondent. I knew that she needed to be on medication, but she was fighting that. She'd been depressed many times in her life and had never been helped by antidepressants. And now she was nursing and worried about side effects to the baby.

One day I called her, and she sounded worse. She told me she was scared, thinking she should be in the hospital, but she was reluctant to do anything. You know, when you get depressed, you are just stuck, and she was frozen. It seemed she couldn't do anything to help herself, so I asked if I could call her doctor for her, and she gave me permission. I called and they got her right in that day and put her on medication. They also assigned a counselor who started seeing her daily.

The outcome was a success. She thanked me many times for doing the right thing and helping her to feel that someone cared, for calling her doctor that day and getting in touch with a counselor. I had also contacted her husband to make sure he understood the severity of her situation, because at that point she'd been talking about leaving her family. Her self-esteem was low, she felt like her kids would be better off without her, and she was ready to take off. It was real scary, for her and me. She was really in crisis and needed somebody to intervene for her. And it was great, because we had good rapport. Even though she's somebody who doesn't trust real easily, she trusted me. It was gratifying to be able to get her the help she needed.

Adapted from Home Health Nurse, Interviewee 3 in Katz, 1996.

Many women and men choose to become nurses because they admire and would like to emulate characteristics that they see nurses exemplify. Many nurses, like Elena D'Amico, are caring, compassionate, and nurturing. They are people of integrity and competent problem solvers who serve as resilient advocates and mediators for their patients. To be an effective nurse requires not only education, mentoring, and the acquisition of skills, but also the development of character. Becoming a nurse is a process of joining the community of nurses—a community whose members are distinguished by characteristic traits.

Virtue ethics focuses on the development of character, our core identity as individual human beings. ***Character*** is a configuration of innate dispositions, shaped by environmental influences, as well as traits acquired through habitual behavior and choices (McKinnon, 1999). Our character will determine what we care about, what choices we make, what behaviors will be characteristic of us, and what kind of lives we live. Each of us has a unique moral identity—a unique character. This unique character is formed by the choices we make and the habits or patterns of behavior that we develop (Connors & McCormick, 1998).

All persons are born with certain temperaments or dispositions. Character develops as individuals interact with their worlds, responding to various opportunities and challenges. These responses and choices shape character. As people make choices and develop characteristic habits, they are choosing what kind of people they want to be. Character integrates choices and habits into a coherent and consistent whole that is a unique self.

Human beings evaluate their own lives and the lives of others around them. We assess people's character as good or bad, morally praiseworthy or not. These assessments depend on shared conceptions of good or flourishing human lives. These shared conceptions emerge from ongoing dialogue within particular communities. ***Virtues***, or strengths of character that promote human flourishing, and ***vices***, deficiencies or weaknesses of character that undermine human flourishing, are also defined through this communal dialogue.

Although each person's character is unique, individuals live in communities that significantly affect their character development. Persons can be nurtured or marred by their communities. Consequently, virtue ethics asserts that we are not only responsible for developing good character as individuals, but that we also have responsibilities for the kind of communities that we collectively develop.

From this brief sketch of virtue ethics, we see a clear shift in focus from rule ethics. While the primary question posed by rule ethics is "What is the right thing to do?", the primary question for virtue ethics is "What kind of people and what kind of community should we be?" In virtue ethics, character is primary and behavior is secondary. When she responded to Kirsten's needs, Nurse D'Amico's actions were motivated and shaped by her character.

The priority of character in virtue ethics emerges in three ways. First, appropriate behavior flows from good character. Persons of good character do good things because of who they are—because they are honest, generous, and compassionate—not simply because they believe that doing good deeds is their duty or the right thing to do. Second, character shapes our capacity for making moral judgments. Everything we need to know about living a good life cannot be summarized into a set of moral rules that we can apply to all situations. We need a more complex capacity for moral judgment that will enable us to discern how to feel and how to act in response to particular situations. Third, even in cases in which moral rules can direct our behavior, we need good character and judgment to know how to apply these moral rules to guide our actions.

Virtue ethics recognizes people as social beings who live and act in the context of various communities. Each community has its own characteristic goals and purposes. Some communities are defined by goals that are explicitly moral, which means they commit to goals that transcend the personal interests of their members. Nursing can be viewed as a moral community pledged to pursue goals that extend beyond the personal interests of nurses and distinguished by characteristic nursing virtues. Each moral community determines through an ongoing conversation what virtues are needed to enable its members to promote and sustain the values and goals of this community. A set of nursing virtues is outlined in this chapter, and readers are encouraged to evaluate the adequacy of this list. Like other virtues, nursing virtues are developed and preserved through mentoring processes. This chapter will emphasize the importance of mentoring and of critical reflection by nursing communities about their values, virtues, and concrete moral judgments. Furthermore, since the role of communities in developing and sustaining individual character is an essential theme in virtue ethics, this chapter also will explore how professional nursing communities consider and develop policies, practices, and organizations that develop and sustain character.

Human Flourishing and Virtues

Virtue ethics clearly approaches ethical issues in a dramatically different manner than rule ethics does. Thinking about ethics in terms of rules and what is right or wrong is so familiar to us that we easily forget that, before the seventeenth century, virtue ethics predominated in most cultures. The roots of this philosophical tradition in the West are found in Plato and Aristotle's Greece in the fifth and fourth centuries B.C.E. Other Asian traditions of virtue ethics—Buddhistic moral theory, Confucianism, and Taoism—emerged at about the same time. Judaism and many Native American tribes also claim rich virtue ethical traditions.

Chapter 2 (pp. 28–30) presented developments in modern Europe that inspired the shift from virtue ethics to rule ethics. An awareness of the historical and cultural context of Aristotle's virtue ethics will help us to understand this earlier ethical theory.

Aristotle on Human Flourishing

Aristotle's immersion in biology is key to his work and exerted considerable influence on his approach to ethics. A careful observer of flora and fauna, Aristotle laid down the foundations of biological classification. He introduced the concept of empirical science to the ancient world, developing the empirical methods of gathering evidence, making hypotheses, and testing theories against experience. Aristotle's philosophical method always began with setting down what he called "the relevant appearances," and virtue ethics reflects this commitment to contextuality. Aristotle also advocated the process of reviewing how previous wise men, whether scientists or philosophers, treated the relevant issues. Aristotle believed that though theorists should critically evaluate previously imparted wisdom, they must ultimately return to their initial observations about how human beings live, act, and perceive (Nussbaum, 1986). Virtue ethics also reflects an appreciation for the important role of "wise men."

Community and relationships play central roles in virtue ethics. During the time of Aristotle, Greek citizens lived in what were called city-states. The Greek city-state was not merely a political community; its citizens were unified on other levels as well. These included geographic boundaries, shared familial and cultural histories, and religious traditions. Political and cultural institutions varied from one to another city-state. Athens, a democracy, allowed free men without property to participate in government. In contrast, some city-states were monarchies, and most limited citizenship to property owners. All except Sparta had slaves, and while all limited the roles of women, the nature of these limitations varied from one city-state to another. Aristotle grew up in Macedonia, a rural community more socially stratified than the urban, democratic Athens where he spent much of his adult life. All Greek city-states shared, however, the concept of human life as essentially communal. A person's identity was defined through relations and roles within the community. Those who lived outside these political/cultural communities were considered uncivilized barbarians.

The Search for Universal Virtues

When Aristotle applied his philosophical, empirical method to ethics, we can hear the biologist in him asking questions: What is the purpose of human existence? How are human beings unique? What do they do best? What do flourishing, healthy human beings look like? What do human beings need in order to function well? To Aristotle, it seemed obvious that if olive trees and spiders have a purpose in nature, then human beings must as well. From his careful observation of human beings, Aristotle concluded that we have two distinct functions: (1) to build and maintain a fruitful communal life together and (2) to engage in rational reflection. From these functions, Aristotle derived his list of necessary human virtues.

Critics of virtue ethics, however, note that today's pluralistic societies do not share the cohesion and homogeneity of Aristotle's city-states. As a result, we find disagreement about the purpose of life and which virtues are desired. Furthermore, critics suggest that Aristotle's virtues are not universal as he supposed, but instead that they are culture-bound (Williams, 1985; MacIntyre, 1981). Aristotle's mistake, critics argue, rests on his reliance on *the craft analogy.*

THE CRAFT ANALOGY

Flourishing, as we have said, means functioning or living well. Relying on a craft analogy (Wallace, 1988a), Aristotle and later virtue theorists assume that human beings have distinct, readily recognizable functions. Just as we can identify the purpose or point of a craft—like flute playing, sculpting, or healing—the craft analogy proposes that we can also identify the unique goals or functions of human life (cf. Aristotle, *Nichomachean Ethics*, Book Two). Consequently, good human persons are those who perform their functions well, just as good bakers and good carpenters are those who are recognized as expert practitioners of their craft. Furthermore, because we can study these experts to identify the skills needed to perform these crafts well, we should also be able to uncover the virtues and standards of excellence in good human lives.

The concept of human flourishing, however, has been controversial throughout human history, inspiring many different accounts of human function. Some concepts of human flourishing have been based in religion; for example, "to achieve a state of nirvana in which suffering has ceased." Some theorists define human flourishing in terms of achieving economic goals that maximize opportunities for entrepreneurial success. Others describe this concept in psychological terms, such as the ability to balance one's id, ego, and superego. Thus, no universal agreement exists about the function of human life, and reflective people of good will disagree about what makes a good life. For the human being, no clear function or purpose appears to exist as it does for the flute player, the carpenter, or the baker.

Most contemporary virtue ethicists do not envision a singular, universal account of human flourishing or the good life. Human flourishing is understood pluralistically as having a wide variability (MacIntyre, 1981; Pellegrino & Thomasma, 1993; Wallace, 1988b; Hauerwas, 1981; Hinman, 1994). Our concepts differ as to what constitutes a good human life, a good human community, and a good person. Attempting to extract from these diverse views a general idea of what makes a good life gives us an account so abstract that it is of no practical use. For instance, we might reasonably argue that "inner peace" is an essential element of a good life. Clearly, however, the meaning of inner peace varies dramatically among Freudian, Buddhist, and Navajo conceptions. Each would prescribe distinctly different individual and social practices.

MORAL CONSIDERATIONS AND VIRTUES

The conclusion we can draw, then, is that human life is much too complex and its contexts too varied for us to identify a single fixed goal for human living. The standards for living a good human life or being a good person are not as well defined and discernible as standards for the crafts of sculpting, healing, or parenting. Because no single, fixed goal is shared by all members of the human community, we cannot derive a single set of virtues that will define and promote human flourishing in all contexts. Consequently, virtue ethics does not provide us with a list of universal human virtues that we can then apply to the nursing context.

But pluralistic accounts of virtue ethics do recognize our abilities as human persons and human communities to identify, interpret, prioritize, and adapt relevant moral considerations in particular contexts. All communities will face some common concerns and problems as they try to develop and sustain a communal life. *Moral considerations* are practical concerns that arise as communities consider how to promote mutual human welfare, growth, and meaning in their particular communal contexts. These moral considerations require some response or resolution by the communities (Wallace, 1988a). These considerations are practical because they are "how to" considerations, but they are distinct from technical considerations of communal living such as how to build bridges that resist earthquakes or how to preserve sterile conditions in an operating room.

Moral considerations will arise as communities address common problems such as how to raise children, how to support the disabled and infirm, how to balance privacy and public welfare, how to provide basic security against violence and natural disasters, and how to provide education, economic opportunities, and health care. Although they will face these common responsibilities, how communities conceptualize and address them will differ depending on specific circumstances, histories, and traditions of each community. And how a community resolves these moral considerations will define its character.

The particular goals and purposes of individual communities will determine what sort of moral considerations they will face. Examples of moral considerations in nursing include such challenges as how to respond to those who are suffering or ill; how to balance one's responsibilities to patients, families, physicians, employers, and one's profession; and how to determine when medical treatment should be considered futile.

A community's moral considerations will not be static but will modulate with the community's changing contexts and conditions. This dynamic nature of communities means that virtues are essential for making moral judgments. As indicated earlier, virtues are character strengths. More specifically, *virtues* are complex, learned dispositions that enable individuals to perceive, feel, and act appropriately in response to the challenges and circumstances of their communal lives. Instead of focusing on rules to direct our responses, virtue ethics emphasizes the development of the ability to perceive, feel, and act appropriately in changing and complex circumstances.

Defining the Good Life

Each community develops characteristic goals and purposes. To achieve their defining goals, communities must acknowledge and respond to a number of moral considerations. Through collective experience and dialogue, each community discovers that certain strengths of character—or virtues—will enable its members to respond appropriately to the moral considerations that confront them. Communities that foster these virtues achieve their goals and enable their members to flourish.

As discussed in Chapter 1, not every vision of human flourishing is morally acceptable. A community must support its vision with good reasons and must test that vision against its collective human experience. A proposal that such-and-such promotes human flourishing must be supported by empirical observations about actual human lives. Every proposal or vision of human flourishing involves interpretations of particular human experiences that must be credible and meaningful. Visions of the good life are not simply "made up": They emerge from thoughtful community dialogues in which community members reflect on and make sense of their collective human experiences.

Developing a Nursing Virtue Ethics

A key step in describing a nursing virtue ethics framework is identifying the communities that are relevant to nursing. The term *community* is defined in a variety of ways depending on context. Nurses may refer to a group of people all of whom have arthritis as a community of interest. In this context, community designates people who share a common characteristic and, consequently, who have some shared interests in health care education and services.

Community has a more specific meaning, however, in the context of virtue ethics, which defines *community* as a group of people bound together by a common purpose or goal. Members of a community interact with one another and coordinate their actions in order to achieve their goals.

A community is not merely a group of people who happen to be together or who share a common characteristic. Thus, riders who share the same commuter bus each day or people in Illinois with arthritis are not communities. People riding a bus do have a common purpose—to reach a destination. But they do not consciously coordinate their actions to achieve this goal; they each independently choose their own goal and actions.

Because they work together to achieve common goals, people who design the bus routes, maintain and staff buses, and obtain funding for these projects are a community. The riders could become a community if they consciously chose to work together on common concerns, such as organizing and participating in a bus boycott to protest proposed changes in bus routes. Similarly, the aggregate of people in Illinois who have arthritis could become a community by forming an association to work for increased medical research on arthritis.

While geopolitical communities are probably most familiar to us, mere geographic proximity is insufficient to constitute a community in the ethical sense. Beyond geographic location, communities with defined geographic and jurisdictional boundaries such as cities and counties share a variety of common goals and projects, which require conscious coordination of actions. These shared goals may be educational, political, economic, health-oriented, and recreational.

Communities must engage in ongoing discussion about what they value and in light of these values, what they should do. Virtues, community practices, and institutions will be developed that reflect and support these values. Every community will develop wisdom and collective traditions that emerge from its pursuit of shared goals and problem solving.

Nursing as a Moral Community

Individual nurses belong to multiple nursing communities, including the organizational community within which they work, professional nursing organizations, their national nursing profession, and the worldwide community of professional nurses. Each of these communities develops its own specific goals that reflect the needs of the particular patient community that it serves and the needs of its professional members.

Its interpretation of nursing goals and values guides each of these communities. Each community's understanding of these values emerges from ongoing dialogue among its members. But these conversations extend also to dialogue with the broader nursing communities and are also influenced by nursing traditions with which these individual communities identify. For nurses in the United States, Canada, United Kingdom, and Australia, this tradition of nursing values has Victorian roots and names among its founders Florence Nightingale, Isabel Robb, and Lillian Wald.

HEALTH AND CARING AS COMMON MORAL PURPOSES

Moral communities are engaged in a moral enterprise. As such, these communities are guided by goals that transcend personal interests or gain and promote respect for the well-being of others. Members of these communities, bound together by their common moral purpose, have collective as well as individual moral responsibilities and obligations. Within the broader moral community of health care, nursing is one of a number of specialized communities that share the common moral purpose of promoting health and alleviating suffering with caring and compassion (Aroskar, 1995; Pellegrino & Thomasma, 1993). This view is consistent with the claims of Benner (1991), Bishop & Scudder (1991), Leininger (1990), Ray (1994), and Watson (1985) that nursing ethics is an ethics of care. Each of the health and caring communities will have characteristic virtues as well as overlapping virtues. Within the nursing community, virtues will define what it means to be a good nurse and will encourage nurses to do well their work to promote and restore health.

NURSING AS A PROFESSING COMMUNITY

The role of providing health care requires professional health care communities to make a commitment to society. The *Code for Ethics* (8.1–9.4) recognizes nurses collective responsibilities and accountability to the societies they serve (American Nurses Association [ANA], 2000). The focus of mainstream medical ethics on the doctor–patient relationship as the locus of ethical decision making has tended to obscure this larger social context of health care ethics. The same is true in much of nursing ethics, which concentrates on the nurse–patient dyad. Of course, health care professionals are committed to the care of individual patients, but they are also committed to the care of the communities they serve. Service to the community has always been, in fact, an essential part of nursing care and nursing ethics (Davis et al., 1997). This commitment is reflected in nursing's advocacy on issues ranging from public health and poverty to child labor laws and domestic violence.

Professions enter into a special trust relationship with their communities: a covenant with society (Pellegrino & Thomasma, 1993; Moline, 1986). To be a professional means "to profess." Professionals declare aloud or accept in public a special way of life, one that promises that the profession can be trusted to act in the interests of those served. Patients and society entrust themselves to the care of health professionals who commit to serve the interests of those needing care. In return for their commitment and service, health professionals receive certain benefits from society. One of these benefits is the right to be self-regulating or autonomous in setting the requirements and standards for practice and in policing the competence of their own members. A second benefit is society's support of health care education, including financial subsidies of research and education (Aiken, 1995) as well as considerable freedom for students and practitioners to develop their knowledge and skills by "practicing on" patients.

This act of "professing" is not simply a matter of taking an oath such as the Nightingale Pledge, which most student nurses, at one time, repeated at graduation (Calhoun, 1993). Although many health care professionals no longer literally take a professional oath when they complete their education, when they enter practice they profess their commitment to serve and to be competent and trustworthy. An important element of BSN-level education is the development of this sense of professing through mentoring and internships that go beyond skill-based education.

Concrete oaths, like the Nightingale Pledge and the Hippocratic Oath, are symbols of health care professionals' fundamental commitment to healing (Calhoun,

1993). A complex web of laws, public policies, and ethical traditions maintains this fiduciary (held in trust) relationship between professions and societies. The commitments of the profession and of the society it serves must be continually affirmed and validated by trustworthy behavior.

Nurses have had less control than physicians have had over the policies, practices, and organizations that define their practice environments. Under various forms of managed care, however, physicians and other medical professionals are finding that insurers and health care corporations increasingly control their work environments. It is worth noting that physicians traditionally have enjoyed a greater degree of independence and control of their work environments than have many professionals. Teachers, engineers, accountants, and many attorneys work for organizations that, to a large degree, define their work environments. Medical professionals may find that the expectations of their employers conflict with those of their professional communities. This tension should remind health care professionals that they are not merely employees and their patients are not merely consumers. As professionals who have committed themselves to moral goals and purposes that go beyond the economic and organizational interests of their employers, they must continually educate their employers about their professional commitments. They must be politically active in the workplace so that they have a strong voice in defining the policies and practices that are needed to support their professional virtues.

Clearly, nursing professes its commitment, competence, and trustworthiness to meet society's needs for nursing care. Nurses individually and collectively accept responsibility for their professional actions. Nursing is a profession in the sense that it is a moral community bound together by its common moral purpose and its covenant with society. Nursing educators need to develop and affirm this communal moral identity in their students. They must also prepare their students for the dual roles they will play as employees and professionals. It is also critical that practicing nurses look beyond their educational differences and cultivate their collective professional identity if they hope to be effective in shaping their workplace environments.

Nursing Virtues

It is clear why a virtue ethics approach to nursing is character-oriented rather than rule-oriented. Thus the critical question in virtue ethics is not "what as a nurse should I do?" but "what kind of nurse should I be?" Nursing is a moral community in which its members are individually and collectively committed to the promotion and restoration of health. Effective promotion of the well-being of others requires the cultivation of virtuous character. Nursing professionals enter into a special trust relationship with their communities; they commit themselves to serve the interests of those who need care. The community and its citizens expect more from nurses than intellectual knowledge and technical competence; they also expect good character. Good character includes virtues such as compassion, integrity, fidelity, courage, justice, mediation, self-confidence, resilience, and practical reasoning.

Nursing Virtues Emerge from Communal Dialogue

Virtue ethics focuses not only on the kind of character essential to good nursing but also on what kind of policies, practices, and organizations are needed to develop and sustain this character. This is clearly a significant departure from the primary focus of rule ethics on the analysis of individual cases and practical dilemmas. On the other hand, the virtue ethics approach is consistent with the traditional emphasis in professional education on emulating excellent role models. Professional internships aim to develop through the immersion of interns in practice not only knowledge but also professional values and virtues.

In her classic work, *From Novice to Expert*, Benner (1984) reflects on the work of nurses who are recognized as expert practitioners by their colleagues. She provides a rich description of expert nursing practice and how it is distinguished from other levels of nursing competence. As Benner notes in her Preface, however, the process of defining the characteristics and standards of expert practice is not merely one of description; it is also a process of reflective dialogue among expert practitioners and between practitioners and nursing theorists. Theorists contribute to this dialogue by describing and articulating what practitioners do. They also reflect back to these experts any unnoticed connections, patterns, inconsistencies and ambiguities in their practice, and questions for further development of practice. The dialogue about what virtues are essential to good nursing will also be characterized by this reflective interaction of practitioners and theorists.

Definitions of selected nursing virtues are presented in Box 4–1. The list of nursing virtues offered here is intended to be suggestive, not exhaustive. It is drawn primarily from the experiences of expert practitioners in the Anglo-American community of nursing. The list needs to be considered by various nursing communities. Readers are invited to participate in this dialogue. Are these the important virtues that constitute good nursing? Nurses as a community must determine the adequacy of this list or other summaries of nursing virtues, which requires an ongoing evaluation of how well the identified nursing virtues promote the goals of the nursing community and enable its members to live fruitful lives.

A thorough discussion of each of these virtues would require us to examine how each is embodied and interpreted within various nursing communities. Although space restricts comprehensive discussion of each virtue here, the nursing virtues of compassion and practical reasoning are discussed in this chapter, and others will be explored in the next chapter.

Cultural Context of Nursing Virtues

Community practices, such as nursing or teaching, are socially constructed. Their virtues and standards may vary over time and from one culture to another. The practice of nursing flourishes in societies with different interpretations of the virtues of nursing care. Leininger (1990) observes that "ethical and moral care behaviors are deeply rooted in the culture's social structure, language, and environmental contexts" (p. 49). Although nursing is committed to the promotion and restoration of

Box 4–1   Definition of Nursing Virtues

Nursing Virtue	Definition
Compassion	Empathetic understanding of health challenges, sympathetic response, and a disposition to alleviate suffering or to comfort.
Fidelity to trust	Consistent honesty and promotion of patient well-being such that patients' trust in the nurse's benevolence and character is developed and confirmed.
Moral courage	The willingness to risk personally in the effort to protect patients' safety and to promote patient well-being without retreating too soon or pointlessly continuing on.
Justice	Giving what is due to each person including equal respect and promotion of patient well-being. Commitment to fair distribution of communal health care resources and costs.
Mediation	A disposition to facilitate cooperation and communication among the nursing web of patients, families, and health care providers to promote human healing.
Self-confidence	Appropriate respect for one's own professional abilities and knowledge. Positive regard for the central role of nursing to promote healing.
Resilience	The ability to recover from loss or stress; to see oneself not as a victim of institutions or policies, but as an advocate for one's patients, one's profession, and oneself.
Practical reasoning	The ability to identify relevant moral considerations within the context of particular situations, and to actively interpret and adapt these considerations to new situations. The active embodiment of virtues in particular cases.
Integrity	The ability to integrate the various dimensions of one's personal and professional life in such a way that the nurse is morally whole, consistent, and trustworthy.

health and caring in all cultural contexts, there is substantial evidence that particular cultures interpret and explain their nursing virtues differently.

In Anglo-American culture, individualism and self-reliance are values that have permeated health care and significantly shaped nursing virtues (Leininger, 1990). Individualism is reflected, for instance, in the emphasis placed on the role of nurses as advocates who assert the rights of their patients to be active decision makers in the health care setting. Moral courage, self-confidence, and resilience are all nursing virtues that reflect the need for nurses to defend patient rights and interests, sometimes in the face of physician, institutional, or familial opposition. The virtue of mediation reflects the fact that in a culture that promotes individual rights, conflicts will occur and mediation will be necessary. In contrast, in the People's Republic of China, the collective societal good is the primary consideration in decision making and individual rights are subsumed under communal obligations. Consequently, we would expect to see distinctly different nursing virtues, such as loyalty and self-sacrifice, in a culture where obedience and compliance are highly valued (Leininger, 1990).

Self-reliance is also a key value in Anglo-American culture. It is reflected in the increasing emphasis on the nursing role of educating patients to empower them to engage in self-care. In cultures that do not place a similar emphasis on self-reliance, different expectations arise for nurses. Leininger notes how efforts by Anglo-American nurses to encourage self-reliance and self-care were resisted by elderly Vietnamese and Chinese patients. These values sharply clashed with their cultural value of filial respect for the elderly and their consequent expectations that younger members of their communities would provide for their needs (Leininger, 1990).

With modern modes of communication and transportation, differences and similarities in cultural beliefs, virtues, and social practices are becoming more apparent. In nursing ethics these differences have been insufficiently acknowledged. This is due, in part, to a fear that acknowledging these differences commits us to a hopeless ethical relativism. The ethical relativist notes the significant variation in cultural values and virtues and concludes that ethical beliefs are completely subjective and arbitrary. But pluralism in values and ethical theories need not be equivalent to this relativist view. Diverse cultures may have different conceptions and interpretations of nursing virtues, but the ideals in each community are not arbitrary and groundless. Each community should be guided by its historical tradition that is itself grounded in ongoing critical reflection on the experiences of expert practitioners within that cultural context. Each culture's dialogue about virtues does not take place in a vacuum; the dialogue transpires within the context of the concrete physical, social, and economic circumstances of a particular community. As the diversity of cultures is recognized, however, cross-cultural conversations and reflection can enrich the standards of nursing practice. Box 4–2 provides an interesting example of how culture can influence community practices.

Although practices are constructed in particular social contexts, changes in the context do not automatically lead to correlative changes in the virtues of those practices. Revising the virtues of a practice requires time, reflection, and experience in order to critically appropriate (or reject) the cultural changes. Recent nursing ethics is an excellent example of this sort of reassessment of virtues. European American nurs-

Box 4–2   Communities in Dialogue:

Intubation of the Recently Deceased

Moral considerations are embedded in particular cultures with their own histories, stories, and traditions. In a pluralistic society, health care providers must be especially sensitive to the fact that ethical problems may be the result of conflicting cultural understandings of moral considerations.

Paramedics in a major U.S. city practice intubation in the emergency room (ER) on the bodies of recently deceased persons. This practice is considered a vital avenue for paramedics to develop and maintain their skills, but after some objections were raised, a committee was formed to develop a uniform policy to be followed in all hospitals in this city. To avoid the awkwardness of seeking consent from grieving relatives, paramedics proposed practicing on bodies that were not claimed by relatives. Civil law seemed to support this policy. Civil law traditionally grants the custody and care of a dead person's body to the next of kin. Consent for autopsies, other than those mandated by the medical examiner, must be obtained from the next of kin. Bodies that are unidentified or unclaimed, however, are generally considered available for autopsies or research that will improve medical knowledge and practice. The paramedics argued that practicing intubation on unclaimed bodies is analogous to doing autopsies or research. Community discussion of this issue revealed, however, that restricting this practice to unclaimed bodies did not resolve all ethical issues.

One of the strongest objections came from members of the Jewish community who were appalled by the proposal. The bodies of those who die without family enjoy not less but more protection from Jewish law. Autopsies generally are not permitted under Jewish law, since the human body is regarded as divine property and therefore inviolable. After death, custody and care of the body is assumed by the next of kin, or in their absence, by the community. Jewish law provides for special protection of unclaimed bodies because they are even more defenseless than others are. The community has special obligations to ensure that the integrity of the corpse is preserved and that proper burial occurs. Permitting autopsies, research, or the practice of intubation on unclaimed bodies would be a grave violation of these special obligations.

Questions

1. Describe the relevant moral consideration in this case.
2. How was this moral consideration interpreted differently within the two cultural communities, and how might these conflicting perceptions affect the ER policy making regarding intubation of the recently deceased?
3. How might a policy accommodate both cultural traditions?
4. What other kinds of health care issues might produce similar conflict between communities?

ing emerged as a practice in the context of Victorian society. Early nursing virtues of submissiveness, self-sacrifice, cleanliness, and loyalty reflected the Victorian understanding of women's moral nature (Calhoun, 1993; Reverby, 1987). Yet, though this conception of womanly virtues was seriously called into question in the 1920s, the 1940s, and the 1960s in North American and European cultures, nursing did not systematically rearticulate its goals and values until the late 1970s and 1980s. This period of reflection has been extraordinarily fruitful. Nursing's understanding of the virtues that constitute good nursing has evolved along with this clarification of goals and values. As the model of nursing has shifted from one of the physician's helpmate to that of care provider and coordinator, earlier virtues of submissiveness and loyalty have been replaced with virtues such as courage, self-confidence, mediation, and justice. Other virtues such as compassion, trustworthiness, and integrity have been reinterpreted in light of the revised nursing role.

Virtues as Habitual Patterns

Aristotle described *virtues* as habitual patterns of perception, affective response, and action. Virtues manifest themselves in predictable and regular behavior. Like ordinary habits, virtues must be learned or acquired. We are not born with virtues, though some persons may by temperament be more inclined to act in certain ways than are others. Virtues are not *mere* habits or tendencies to respond in predictable ways. To possess a virtue requires that one wants to act in certain ways and not simply that one does act in certain ways. Someone may regularly make contributions to charitable causes but may not possess the virtue of generosity. If the person is motivated simply by a sense of duty or by a tax deduction, this habitual behavior is not evidence of generosity. Similarly, nurses who perform nursing tasks simply because it is their job or even out of a sense of pride in technical excellence lack essential elements of nursing virtues.

One of the strengths of virtue ethics is the integration of seeing, feeling, and acting. Possessing a virtue is more than just acting in certain ways. It also means that one desires or wants to act in those ways. As we noted in Chapter 2, the Enlightenment period stressed the role of reason in ethics. But it also devalued emotions as fickle, unreliable disturbances that distort rational thinking. Although our emotions can be unreliable guides that make it difficult for us to understand clearly, if properly developed, they can also be rational, reliable sources of intuition and knowledge. Properly trained emotions can direct our perceptions and our actions. They also provide motivation for good actions. The term *affective response* is used here to emphasize that it is not only how one feels that is important, but also one's affections—what one cares about, what one is attached to. An affective response reveals a person's heartfelt commitments and attachments that motivate his or her actions. Consequently, affective responses provide a bridge between perception and actions.

Morally, it matters not only what you think is the right thing to do but also what moves you, what you are drawn to or repulsed by. Virtues are states of character that motivate and reinforce the kinds of desires and actions that promote human flourishing (McKinnon, 1999). Consequently, virtues entail patterned ways of acting, but they also include commitments to be a certain kind of person or to create a certain kind of community.

The scenario that opens this chapter illustrates the integration of perception, affective response, and action in the virtue of fidelity to patient trust. Nurse D'Amico is able to help her patient, Kirsten, because they developed a relationship of trust. Nurse D'Amico exhibited the virtue of fidelity to trust. She promoted Kirsten's well-being in such a way that Kirsten's trust in the nurse's benevolence and character was developed and confirmed. Fidelity to trust was a part of this nurse's character—part of who she was, part of her characteristic behavior. Because of this virtue, this nurse was inclined to promote her patients' well-being in ways that confirmed their trust in her. While much has been said about the central nursing role of patient advocate, the interdependence of patient trust and patient advocacy is less frequently noted. Trust is essential in human relationships and, yet, trusting is difficult, especially when we are in positions of dependence and vulnerability.

Though her history of childhood abuse made it difficult for her to trust others, Kirsten was able to trust this nurse. In this vignette, we see how Kirsten's trust in her nurse is confirmed. The nurse anticipated that Kirsten might suffer postpartum depression and took steps to prevent it. Her first and foundational action was to communicate with Kirsten about her needs. The ongoing dialogue and open communication allowed Nurse D'Amico to evaluate Kirsten's need for additional support. This communication led to several further actions: She got both Kirsten and her doctor to agree to continue the First Steps program, sought advice from other professionals, kept in touch with Kirsten, increased her visits, intervened at a critical moment to obtain necessary medication and counseling, and educated Kirsten's husband about his wife's condition.

Virtuous persons have the capacity to perceive what is morally relevant in a particular situation and then to act appropriately. The nurse's character is revealed here not simply through her actions but also through her perceptions. She picked up on perceptual cues like the sound of Kirsten's voice—she sounded as if she was going to hurt herself, she sounded scared. She noted that Kirsten was not comfortable with unfamiliar nurses who visited her and that Kirsten was "frozen" in her depression and needed the nurse to take charge. Certainly, there was a delicate balance that the nurse needed to preserve between remaining vigilant, staying in touch, without triggering Kirsten's learned guardedness. Maintaining this balance required being acutely attuned to these perceptual clues.

Finally, although the nurse does not specifically describe her affective response to Kirsten's situation, it is clear that she is compassionate. It is unlikely that trust would have developed if Kirsten had felt that the nurse's actions were merely a function of doing her job. Clinical experience likely enabled Kirsten's nurse to pick up on important perceptual cues, but her concern and compassion for Kirsten also heightened her perception. Emotions and intuitive hunches can enable us to attend to critical perceptual clues in particular situations. They also can challenge our imagination to consider a wider range of creative, moral options.

In virtue ethics, affective responses provide critical motivation for our actions. Perceptions, affective responses, and actions are interrelated. Consequently, the development of character leads to wholeness of self. In virtue ethics, affective responses are a vital resource that enriches perceptions and motivates actions, rather than being alienated aspects of our personality that must be suppressed. Box 4–3 summarizes this discussion of the virtue of fidelity to patient trust.

Box 4–3   *Exploring the Virtue of Fidelity to Trust*

Recap of Case Scenario

Elena D'Amico, RN, shows caring and respect for Kirsten's feelings and seeks her approval to intervene for postpartum depression. Because she trusts the nurse, Kirsten confides in her and accepts her help.

Moral Consideration

How to cultivate a patient relationship conducive to patient advocacy?

Characteristic Elements

◆ **Perception:** Nurse D'Amico is attuned to key perceptual cues which alert her to patient's fearfulness about relationship, anticipation of recurrence of depression, and concern about hurting herself.
◆ **Affective response:** Compassionate response helped patient to trust and heightened nurse's perception.
◆ **Action:** Nurse D'Amico communicated with Kirsten about her needs, sought approval for First Steps program, obtained advice from professionals, kept in touch with Kirsten, increased her visits, and intervened in a critical moment.

The Virtue of Compassion

Compassion is central to nursing's commitment to care for patients. Like all virtues, compassion integrates perceptions, affective responses, and actions. Compassion includes at least three elements: (1) empathic understanding of conditions that cause suffering, limit functioning, or create health challenges; (2) appropriate affective response; and (3) a disposition to alleviate the suffering, to enhance functioning, or to comfort (Blum, 1987; Hinman, 1994; Pellegrino & Thomasma, 1993; Piper, 1991).

EMPATHIC UNDERSTANDING

Compassion is embedded in a personal dynamic relationship with a particular patient. To be compassionate is to be disposed to see and feel what it is like for this particular person to feel, live with, and endure his or her suffering or impaired health. Empathic understanding of a patient's condition requires imaginative dwelling on this person's situation (Piper, 1991; Blum, 1987). A good nurse comprehends the patient's condition, imagining what the patient is experiencing given his or her history, beliefs, and values. It is easy to misread patient needs, feelings, and experiences when nurses imagine how they themselves would experience the conditions rather than imagining the situation from the patient's perspective. Communicating with patients to validate assumptions about their experience is essential. Empathic understanding enables a nurse to comprehend, assess, and weigh the uniqueness of a patient's condition. Consequently, empathy has an important cognitive function because it can help the nurse to tailor interventions to a patient's unique experience.

APPROPRIATE AFFECTIVE RESPONSE

Compassionate nurses imagine what it is like for someone to cope with health challenges and display an appropriate affective response to their patients' suffering or impairment. Sympathy is an appropriate affective response, if it is distinguished from feeling pity. Feeling sorry for patients may actually inhibit their recovery rather than enable them to assume an active role in their recovery process. Pity suggests an inclination to help and implies that on some level one has more power and thus looks down on the one who is suffering. Commiseration, on the other hand, may imply that one accepts or encourages self-pity in one's patient. Compassion, however, is not the same as pity or commiseration.

Compassion fundamentally depends on a sense of shared humanity or "fellow feeling." As Blum (1987) notes, compassion promotes the experience of equality. The compassionate identification with others should be based on what Hampl (1995) calls "the acknowledgment of connection, the refusal to see the world as divided into distinct units that can do without one another" (p. 298). Compassion is not generosity or mercy. It is a sharing in the sorrow of those that we recognize as connected, attached, and intertwined with us (Hampl, 1995). We acknowledge that we are all vulnerable to suffering and misfortune, and we feel sorrow for the unique pain, impairment, or suffering that an individual experiences. More than empathic understanding of a patient's suffering, compassion adds an affective response. Compassionate nurses express concern for their patient's feelings through verbal support, active listening, and comforting touch.

DISPOSITION TO PROMOTE COMFORT AND ALLEVIATE SUFFERING

Responsiveness is the essence of compassion. Empathic understanding and appropriate sympathy are part of this response, but compassion also implies a disposition to provide comfort and alleviate the suffering of those who experience it. Their professional commitment already disposes nurses to give aid to their patients. This commitment to aid, however, is enhanced and strengthened by compassion for individuals. The steps nurses take to aid their patients will be guided by their imaginative reconstruction and concern in each case. Their professional skills, judgment, and experience will also guide their care.

We earlier described the affective response as a motivational bridge between perception and action. Sympathy is an appropriate and essential element of compassion even when a patient is not suffering pain or significant disability. Consider, for instance, the situation of a patient with asthma who is addicted to smoking. Her cholesterol is elevated and she is beginning to experience some cardiac symptoms. Her doctor has given her three months to get her cholesterol down before he puts her on medication. Two months later she visits you, a nurse practitioner. She states that she does not want to go on drugs, but her cholesterol has not come down.

This patient is not suffering in the usual sense of experiencing pain or discomfort, but compassion is no less essential in this case. You may feel some annoyance or disgust with her continued smoking. You may think that it is irrational for anyone to continue such health-destroying behavior. Because of this you may feel impatient with her concerns about taking the cholesterol medication. The bridging affective response of compassion will help to effectively support this patient and assist her in managing her health care problems. This patient needs you to understand her reluctance to begin taking medication. She also needs you to appreciate that this option feels limiting rather than empowering to her. An appropriate affective response to her experience is sympathy and shared fellow feeling—we all know how it feels to be disempowered. Your affective appreciation of her feelings of disempowerment can enable you to move from a cognitive awareness of her concerns to take actions to explore other strategies for attenuating, improving, and reducing her cholesterol problem.

LIMITS TO COMPASSION

To be compassionate requires a certain vulnerability. Allowing themselves to feel sorrow for the suffering of others exposes nurses to the risk of being overwhelmed by suffering. This risk is a reason nursing educators have traditionally encouraged students to empathize with, but not to sympathize with, their patients. Nurses cannot be effective if, day in and day out, they take on the full weight of their patients' suffering. They must preserve some emotional distance for the sake of professional objectivity as well as to prevent their own burnout and depression. Sympathy is an essential element of compassion, but there are appropriate limits. More compassion will not always be better than less. Mature expert practitioners develop an appropriate balance between professional distance and compassion. Box 4–4 further explores the virtue of compassion in the context of a case scenario.

The Virtue of Practical Reasoning

The virtue of practical reasoning occupies a special place in virtue ethics. Aristotle understood *practical reasoning* as the capacity for moral insight in response to a particular set of circumstances. Practical reasoning enables us to discern what the appropriate goal of our action should be and to assess the most appropriate means to achieve that goal in a given context. Practical reasoning is not merely cleverness or knowing how to get things done. It is an intellectual, perceptual capacity, which is inextricably interwoven with the other virtues of moral character (compassion, courage, fidelity, etc.) Practical reasoning shapes the other virtues and is shaped by them. All virtues incline or dispose us to good ends. Practical reasoning enables us to determine concrete measures that will attain these ends. In addition, the other virtues enhance the insight that fosters practical reasoning.

Box 4–4   Exploring the Virtue of Compassion

Case Scenario

Bernard Pesaro, RN, works on a medical-surgical unit of a community hospital. One of his primary patients, Kelly, is recovering from a sex-change operation. Bernard is repulsed by this patient's condition and uncomfortable in providing care. He feels confused about whether this surgery is ethical or an unnatural intervention.

Moral Consideration

How to respond to and provide competent care for a patient whose choices are personally offensive to the nurse?

Characteristic Elements

♦ **Perception:** Bernard seeks information and understanding about the surgery to facilitate imaginative, empathetic understanding of this patient's history and experience of suffering.

♦ **Affective response:** Bernard cares about this patient's needs even if he is unable to truly imagine or approve of the patient's perspective; responds positively based on sense of shared humanity.

♦ **Action:** Bernard uses his professional skills and experience to alleviate patient's discomfort guided by his imaginative reconstruction and concern for this patient's condition.

Practical reasoning is more than a rational or logical capacity—it is an embodied practical knowledge. Practical reasoning requires the perceptual abilities that are developed through role modeling and experience. Furthermore, this intellectual, perceptual capacity is deeply connected to affective and behavioral dispositions that are essential aspects of a person's character. Consequently, a nurse who has the virtue of practical reasoning does not simply apply practical reasoning—she or he will exemplify it. Thus practical knowledge is embodied in this nurse's character. Benner's *From Novice to Expert* (1984) describes several aspects of the embodied practical knowledge of the expert clinician. Exploring the parallels between this embodied clinical knowledge and embodied moral knowledge will help to further reveal the nature and function of the virtue of practical reasoning. Clinical knowledge and the virtue of practical reasoning are both forms of embodied knowledge.

Perceptual, Recognitional Ability

The first aspect of clinical knowledge, which Benner describes, is a perceptual, recognitional ability. Expert nurses are able to recognize subtle physiological and psychological changes that take on significance only in light of a particular patient's history and current condition. The ability to recognize early stages of septic shock, a pulmonary embolus, or impending shock and the need for prompt resuscitation efforts before documentable changes appear in vital signs are examples Benner notes of this recognitional ability (1984). In one example, Benner notes how perceptual knowledge is embedded in the nurse's hands: A patient is ventilated by hand, allowing the nurse to <u>feel</u> the degree of resistance in the lung. The nurse "knows in her hands how different resistances feel" (p. 19). This knowledge is shared by having the beginning nurse feel the resistance and compare cases over time in dialogue with a mentor.

Perceptual, recognitional ability is a component of practical reasoning. This ability is demonstrated by Randy Parker in her narrative of "Mike's Story" (Parker, 1990). Mike suffered from emphysema, diabetes, and the effects of a stroke. Over a period of several years, Mike underwent an above-the-knee amputation of both legs and, eventually, a right hip disarticulation that left him with a cavernous wound extending from his rib cage to his pelvis. The dressing changes and debriding of the wound that followed his surgery were terrifying experiences for Mike and distressing for Parker. Mike suffered from aphasia, making communication with him extremely difficult. While other caregivers believed that Mike was disoriented and could not communicate, Parker perceived a man who was desperate to communicate. Compassion sensitized her to Mike's high-pitched moaning and to the terror in his eyes. Practical reasoning guided her compassion. Parker didn't merely perform her nursing tasks (changing dressings, turning Mike religiously, and monitoring vital signs), but she also genuinely listened to and shared with her patient. Paying close attention to essential perceptual cues enabled Parker to find ways to communicate with Mike. These cues were found in Mike's eyes, in the tension and relaxation of his muscles, and in garbled utterances and guttural groans. Because Parker allowed herself to perceive and to recognize Mike's pain and frustration as well as his courage and hope, she and Mike were able together to construct some meaning in his excruciating experience. Her perceptual, recognitional ability enabled Parker to respond with genuine compassion embodied in her words, her touch, and her presence. It also enabled her to advocate for a patient who clearly could not speak for himself (Parker, 1990).

Aspect Recognition

The transition from novice to expert reflects an important change in the abilities to determine what is relevant and to set priorities. Benner (1984) calls this aspect recognition; it is another component of embodied practical knowledge. Initially, for the novice, situations are simply compilations of equally relevant bits of information. Beginners often are overwhelmed, even paralyzed, in crisis situations because they lack developed aspect recognition. As a nurse develops competence and moves toward expert status, complex situations are more and more seen as complete wholes in which only some parts are relevant and some aspects take priority over others.

Identifying and Prioritizing Moral Considerations

The development of the virtue of practical reasoning similarly enables morally mature persons to identify certain aspects of a situation as morally significant and to give appropriate weight to various moral considerations. Rarely do experiences come to us as neatly and clearly delineated as the typical cases presented in ethics textbooks. Most of these cases are limited to one or two moral considerations that are clearly identifiable. For instance, we may be asked whether we should break a *promise* to a friend in order to <u>aid</u> someone in an <u>emergency.</u> But life rarely presents itself with the morally relevant aspects underlined. Nurses in practice frequently find it difficult to distinguish what is morally significant in complex situations from what is sociologically, politically, or theologically relevant.

Furthermore, complex situations requiring moral judgment often involve several moral considerations that must be prioritized. This requires character and good judgment—embodied expert knowledge. The application of the criteria of disproportionate care discussed in Chapter 2 (pp. 52–54) requires this embodied knowledge of aspect recognition. One must identify which physical, social, psychological, and economic factors are relevant, and then prioritize and weigh the burdens and benefits of the proposed treatment. This is more than simply a mathematical process: It requires the aspect recognition of practical moral reasoning.

Aspect recognition includes the ability described by Wallace (1988b) as the use of practical reasoning to identify relevant moral considerations within the context of particular situations and to actively interpret and adapt these considerations to solve new practical moral problems. This ability is a critical one for nursing ethics. The rapid technological changes in health care repeatedly present new moral problems about how to use this technology in ways that genuinely promote human healing. The development of advanced resuscitation techniques, artificial respiration, neonatal intensive care, organ transplantation, and artificial hearts have created practical moral problems in bioethics. Furthermore, the commercialization of health care and the current restructuring of health care delivery have also created practical moral problems. These include the difficulty of maintaining patient trust in a system that provides financial incentives for health care providers that may conflict with the best interests of patients. Managed care and workplace redesign also raise new concerns about adequate staffing of nurses and the possible undermining of patient safety.

Artificial Nutrition and Hydration

The withdrawal of artificial nutrition and hydration is an example of a decision that requires moral aspect recognition. We must identify the relevant moral considerations, understand their origins, and determine how they can be appropriately adapted to this new technological circumstance. One moral consideration that seems relevant is the concept of disproportionate care: Are the burdens of artificial nutrition and hydration disproportionate to the benefits of this treatment for dying patients or for those in persistent vegetative states (PVS)? If so, the decision to withdraw artificial nutrition and hydration (ANH) would be like decisions about discontinuing use of a ventilator or renal dialysis.

Others argue that artificial nutrition and hydration are not medical treatments in the same sense as dialysis or the use of a ventilator (Callahan, 1983; Meilander, 1984; Weisbard & Siegler, 1986). These authors argue that food and drink are more than mere medical treatments because they play a deep symbolic role in our culture. Offering food and drink represents one of our most basic human responses of caring, human connectedness, and human community. For some, the withdrawal of artificial nutrition and hydration from vulnerable patients represents the denial of regard and care by the human community. Consequently, the primary moral consideration in these cases is not whether ANH represents disproportionate care, but whether withdrawing it amounts to communal abandonment of these patients. Box 4–5 explores aspect recognition as a component of the virtue of practical reasoning.

Others disagree with the claim that withdrawing ANH is an act of abandonment, neglect, or abuse (Carson, 1986; Lynn & Childress, 1986; Zerwekh, 1997). In some circumstances, such as the last days of the dying process, patients simply do not benefit from the medical treatment of hydration and nutrition. It is critically important to abide with and attend to dying patients—to do what we can to provide comfort through the dying process. In near terminal patients, however, continuation of ANH often adds discomfort by increasing terminal pulmonary edema, nausea, and mental confusion (Zerwekh, 1997). More appropriate forms of care may include offering ice chips for a dry mouth, analgesics for pain, antiemetics for nausea, and backrubs for comfort and human connection (American Medical Association, [AMA], 1988).

Box 4–5   *Exploring the Virtue of Practical Reasoning*

Case Scenario

The ethics committee at a community hospital responsible for reviewing the policy on withdrawal of life-sustaining treatment has been asked by several nursing staff to consider the issue of withdrawing artificial nutrition and hydration (ANH).

Moral Consideration

Is ANH in the same or in a different moral category than medical treatments such as cardiopulmonary resuscitation or dialysis?

Characteristic Elements

- **Perception:** Committee members recognize that the relevant moral concepts here are disproportionate care and patient abandonment.
- **Affective response:** Concern for patients and their families facing this issue heightens moral aspect recognition and motivates nursing staff to raise this issue.
- **Action:** Nurses encourage ethics committee to analyze relevant moral concepts and to develop/revise appropriate hospital policy and practice guidelines.

The care of patients in a persistent vegetative state is a central concern for many who oppose the withdrawal of ANH. Some authors acknowledge that while ANH may impose significant burdens on the terminally ill, feeding an unconscious patient through a gastrostomy or jejunostomy tube is burdensome neither to the patient nor to the nursing/medical staff (Derr, 1986). The provision of ANH does not *reduce* the quality of the patient's life in this case. It is not the fact that the *treatment* is burdensome, but the perception of family, caregivers, or society that this patient's *life* is too burdensome that is driving the decision to withdraw ANH. And this clearly is then an act of abandonment of these patients: Their lives are considered so lacking in value that they do not warrant continued human care. The withdrawal of ANH from PVS patients is not, in this case, based on a judgment that ANH imposes burdens that are disproportionate to the anticipated benefits of this treatment.

Other authors disagree with this conclusion. While agreeing that feeding is a deeply symbolic human act, they note that its symbolic significance is tied to the mutuality of giving and taking food and water (Cranford, 1988; Carson, 1986). Feeding is a reciprocal act through which a human connection is made and affirmed. In the case of PVS patients, who are unaware of the gift of food and water, there is no reciprocity, no mutuality possible. Without the possibility of response to human touch or to the presence of another human being, human connection and interaction is no longer meaningful. Consequently, these authors conclude that for PVS patients, the idea of attending and abiding with them is no longer meaningful and the withdrawal of ANH may be the final appropriate act of caring.

Clearly, removal of ANH from PVS patients is a controversial and complex issue. How can the aspect recognition of practical reasoning help us think about this issue? It can help us to identify which moral considerations are relevant to this case and then to interpret and adapt these to this new moral problem. This is not, however, simply a matter of thinking logically and clearly. Deciding what is relevant, interpreting, and adapting moral considerations are all processes that include value judgments. Value judgments in such complex cases require a communal dialogue that draws on the accumulated wisdom from a community's history and on the wisdom embodied in mature members of the present community. Our communities are still engaged in this process with regard to the issue of ANH. This author alone cannot settle this issue, but some observations on the communal dialogue can be made.

In the case of terminally ill patients, it is clear that ANH is sometimes a burdensome treatment, adding only further discomfort with no real benefit to the patients. Comfort and care can be provided in other ways that demonstrate the commitment to accompany these patients through the dying process. The decision to withdraw care in these cases is an appropriate extension of the moral consideration that one need not preserve life when the necessary medical treatment imposes burdens that are disproportionate relative to the anticipated benefits.

The case of the patients in a PVS is not so clear. ANH does not cause discomfort for these patients, nor does it require excessive effort for caregivers to provide. The difficult judgment here is whether these patients genuinely benefit from this treatment. Physiologically, their bodies receive nutrients, but the human beings have no subjective capacity to experience any treatment as beneficial. This lack of subjective capacity is related to the point that they cannot in any way appreciate, acknowledge, or respond to the deeply symbolic human gift of feeding. This point cannot be considered irrelevant to our communal value judgments in these cases. But we should acknowledge how far-reaching this observation may be. Some persons who are severely demented or profoundly retarded also seem incapable of appreciating or even responding to the efforts of others to care for them. There may be no authentic sense in which these human beings can interact with other human beings.

Other moral considerations are relevant here. First, what does it mean to be a person whose intrinsic value demands our respect and grounds our moral obligations? Are all human beings persons in this moral sense? Have those human beings who are in a PVS lost some essential element(s) of personhood? A second moral consideration is what it means for a human person to die. Is the persistent vegetative state actually a state of being dead and not simply debilitated or damaged? Obviously, this is not merely a physiological question, but a value question with profound implications. These questions must be answered before we can know clearly how to apply the moral consideration of disproportionate care to the issue of withdrawing ANH from patients in a PVS. Answering these questions will require further communal reflection and dialogue.

Holistic Reasoning

A third aspect of embodied practical knowledge is the ability to approach complex situations from an experience-rich, holistic basis rather than from a rule-governed one. Benner (1984) suggests that the decision making skills of proficient and expert nurses are qualitatively different from those of nurses at the earlier novice and competent stages of development. At these earlier stages, nurses rely on rules and formulas to guide their performance. In later stages, a more holistic and intuitive process generates experienced judgments.

EXPERIENCE AND CONTEXTUAL JUDGMENT

With experience and mastery of skills, proficient and expert practitioners do not simply apply rules more rapidly and accurately than beginners. Rather, their skills of perception, assessment, and judgment are transformed. In advanced practice, nurses call on their accumulated experience and understanding of the context and meanings inherent in similar situations to approach new situations in a more holistic manner. Because they have learned from experience what happens in a "typical" situation, they can rapidly recognize whether or not a current situation is customary. Their intuitive grasp of whole situations enables them to quickly identify and assess the most relevant factors.

Virtue ethics makes similar claims about the relationship between moral rules and the moral judgments of persons of mature character. Like many areas of nursing practice, human moral experiences are frequently too complex and context rich to be assessed by applying rules. Many situations require discretionary judgments that cannot be summarized in a set of rules. We need practical knowledge that is developed through reflective appropriation of past concrete experiences in dialogue with other morally mature community members.

ROLE OF RULES

Rules are not completely irrelevant, however, in virtue ethics. Rules have an important pedagogical value: They provide a structured way to begin to think about ethical decision making. Beginners who lack experience start with context-free rules to guide their performance. In educating our children about ethics, we usually begin with rules. As these beginners develop life experience, however, we encourage them to consider the relevance of context, the complexities of real cases, and the ambiguities of genuine moral dilemmas. As they gain experience, they also learn that some areas of moral judgment lend themselves more readily to satisfactory codification into rules.

The area of justice which forbids certain behaviors is more readily codified, for instance, than the areas of benevolence or self-development that require us to consider a much wider range of alternative actions. Rules such as "do not steal" or "do not intentionally deceive someone" are general moral rules that have emerged from our communal reflection on our shared human experience over time. These rules are usually reliable guides for action. Rules thus set some boundaries for moral behavior. Yet even in these areas where rules are relatively adequate guides for action, rules are at best mere approximations and not complete substitutes for good judgment.

In addition, we need character and good judgment to help us interpret and apply rules. In more complex areas where rules are less adequate, experience, character, and contextual judgment are more essential to good ethical decision making. The development of nursing virtues will dispose nurses to perceive, affectively respond, and act in ways that will tend to promote health and alleviate suffering in their communities. Nurses who embody these virtues—who possess a mature moral character—will be able to bring this "big picture" to their interpretation and application of rules in particular contexts. Thus, the commitment to promoting health and alleviating suffering will guide the adaptation of rules to cases, rather than allowing rules to rigidly dictate actions.

HOLISTIC JUDGMENT AND MORAL COURAGE

Nurses often rely on holistic moral judgment in their role as patient advocates. At times, for instance, nurses must assess when incompetent/impaired practitioners or unsafe working conditions endanger the safety of their patients. Rarely will these judgments be easy or simply deductive. Generally, these judgments require the nurse to determine the degree of risk to patients, the likelihood that the nurse's complaint will be effective or that others will support it, and the personal and professional costs of making a complaint. Situations in which a nurse must question physician authority or institutional authority often require moral courage. But courage itself requires judgment; courage enables us to act in spite of fear, but it is not rash or foolish. Moral courage requires a holistic judgment of the particular situation so that the nurse will not retreat too quickly but also not risk more than the potential danger would justify. Using holistic judgment is qualitatively different than working through the steps of a protocol—that is, of applying rules to a particular situation. Holistic judgment requires an embodied moral knowledge or character.

How Moral Character Is Developed and Sustained

How are virtues—that is, character—developed? Remember that virtues, including practical reasoning, are habits of perception, affective response, and action. Habits are developed through observation and repetition. As anyone knows who has tried to learn to play an instrument, develop an athletic skill, or speak a new language, practice alone does not guarantee a good result. A person can practice for hours, performing the action incorrectly, and the result will be bad habits, which have become ingrained through the long practice sessions. To develop the habitual patterns that will lead to excellent practice, one needs good models and attentive feedback to guide one's performance.

Mentoring and Co-Mentoring

Embodied knowledge can be learned only by being immersed in the context of practice with other thinking, feeling people who know what they are doing. To develop virtues, we need mentors who are expert practitioners. Mentoring is a key component of the method for teaching nurses the embodied knowledge of clinical skills and judgment. Clinical skills and judgment cannot be taught solely in a classroom or learned only through reading books, because this embodied know-how requires discretionary judgments that cannot be reduced to the application of rules (Alderman, 1982). So nursing students and novice nurses are assigned preceptors who are responsible for mentoring these beginners in the clinical context. Students begin by observing their mentors and continue to learn by imitating them.

The mentoring process requires ongoing critical reflection about practice. Mentors share with students the reasons for various responses and decisions or for the particular manner in which actions are taken. Students must understand the point of various considerations that go into a nursing response. As students practice and become more independent, the mentor will critically reflect with them on how and why they have responded to particular situations. As Benner demonstrates, this process of mentoring continues beyond the student level as nurses gain experience and mature in their judgment. Most will become competent nurses, some proficient, and some will become expert practitioners. But the process of modeling and critical reflection continues even with proficient and expert practitioners as they co-mentor one another in daily practice.

Character is developed through the same sort of *mentoring process*. It requires the same three elements of mentoring that are needed in the development of clinical skills and complex judgments in clinical situations:

1. *Immersion in the context of practice*
2. *Imitation of good models*
3. *Ongoing critical reflection*

The goal of professional internships in health care has always included the development of professional moral virtues as well as clinical skills and judgment. Early nursing textbooks, such as Isabel Robb's *Nursing Ethics: For Hospital and Private Use* (1911, 1916, 1920) clearly reflect an expectation that nursing education includes character development. Although much of the discussion about nurses being "formed morally" was expressed in flowery, high-Victorian language that might obscure its substance and insight, early educators recognized that a nurse's professional behavior could not be separated entirely from a nurse's character and that both would be shaped by good mentoring (Fowler, 1997).

The goal of mentoring relationships is to allow the apprentice to walk, as closely as possible, in the mentor's shoes. The student learns to imitate the mentor by seeing as the mentor sees, hearing as the mentor hears, and feeling what the mentor feels in order to embody the virtues, values, and practical moral judgment of the mentor. Through the mentor, the student learns how to respond appropriately with words, feelings, touch, attitude, presence, and action.

Experts and Everyday Exemplars

The idea of mentors and expert practitioners is commonplace in the context of a professional practice. We may be less comfortable with the idea of expert practitioners in ethics. Most will agree that a significant part of our moral education comes through our observation and imitation of early role models. In this early apprenticeship, we begin to develop our character, embodying values, dispositions, and commitments of the models and traditions within which we are socialized. In our homes, in our schools, and in our religious and community organizations, we begin to develop virtues such as fairness, promise keeping, courage, generosity, accountability, friendship, and loyalty. We readily accept the necessity of good models in educating children and young adults. However, we are less likely to think that adults should look to experts or mentors in matters of ethics. After all, we consider the capacity to make autonomous decisions for oneself and to be accountable for one's own actions to be indicators of adulthood.

RECOGNIZING EXPERT PRACTITIONERS

In European American culture, the paradigm of moral maturity is of persons who critically choose their own values, think for themselves, and respect the choices of others. Parents want to raise their children to be capable of making their own decisions and being accountable for them—to be able "to stand on their own two feet." Adolescence, the period of transition from childhood to adulthood, is anticipated as a time when young adults critique and sometimes reject their parents' values. Consequently, it is with both dread and satisfaction that parents anticipate this time of rebellion; it is unpleasant to be the object of critique, but it is accepted and welcomed as evidence of the maturing process.

Within this paradigm, the idea of experts in moral practice is suspect. We are always on guard against attempts by others "to tell us what we ought to do," whether those others are political or religious authorities or self-righteous individuals. We pride ourselves on our enlightened rejection of moral authority based on privileges due to birth, inheritance of wealth, or social position. The eighteenth and nineteenth century Enlightenment tradition, discussed in Chapter 2, was precisely about the assertion of the equal dignity of all free men (the recognition of the equal status of slaves, common laborers, and women came later) and the rejection of the economic, political, and moral tyranny of privileged classes. The rule-oriented model of ethics emerged from this social context. The codification of moral judgment into a universal set of rules reflects the Enlightenment commitment to level the moral playing field. The ability to reason places all moral agents on an equal footing; the same rules apply to all and can be applied by all rational persons. Public education becomes a hallmark of this democratic commitment to equal access of all citizens to the moral, political, and economic life of the community.

From this perspective, the idea of expert practitioners in ethics seems wrong-headed. In fact, the virtue ethics approach often is dismissed on the grounds that the search for models or experts in ethics is either misguided or fruitless. Who could presume to be such a model? The long history of religious wars demonstrates the futility of achieving any consensus on who our moral leaders should be. Is it Buddha or Jesus or Mohammed? Actually, we need a gestalt shift here. Let us return to Benner's concept of an expert practitioner. What sort of people was she looking for, and where did she expect to find them? It is clear from her methodology that Benner was not looking for flawless, one-in-a-million practitioners so expert in their practice that they were barely recognizable as human. Participants in Benner's (1984) study were instructed to select fellow nurses "with at least five years of clinical experience currently engaged in direct patient care, and who were recognized as being highly skilled clinicians" (p. 15). Apparently it was not difficult for supervisors and peers to agree on the selection of these experts. When nurses were asked to identify people working in the trenches with them whose skills and judgments they respected and trusted, there was considerable consensus. They were not omnicompetent "super nurses," but respected colleagues—people others would go to for advice and would want working on their units.

CO-MENTORS IN EVERYDAY PRACTICE

Certainly, there are such exemplars in our moral lives as well. It is clear that, as adults, our character and our moral judgment continue to be shaped by the company we keep. The expert practitioners we are looking for are people who share common experiences with us. They will be people with whom we work, play, and share our domestic lives. They will be people who are immersed with us in the practice of living morally: choosing values and commitments, making choices, constructing worthwhile lives, living authentically. Our mentors become our friends and our colleagues (Volbrecht, 1994). The process will be more mutual than in traditional apprenticeships—it will, consequently, often be a *process of co-mentoring*.

Just as expert nurses are not expert in all areas of practice, some persons will have greater strengths and insight in some aspects of the moral life than in others. In co-mentoring relationships, the mentee and the mentor may shift roles over time: In some contexts, one person will be the advisor/model while, at other times, the other person will assume this role. Co-mentors are collaborators laboring together, showing each other the way (Bona, Rinehart, & Volbrecht, 1996). A community will have a variety of mentors who will each bring their own strengths and perspectives to the community's dialogue. It is important for members of the community to listen to the dialogue among these "wisdom people" in the community and to see how each one embodies the community's virtues.

A diversity of relationships with people from a variety of backgrounds, races, religions, and lifestyles can provide needed perspective and checks against individual or group biases. But we need as well to have close friends and colleagues with whom we share details of our lives and whom we trust enough to help us examine our motives, mistakes, and struggles. All of these relationships provide contexts for the essential critical self-reflection that is necessary for continued moral development.

Institutionalizing Co-Mentoring

The development of character must be nurtured in nursing education and practice. The bulk of mentoring and co-mentoring in moral development will not occur in the classroom or in ethics seminars and workshops. The primary context for mentoring will be the context of nursing practice. The formal study of ethics does play a critical role in the process of nursing ethics education. Ethics courses and seminars provide the opportunity to systematically study a variety of ethical theories and moral considerations. It is important for us to understand how these theories and considerations have shaped contemporary dialogues about moral issues. We need to understand the contexts and issues from which these theories and moral considerations emerged and how they have been modified and adapted to address changing circumstances. Similarly, courses in applied ethics enable us to explore particular issues in applied areas and to consider how the unique circumstances of diverse practices generate new insights and revisions of traditional moral considerations.

CRITICAL REFLECTION IN EVERYDAY PRACTICE

As valuable as this formal study of ethics is, it is a supplement to and not a substitute for ongoing critical reflection in our practice communities. Individual nurses and nursing organizations must "build in" space and support for this process of co-mentoring. Embodied knowledge is more than a collection of accumulated experiences. The development of embodied knowledge requires reflection on these experiences. In formal mentoring relationships, the mentor systematically guides this critical reflection. In the context of everyday practice, there still must be opportunities to reflect on observations and outcomes. This reflection frequently occurs informally by sharing and comparing stories with co-workers. Benner notes that most expert nurses have little opportunity to compare experiences and to develop consensus with other nurses. She argues that more systematic discussion among expert nurses would enhance performance. The same is true for the practice of ethical decision making in nursing.

Although casual discussion of ethical issues occurs in employee lounges, cafeterias, and report areas, nurses need to institutionalize more systemic discussion. Nurses need opportunities to tell one another stories, for continued mentoring and co-mentoring, for review of current and past decisions, and for more continuing education on ethical issues. All of these provide contexts for the ongoing critical reflection and dialogue about the goals and values that should characterize their moral community.

INCENTIVES AND IMPEDIMENTS

Critical reflection and dialogue should focus on more than just the individual moral agent. One of the most critical tasks in virtue ethics is ongoing analysis of the environment of relevant moral communities. Communities need ongoing dialogue not only about what goals and values they will embody, but also about how support for the characteristic virtues of this community is institutionalized. Communities should ask themselves how well the policies, practices, and reward systems of their organizations promote the continuing development of character, practical reasoning, and moral judgment. Are there impediments that hinder or undermine the virtues that this community desires to embody? If so, how can these be decreased or removed? Finally, how can positive incentives and supports be institutionalized? If virtues are to be more than ideals articulated in mission statements, then the organizational environment needs to nurture virtues and allow them to flourish.

The case in Box 4–6 reminds us that impediments to character development are not all external to nursing; sometimes, they are created by nursing peers. Critical reflection and analysis of the environments that either support or hinder the development of nursing virtues must include an internal critique of nursing communities themselves.

Box 4–6 *Challenges to Resilience and Self-Confidence*

Dale Erkes was hired in the emergency department (ED) of a 200-bed hospital as a new graduate nurse. He was to be precepted by a clinical nurse specialist (CNS) during his six-month probationary period but the position was eliminated prior to his start date. The charge nurse who became his preceptor was ambivalent about new grads working in the ED. She assisted when he requested it but didn't go out of her way to be helpful.

Dale's second preceptor, a staff nurse, had no ambivalence about new grads in the ED. During Dale's first days in the department, she pounded her finger into his chest and stated that "I never wanted a new grad in the ED, I don't want one here now, and I'll make sure that our hiring committee never hires a new grad again." This nurse pointed out Dale's mistakes to other RNs. When Dale administered a medication at too slow a rate for a therapeutic effect (but without potential for causing harm to the patient), she exclaimed loudly for other staff to hear, "You won't be satisfied until you kill someone."

Although not as hostile, other nurses were also unhelpful. When Dale asked questions, some of the nurses ignored him as if he wasn't there, even if he repeated the question thinking that they hadn't heard him. Other nurses answered his questions but left out critical information. When he asked, for instance, how to calculate the drip rate for a specific medication, one nurse

continues

Box 4–6   Challenges to Resilience and Self-Confidence (cont.)

answered but did not tell him that he should never run that medication through regular tubing or into a peripheral vein.

The ED supervisor was either unwilling or unable to provide Dale with the support he needed to successfully complete his orientation. He was let go at the end of his probationary period and was not considered for another nursing position in the hospital.

Questions

1. Have you had or observed similar experiences in which nurses undermine the self-confidence and resilience of new nurses? If so, describe one of these experiences. Why do you think that some nurses relate this way to new (and not new) nurses?

2. Some veteran nurses defend this sort of initiation of new grads by claiming that it helps them to become self-reliant and prepares them for the difficult challenges they will face in nursing. Do you agree?

NURSING ETHICS GROUPS AND PEER MENTORING

Formation of nursing ethics groups provides an important forum for nurses to share their stories of moral development and to explore unique insights and perspectives that nurses bring to the promotion of human healing (Scanlon, 1994; Parker, 1990). Many hospitals and extended care facilities have multidisciplinary ethics committees that educate, develop and review policies, and often conduct case reviews and consultation. It is critical that nurses participate in these multidisciplinary dialogues, contributing their own experience and points of view to these conversations. Multidisciplinary forums are not a substitute, however, for ethics groups composed only of nurses. It is important that nurses have their own space to explore ethical decisions and moral development with their nursing colleagues. The politics and the hierarchical nature of health care institutions make it unlikely that multidisciplinary ethics committees will be a place where nurses (or, for that matter, physicians) will feel free to explore their questions, frustrations, and insights. As Ray (1987) notes, nurses need to provide "life support" to one another so that they can "share, rather than deny or hide their support needs" (pp. 171–172).

Although nursing ethics groups may be most appropriate at the unit level, it is essential that these groups provide the opportunity for reflection on participants' moral experiences and not only for the discussion of pressing cases calling for imme-diate decisions. Many nurses work in contexts where they are isolated from other nurses or where they have too few opportunities for interaction with other nurses. School nurses, nurses working in physicians' offices, occupational health nurses, home health nurses, and nurse practitioners may belong in this category. Organizing a nursing ethics group with others who practice in similar settings could provide a critical context for support and reflection.

A formally developed mentorship program using peer-to-peer relationships could provide another institutionalized context for critical reflection on ethical issues and on nurses' moral experiences. Preceptors are available for new nurses, but experi-enced nurses also need mentoring relationships within which they can explore their struggles with ethical decisions (Ray, 1987). Addressing this need might involve pair-ing a nurse who is more mature in character and moral judgment with a less mature nurse, or it might mean developing peer co-mentoring relationships. What is critical is that these are relationships of respect and trust.

Nurses need to discuss the goals and values of nursing within the context of regional and national professional associations as well. The document *Nursing's Agenda for Health Care Reform* (ANA, 1992) is tangible evidence that nurses are committed to this dialogue. Yet this document represents a level of collaboration among professional nursing groups that is much too rare. Professional associations must do more to institutionalize dialogue about shared values, decision-making processes, and desired ethical outcomes so that this dialogue becomes an estab-lished part of the ongoing work of these organizations and not a response to crisis situations.

Nurses must develop a personal practice of critical reflection by embodying dis-positions and skills that will enable them to participate in debates within their profes-sion and their communities. Nurses must exchange ideas about what kinds of people they want to be with regard to health care and must consider concrete controversial issues such as whether to continue treatment of a patient with multiple organ failure, how to fund treatment for an indigent illegal immigrant, or how nurses can educate young people about date rape. Nurse educators have a special responsibility for mod-eling the process of critical reflection. Students need to witness nurses initiating, facil-itating, and participating in ongoing critical reflection in the classroom, workplace, and other community forums.

CREATING OPPORTUNITIES FOR DIALOGUE

It is, of course, a simplification to say that dialogue will lead to better ethical decision making. The political reality is that nurses are not fully autonomous with regard to patient care decisions. It may seem at times that it doesn't matter if nurses discuss val-ues because not all of the decision making is in their hands. Furthermore, with the growing pressures of cost containment, it will be increasingly difficult to persuade institutions to free up time for nurses to dialogue about ethics.

Although nurses are working to achieve greater professional autonomy, they should also recognize that all individual moral agents live and work in community with others. Most people work within institutions where their participation in decision making is limited by hierarchical power structures. This is not ideal, but it does not mean that workers who are not vice presidents have no responsibility for their actions. Nurses can still seek opportunities to discuss and influence the values in their organizations. They also should discuss how to preserve their own values in contexts where compromise and dissent will be common.

Nurses have developed more collaborative models of ethical decision making in contexts outside of the traditional hospital setting. Hospice units, home health, midwifery, and chronic care are areas where more collaborative models are common. Some special units such as neonatal intensive care units also often exhibit more collaborative decision making. These health care communities can provide critical insights and support for nurses practicing in more traditional settings. They may provide important models for how people with common goals can make good moral choices together.

Finally, even when their institutions provide little support for ethical dialogue and co-mentoring, nurses need to create space for these for the sake of better patient care, as well as for the individual and professional well-being of nurses. Human beings are social beings; working together and reflecting on what we do and why is energizing and restorative. Often, we may not be able to control the circumstances in which we work. We can, however, decide what kind of responses we will make to these circumstances and, ultimately, what kind of persons we want to be.

The key features of Virtue Ethics are summarized in Box 4–7.

Box 4–7   Virtue Ethics Summary

Primary Questions

What kind of person should I be?
What kind of community do we want to be?

Key Features

♦ Concerned with character, virtues, and good judgment.
♦ Integrates reason and emotion: doing the right things because one cares about these things.
♦ Virtues are determined through ongoing communal dialogue.
♦ Virtues are strengths of character that promote human flourishing.
♦ Moral judgment cannot be reduced to a set of rules. Experience, character, and good judgment are assets to be cultivated for moral decision making.
♦ Virtues and good judgment are developed through a mentoring process.

Rebirth of Virtue Ethics

Contemporary ethics has witnessed a renaissance of interest in virtue ethics. We are beginning to see the effects of this renewed interest in the writings of bioethicists as well. Pellegrino and Thomasma (1993) and Drane (1988) make strong cases for the place of virtues in medical ethics, reminding us that health professions are moral communities with longstanding virtue traditions. Some authors attempt to combine virtue ethics with rule ethics (Beauchamp & Childress, 1994, 2001; Garrett, Baillie, & Garrett, 1993). Beauchamp and Childress treat virtue ethics with much more care in the fourth and fifth editions of their classic text, *Principles of Biomedical Ethics*, than in earlier editions. Nonetheless, theirs is largely a rule ethics approach to health care ethics. The effort of Garrett and colleagues to blend virtue ethics with principles is more successful, and they emphasize the importance of practical wisdom as the primary virtue in *Health Care Ethics* (1993).

As noted in Chapter 2 (pp. 59–61), several of the criticisms of rule ethics indicate the need for virtue ethics in nursing. Ethicists have pointed to the contextual nature of moral judgments, the significance of emotions and experiences, and the relational nature of nursing practice as areas that should be developed in nursing ethics (Aroskar, 1995; Benner, 1991; Chinn, 1990; Cooper, 1991; Parker, 1990; Ray, 1994). These areas are all emphasized in virtue ethics, which accounts for the fact that virtue ethics is emerging as a significant perspective in nursing ethics.

KEY POINTS

- Virtue ethics focuses on the development of character, which provides a unifying identity and vision of what kind of people and community they want to be.
- Nursing is a moral community with the common moral purpose of promoting human health and alleviating suffering.
- Expert practitioners within each nursing community identify the nursing virtues that promote the goals of the community and enable its members to live fruitful lives.
- Virtues enable individuals to perceive, feel, and act appropriately in response to changing and complex challenges in their communal lives.
- Virtues are developed through mentoring by expert practitioners and co-mentoring among peers.
- Nurses must create space within their clinical settings for critical reflection and ongoing dialogue on ethical issues and their moral experiences as nurses.

REFLECT AND DISCUSS

1. Explain how virtue ethics shifts the focus from action to character. How are virtues relevant to this focus?

2. Describe Aristotle's "craft analogy." Does Aristotle's analogy lead us to a universal list of human virtues? Why or why not?

3. How are nursing virtues determined? Is there one universal set of nursing virtues shared by all nursing communities? If there is more that one set of nursing virtues, is each community's list arbitrary and changeable (at whim or by majority vote) by these communities?

4. Are there nursing virtues that are missing from the list in Box 4–1? Should any of the qualities defined there as virtues be removed from the list? Are you aware of any cultural differences that might alter this list of nursing virtues in other cultural contexts?

5. Do you believe that compassion should include some kind of affective element? If so, describe this element. If not, explain your reasons.

6. Reconsider the opening scenario from Chapter 2 (pp. 23–24), in which a patient with chronic obstructive pulmonary disease refuses ventilator support. Determine the moral consideration(s) involved, the relevant virtue, and the characteristic elements (perception, affective response, and action) of this virtue.

7. Describe two or three of your own experiences of mentoring or co-mentoring of moral judgment in a nursing context. Describe concrete ways in which the processes of mentoring, co-mentoring, and the ongoing development of practical reasoning could be facilitated and institutionalized in your clinical setting.

8. Health care institutions may be more concerned with nurses getting their work done and charted than with their moral development. How would you persuade employers that it is worth creating time for this process?

REFERENCES

Aiken, L. (1995). Transforming of the nursing workforce. *Nursing Outlook, 43,* 201–209.

Alderman, H. (1982). By virtue of a virtue. *Review of Metaphysics, 36,* 127–153.

American Medical Association, Committee on Ethics. (1988). *Guidelines on withholding and withdrawing food and drink.* Kansas City, MO: Author.

American Nurses Association (2000). *Code of ethics for nurses* (working draft #9). Available: http://www.ana.org/ethics/code9.htm [2000, November 17].

American Nurses Association. (1992). *Nursing's agenda for health care reform.* Washington, DC: American Nurses Publishing.

Aristotle. (1985). *Nichomachean Ethics* (T. Irwin, Trans.). Indianapolis, IN: Hackett.

Aroskar, M. A. (1995). Envisioning nursing as a moral community. *Nursing Outlook, 43,* 134–138.

Beauchamp, T. L., & Childress, J. F. (1994, 2001). *Principles of biomedical ethics.* New York: Oxford University Press.

Benner, P. (1984). *From novice to expert: Excellence and power in clinical nursing practice.* Menlo Park, CA: Addison-Wesley.

Benner, P. (1991). The role of experience, narrative, and community in skilled ethical comportment. *Advances in Nursing Science, 14*(2), 1–21.

Bishop, A. H., & Scudder, J. R. (1991). *Nursing: The practice of caring.* New York: National League for Nursing.

Blum, L. (1987). Compassion. In R. B. Kruschwitz & R. C. Roberts (Eds.), *The virtues: Contemporary essays on moral character* (pp. 229–236). Belmont, CA: Wadsworth.

Bona, M. J., Rinehart, J., & Volbrecht, R. M. (1996). Show me: Co-mentoring as feminist pedagogy. *Feminist Teacher, 9,* 24–31.

Callahan, D. (1983). On feeding the dying. *The Hastings Center Report, 13*(6), 22.

Calhoun, J. (1993). The Nightingale Pledge: A commitment that survives the passage of time. *Nursing & Health Care, 14,*130–136.

Carson, R. A. (1986). The symbolic significance of giving to eat and drink. In J. L. Lynx (Ed.), *By no extraordinary means* (pp. 84–88). Bloomington, IN: Indiana University Press.

Chinn, P. L. (1990). Toward the 21st century: Nursing theory, research, and practice. Paper presented at the 1990 23rd Annual Communicating Nursing Research Conference, Western Institute of Nursing, Boulder, CO.

Connor, R. B., & McCormick, P. T. (1998). *Character, choices, & community: The three faces of Christian ethics.* New York: Pavlist Press.

Cooper, M. C. (1991). Principle-oriented ethics and the ethic of care: A creative tension. *Advances in Nursing Science, 14*(2), 22–31.

Cranford, R. E. (1988). The persistent vegetative state: (Getting the facts straight). *The Hastings Center Report, 18*(1), 27–32.

Davis, A. J., Aroskar, M. A., Liaschenko, J., & Drought, T. S. (1997). *Ethical dilemmas and nursing practice.* Stamford, CT: Appleton & Lange.

Derr, P. G. (1986). Nutrition and hydration as elective therapy: Brophy and Jobes from an ethical and historical perspective. *Issues in Law and Medicine, 2*(1), 25–38.

Drane, J. F. (1988). *Becoming a good doctor: The place of virtue and character in medical ethics.* Kansas City, MO: Sheed and Ward.

Fowler, M. (1997). Chapter 2: Nursing's ethics. In A. J. Davis, M. A. Aroskar, K. Liaschenko, & T. S. Drought (Eds.), *Ethical dilemmas and nursing practice.* Stamford, CT: Appleton & Lange.

Garrett, T. M., Baillie, H. W., & Garrett, R. M. (1993). *Health care ethics: Principles & problems.* Upper Saddle River, NJ: Prentice Hall.

Hampl, P. (1995). In the belly of the whale. In C. Buchman & C. Spiegel (Eds.), *Out of the garden: Women writers on the Bible* (pp. 289–300). New York: Balantine Books.

Hauerwas, S. (1981). *A community of character: Toward a constructive Christian social ethic.* Notre Dame, IN: University of Notre Dame Press.

Hinman, L. (1994). *Ethics: A pluralistic approach to moral theory.* Orlando, FL: Harcourt Brace Jovanovich.

Katz, J. (1996). The stories nurses tell: The self-perceptions of working women nurses interpreted through narrative. Unpublished master's thesis, Gonzaga University, Spokane, WA.

Leininger, M. (1990). Culture: The conspicuous missing link to understand ethical and moral dimensions of human care. In M. Leininger (Ed.), *Ethical and moral dimensions of care* (pp. 49–66). Detroit: Wayne State University Press.

Lynn, J., & Childress, J. F. (1986). Must patients always be given food and water? In J. Lynn (Ed.), *By no extraordinary means* (pp. 47–60). Bloomington, IN: Indiana University Press.

MacIntyre, A. (1981). *After virtue.* Notre Dame, IN: University of Notre Dame Press.

McKinnon, C. (1999). *Character, virtue theories, and the vices.* Peterborough, Ontario: Broadview Press.

Meilander, G. (1984). On removing food and water: Against the stream. *The Hastings Center Report, 14*(6), 11–13.

Moline, J. (1986). Professionals and professions: A philosophical examination of an ideal. *Social Science and Medicine, 22*(5), 501–508.

Nussbaum, M. C. (1986). *The fragility of goodness: Luck and ethics in Greek tragedy and philosophy.* Cambridge, MA: Cambridge University Press.

Parker, R. S. (1990). Nurses' stories: The search for a relational ethic of care. *Advances in Nursing Science, 13*(1), 31–40.

Pellegrino, E. D., & Thomasma, D. C. (1993). *The virtues in medical practice*. New York: Oxford University Press.

Piper, A. (1991). Impartiality, compassion, and modal imagination. *Ethics, 101,* 726–757.

Ray, M. A. (1987). Technological caring: A new model in critical care. *Dimensions of Critical Care Nursing, 6,* 166–173.

Ray, M. A. (1994). Communal moral experience as the starting point for research in health care ethics. *Nursing Outlook, 42,* 104–109.

Reverby, S. (1987). A caring dilemma: Womanhood and nursing in historical perspective. *Nursing Research, 36,* 5–11.

Robb, I. A. (1900, 1911, 1916, 1920). *Nursing ethics: For hospital and private use*. New York: E. C. Koeckert.

Scanlon, C. (1994, March). Developing ethical competence. *The American Nurse,* pp. 1, 11.

Volbrecht, R. M. (1994). Careful mutuality: Leadership and friendship in the work place. In E. Buker, M. Leiserson, & J. Rinehart (Eds.), *Taking parts: Leadership, participation, and empowerment* (pp. 195–213). Lanham, MD: University Press of America.

Wallace, J. D. (1988a). *Ethics and the craft analogy*. In P. French, T. Uehling Jr., & H. Wettstein (Eds.), *Ethical theory: Character and virtue* (pp. 222–232). Notre Dame, IN: University of Notre Dame Press.

Wallace, J. D. (1988b). Moral relevance and moral conflict. Ithaca, NY: Cornell University Press.

Watson, J. (1985). *Nursing: Human Science and human care*. Norwalk, CT: Appleton-Century-Crofts.

Weisbard, A., & Siegler, M. (1986). On killing patients with kindness. In J. Lynx (Ed.), *By no extraordinary means* (pp. 108–116). Bloomington, IN: Indiana University Press.

Willams, B. (1985). *Ethics and the Limits of Philosophy*. Cambridge, MA: Harvard University Press.

Zerwekh, J. (1997). Do dying patients really need IV fluids? *American Journal of Nursing, 97*(3), 26–31.

5

Applying Virtue Ethics

As we have noted in previous chapters, nursing theorists have identified a number of weaknesses in rule ethics (Aroskar, 1995; Benner, Tanner, & Chesla, 1995; Benner, 1991; Chinn, 1990; Cooper, 1991; Parker, 1990; and Ray, 1994). Their criticisms of rule ethics include its claim that all ethical decision making can be reduced to the logical application of rules, the emotional detachment it prescribes, and its emphasis of individual autonomy over communal interdependence.

Virtue ethics compensates for these weaknesses through its emphasis on:

- Developing the ability to identify what is morally significant in particular situations and then to respond appropriately
- Integrating emotion as a source of knowledge and a motivational bridge between perception and action
- Recognizing the dynamic role of communal dialogue in developing moral values, mentoring the young, and making moral judgments

131

While nursing texts are giving increasing attention to virtue ethics (Davis et al., 1997; Yeo and Moorhouse, 1996), the following conclusion reached by Yeo and Moorhouse has been characteristic of many in nursing ethics:

> *Virtue ethics has obvious applications concerning the education of health professionals but its relevance to the myriad of problems in contemporary bioethics is less clear. Should the dying client's feeding tube be removed? On what grounds should those in line for a transplant be prioritized? Should consent always be sought for DNR-orders? About such questions virtue ethics offers little guidance . . . (1996, p. 48)*

Certainly, questions such as those raised above are critical in contemporary health care ethics. But, as noted in Chapter 4 (pp. 117–118), virtue ethics does not exclude the development and application of moral rules in ethics.

Some areas of moral judgment lend themselves well to rule making. Rules that summarize obligations not to harm patients (e.g., "Do not lie to patients," "Do not treat competent patients without their adequately informed consent," and "Do not violate patient confidentiality") are reliable guides for action.

Generally, however, rule ethics does not acknowledge the important role that the virtue of practical reasoning plays both in the development and application of rules. Perceptual recognitional ability, aspect recognition, and holistic reasoning are all aspects of practical reasoning that guide rule making and application. We noted in Chapter 4 (pp. 114–117), for instance, how moral aspect recognition enables us to adapt rules to new technological circumstances, such as the withdrawal of artificial nutrition and hydration. James Childress (1994), one of the primary advocates of the rule approach in health care ethics, acknowledges that the process of rule making is less deductive, more complex, and more contextual than he and others initially recognized. In fact, rule making requires the sort of cultivated judgment and perception that virtue ethics outlines.

Interpreting moral considerations and adapting them to changing community conditions is the very heart of applied ethics. Rule development and revision are key aspects of this process, but virtues also play an essential role by enabling individuals and communities to perceive, feel, and act appropriately in response to their communal circumstances.

Yeo and Moorhouse suggest that virtue ethics offers no practical tools to guide health care professionals to make concrete, ethical decisions. Although little has been done in health care ethics to demonstrate it, virtue ethics *can* provide direction for action. This capacity may have been overlooked because virtue ethics focuses on a set of ethical considerations that differ from those emphasized by rule ethics. Whereas the primary question raised by rule ethics is "What is the right thing to do in this situation?", virtue ethics focuses on "What kind of people and community should we be?"

Consequently, virtue ethics emphasizes ongoing evaluation of individual and community or organizational contexts of ethical decision making. To demonstrate this evaluation process, we will apply a virtue ethics perspective to several key issues in nursing.

Moral Distress

Moral distress is a central issue in nursing that virtue ethics can help us understand and ameliorate. *Moral distress* refers to negative feelings such as guilt, anger, frustration, powerlessness, and loss of meaning in one's work. Nurses experience moral distress when they are unable to translate their moral choices into moral action or when they feel that nursing virtues are undermined (Rodney & Starzomski, 1993; Wilkinson, 1987/88). Action and character are interrelated: The ability of nurses to act morally is integrally dependent on their ability to maintain their moral character and their integrity.

Nurses experience a high degree of stress that arises from situational constraints in nursing practice. For instance, hospital policy or physicians' orders may prevent critical care nurses from providing adequate levels of analgesia for dying patients. Or chronic understaffing at a long-term care facility may force a nurse to use restraints for an agitated resident who really just needs more attention. Rodney and Starzomski (1993, p. 24) refer to these situational constraints as ". . . aspects of nurses' structural and interpersonal work environment that impede the implementation of professional standards of nursing." These professional standards include expectations that nurses will adhere to particular rules of professional behavior and will embody shared nursing virtues.

Areas frequently cited as causes of moral distress in nurses include concerns about prolongation of dying, lack of informed consent, impaired or abusive professionals, and difficulties accessing needed resources. Key nursing virtues are at risk in each of these areas. Fidelity to trust and compassion are undermined when a nurse perceives that policies or conflict with a physician may result in an unnecessarily prolonged dying process for a patient. Similarly, mediation and fidelity to trust will be tested when insitutional practices or professional practices create obstacles to obtaining adequately informed consent. A verbally abusive director of nursing or a chemically impaired surgeon will test and undermine nurses' moral courage and resilience if institutional policies do not provide adequate support and remedies for these situations. The lack of an adequate reimbursement system results in less-than-quality patient care and undermines the nursing virtue of justice.

Each of these situations requires moral courage and resilience on the part of nurses to confront, to advocate, and to persist if patient care and safety are threatened. And when serious concerns require nurses to exhibit moral courage and resilience on a daily or weekly basis, then the organizational and interpersonal working environments are in need of reform. When nurses repeatedly feel unable to implement their moral choices on behalf of their patients, they come to feel that they are unable to *be* the kind of persons that nurses should be. Not surprisingly, then, moral distress is strongly linked to stress and burnout in nursing (Barr, 1992; Rodney & Starzomski, 1993; Sundin-Huard & Fahy, 1999). Since Wilkinson conducted one of the first studies of moral distress in nursing in 1987, several further studies in a variety of settings have confirmed that moral distress is a critical issue in nursing.

Moral distress is a critical issue that has often been neglected in organizational ethics. One reason for this neglect is that health care organizations often expect that professionals of good character whom they hire will act ethically. Although the character of employees is an important factor, this expectation ignores the significant role that organizations themselves play in supporting or impeding moral behavior. If health care organizations want employees to act morally and to make good moral decisions, then they must critically assess their organizational culture, policies, and practices. Do they undermine or do they support good choices and behavior? Benign neglect is inadequate. If a health care organization does not actively promote organizational and professional virtues, then it sends a message that these virtues are not a priority in this organization. Complying with health and safety regulations, legal requirements, or billing procedures is encouraged through training, monitoring, and performance evaluation. The ongoing development of a community's virtues must be actively encouraged, supported, and monitored in similar ways. One of the strengths of the new American Nurses Association (ANA) *Code of Ethics* (2000) is its recognition of the important role of the health care environment in either nurturing or thwarting nursing virtues. Virtue ethics encourages us to critically examine the individual and community or organizational contexts in which nurses seek to exhibit moral integrity and to act responsibly as professionals.

To illustrate how virtue ethics can be applied to the current context of nursing, we will follow the framework for ethical analysis outlined in Chapter 1 and shown in Box 5–1. We will use the framework to examine two issues: pain medication in the neonatal intensive care unit (NICU) and the challenge of setting professional boundaries. We will also explore additional issues in nursing that could benefit from the application of a virtue ethics perspective.

Case Study   Pain Medication in the NICU

Baby T was one of in vitro triplets born at 30 weeks' gestation. Melinda, a six-year veteran in the NICU, became his primary nurse. Antiphospholipid syndrome, an autoimmune response during pregnancy that can affect fetal development, caused Baby T to experience intrauterine growth retardation (IUGR). His birth weight was one pound fifteen ounces, while his siblings weighed more than three pounds each. Prematurity caused multiple problems beyond the IUGR for Baby T. He had a heart block with a junctional (atrial ventricular node) heart rate of 50 to 60, and at six weeks, he went into heart failure. When he did not respond to medication to assist his heart function, his physician, Dr. Lyle, decided to insert a pacemaker.

Box 5–1   *Framework for Ethical Analysis*

1. Identify the problem or issue.
2. Analyze context.
3. Explore options.
4. Apply the decision process.
5. Implement the plan and evaluate results.

Baby T's size made this decision a difficult one. Since he weighed only a little over two pounds at this point, his chest wall was too small to accommodate the smallest of pacemakers. As a result, the pacemaker was placed in the anterior abdominal wall on the left side of the abdomen. Unfortunately, it caused inflammation and the baby progressed to sepsis with bowel bacteria. The pacemaker was removed, again leaving Baby T with a junctional heart rate of only 40 to 50. In addition, the wound would not heal, due to poor profusion, poor oxygenation, and overwhelming sepsis.

Baby T went into severe heart failure, his heart rate dropping as low as 25 to 35. He was placed on a ventilator and, due to his labile condition, a subclavian line was placed in the nursery under emergent conditions. Baby T received minimal pain medication for this procedure, because the physician felt that he was too labile to tolerate sedation. An external pacemaker was placed through the subclavian line and sutured to the infant's chest wall with nondissolvable sutures. The pacemaker normalized Baby T's heart rate and eventually he was weaned off the ventilator to oxygen supplementation only with nasal cannula.

Any movement at all caused Baby T pain due to the suture in his chest and the abdominal wound that remained unhealed and infected. He received little or no pain medication at this time because Dr. Lyle believed it would compromise his respiratory effort. The physician decided to open the wound and debride the area without pain medication. Melinda requested pain medication before the procedure, but Dr. Lyle denied the request, stating that the procedure would be brief. The baby's response was not unusual for a premature infant: signs included lack of movement, gaze aversion, splinted breaths, increased oxygen needs, and decreased feeding tolerance (Bildner, 1999).

Dr. Lyle repeated this procedure for two additional days, at which point Melinda refused to assist until pain medication was given. A one-time order was received and, as a result, Baby T tolerated the procedure better. Before the next dressing change and debridement, Melinda again requested a medication order, but Dr. Lyle again denied the request based on the brevity of the procedure. Unfortunately, the NICU had no mission statement or policy regarding pain control. Melinda presented Dr. Lyle with physiological data and research citations to support her claim that Baby T had pain. The two most profound symptoms were gaze avert so severe that Baby T appeared catatonic and emesis with feeding intolerance for nearly eight hours after the procedure (Porter, Wolf, and Miller, 1998). Even with the data, pain medication was again denied.

After this episode, Melinda informed Dr. Lyle that she would not assist with any further dressing changes unless he ordered pain medication. Dr. Lyle again refused the request, stating that the baby would be just fine and would not remember the pain when he was older. Baby T, now three months old, recognized his parents as well as certain nurses. Believing that he would remember, Melinda tried to joke with the physician by suggesting that when Baby T grew up, he would remember and return to seek revenge. Unmoved, Dr. Lyle continued to refuse to order pain medications.

Feeling that direct appeal to the physician had not been successful, Melinda tried another strategy—she enlisted the help of Baby T's parents. They had commented on their baby's behavior after the dressing changes, noting how long it took him to recover. Melinda had assured them that the debridement and dressing changes were necessary. Now Melinda shared with the parents her belief that their baby's behavior was a response to the pain he experienced during dressing changes. When the mother asked what they could do, Melinda suggested they could be present for the next dressing change and request pain medication for their baby.

The parents came the next day for the dressing change and asked the physician to provide pain medication for every dressing change. Dr. Lyle explained why he felt that the baby didn't need medication, but the parents pointed out the symptoms they had observed in their baby and insisted that pain medication be given. The pain medication was ordered. Baby T was more interactive post dressing change with the pain medication. After the parents were gone, the physician confronted Melinda, accusing her of "putting the parents up to this." He was furious, calling her names and ranting at her. This was not untypical behavior for this physician, who was often verbally abusive to nurses. Melinda stated that she had discussed with the parents their concerns about their baby's behavior and had encouraged them to request pain medication when the mother had asked what they could do.

Baby T continued to be more interactive after dressing changes with pain medication. His feeding tolerance increased and he started to gain weight on continuous feedings without emesis.

Step 1. Identify the Problem or Issue

This case involves a physician–nurse conflict regarding the need for pain medication in a neonate. Presumably, both practitioners want to promote their patient's best interests, but they differ about the benefits versus risks of pain medication for this procedure. The value issues in this case are the need for the appropriate use of pain medication for all neonates, processes for resolution of physician–nurse conflicts regarding pain relief, and the appropriate role of parents in treatment disputes of this kind.

Step 2. Analyze the Context

The most crucial contextual factors in this case are (1) the political/organizational aspects of nurses' multiple obligations to their patients, families, physicians, and employing institutions; and (2) attitudes, beliefs, and research about neonates' experience of pain. Both of these issues significantly affect the nurse's perception of her responsibilities and her ability to act effectively as a patient advocate in this case.

NURSES' MULTIPLE OBLIGATIONS

All professionals struggle to maintain their integrity or moral wholeness in the light of multiple obligations. Nurses must not only balance their multiple professional obligations, but they must also contend with their history of subordination to physicians. In fact, nurses may frequently feel caught between nursing ideology, which asserts that their primary commitment is to their patients (ANA, 2000, 2.1), and the realities of their institutional lives. The institutions and those who work within them have been shaped by an earlier ideology that prescribed unquestioning obedience and loyalty to physicians (Yarling & McElmurry, 1986). The *Code of Ethics* states that nurses are accountable for their own judgments and actions in spite of potentially conflicting physician orders or policies of their employing agencies (2.2). Yet, the actions of physicians and employers exert powerful influences on nurses.

NEONATES' EXPERIENCE OF PAIN

There has been a long history of assuming neonates do not experience pain. Until the mid-1980s, major surgery on preterm infants was commonly performed without the use of anesthesia or analgesia (Franck, 1997). Research in the last two decades has documented that neonates do experience pain. Nonetheless, myths regarding neonate pain persist. The following myths are still prevalent:

1. *Infants do not experience pain because their nervous systems are immature.*
2. *Experiencing pain will not harm infants.*
3. *Infants do not have memories of painful experiences.*
4. *Potential side effects associated with the use of narcotics makes their use dangerous in infants.*

(Clancy, Anand, & Lally, 1992; Howard & Thurber, 1998)

Lack of myelination is used frequently to support the argument that preterm or term infants are incapable of pain perception. Research, however, has demonstrated that incomplete myelination merely slows the conduction velocity in neonatal nerves or central nerve tracts (Gilles, Shankle, & Dooling, 1983). A landmark study by Anand and Hickey (1987) further documented that infants are developmentally capable of interpreting pain as early as 24 to 28 weeks. By the late 1980s, other studies had confirmed that neonates are physiologically capable of experiencing pain. Research in the 1990s continued to support this conclusion (Clancy, Anand, & Lally, 1992; Howard & Thurber, 1998).

Several investigators have found evidence of the damaging effects of pain on short- and long-term physiology and development (Als, 1982; Anand & Hickey, 1987; Meinhart & McCaffery, 1983; Shapiro, 1989; Johnston & Stevens, 1990). Potential effects include pulmonary and cardiac insufficiency, cardiac arrhythmias, contribution to a hypermetabolic state, complications, and poor recovery. On the other hand, fears of side effects such as respiratory depression and hypotension from the use of pain medication appear to be clearly inflated. Little objective evidence supports this fear of adverse sequelae when narcotics are administered to infants experiencing pain (Franck, 1997). Actually, evidence of the potential beneficial effects of these drugs in critically ill infants is increasing (Franck & Gregory, 1993). Finally, some research supports the view that infants may remember their experiences of pain (Grunau et al., 1994; McGrath & Craig, 1989).

Step 3. Explore Options

Although the immediate issue of obtaining adequate pain relief for Baby T has been resolved due to the tenacity of this nurse, broader issues remain. Other neonates will also experience pain in the course of their treatment in this NICU. This unit needs to develop a philosophy and protocol regarding pain medication in the NICU as well as procedures for resolving conflicts between nurses and physicians regarding pain relief. Further analysis will be helpful in considering these options. We will explore these issues within the virtue ethics decision process.

Step 4. Apply the Virtue Ethics Decision Process

Box 5–2 outlines a virtue ethics decision process and highlights key aspects of virtue ethics in a useful checklist format.

✓ Identify Relevant Communities

The relevant communities in this case are the community of neonatal nurses and the community of health care professionals in this particular neonatal unit. Neonatal nurses have their own unique challenges and concerns, but they clearly share with other areas of nursing a commitment to quality health care, health restoration, and health promotion. Although this particular NICU lacks a mission statement identifying the specific goals of this unit, the mission statement of the hospital states its goals as respect for the dignity of each individual, care of the whole person, and especially care of the poor within a collaborative, compassionate environment.

Clearly, the neonates in the NICU and their parents become a part of the unit's community while the babies are patients. Their needs and their input should be care-

---

Framework for Ethical Analysis
1. Identify the problem or issue.
2. Analyze context.
3. Explore options.
4. **Apply the Virtue Ethics Decision Process**
5. Implement the plan and evaluate results.

Box 5–2   Virtue Ethics Decision Process

4. Apply the Virtue Ethics Decision Process

♦ Identify relevant communities.

♦ Identify relevant moral considerations.

♦ Identify and apply relevant virtues.

♦ Apply practical reasoning to modify moral concepts.

♦ Remove impediments to character development.

♦ Provide institutional support for character development.

fully considered in the professional dialogue regarding pain relief. Nonetheless, it is the nursing community's virtues that we are interpreting and applying in this context.

✓ IDENTIFY RELEVANT MORAL CONSIDERATIONS

Moral considerations were defined in Chapter 4 (p. 98) as practical concerns that arise as communities consider how to promote mutual human welfare, growth, and meaning in their particular communal contexts. The primary moral consideration in this case is the alleviation of suffering and the promotion of healing and well-being for Baby T and other neonates. A second moral consideration is the development of a more collaborative working relationship among the physicians and nurses in this neonatal unit. Collaboration promotes quality patient care and the well-being of those who provide this care.

✓ IDENTIFY AND APPLY RELEVANT VIRTUES

Virtues enable individuals to perceive, feel, and act appropriately in response to the moral considerations that arise in communal life. The nursing virtues of compassion, fidelity to trust, self-confidence, moral courage, and moral integrity each play a critical role in the nurse's response to the two moral considerations of this case.

COMPASSION AND FIDELITY TO TRUST

The virtue of compassion helps the nurse to perceive and respond to the subtle indications of the baby's pain experiences. Infants cannot express their pain clearly and preterm infants are even less expressive than full-term infants. As noted earlier, many health care practitioners have been educated to believe that neonates are incapable of experiencing pain. The physician in this scenario clearly believed that this was true. No doubt, Dr. Lyle cared about his patient. But his medical beliefs, in this case, blinded him to the physiological evidence that Baby T was experiencing pain. Perhaps the nurse's frequent contact with both the baby and his parents enabled her empathic imagination to override the physiologic theory, one which she also had been taught. She observed the baby's averted gaze, splinted breaths, increased oxygen needs, and decreased feeding tolerance, signs that persisted after the procedure was completed and the physician left the unit.

Melinda had significant experience in the NICU. This baby's condition fit the pain profile documented in reported research (Bildner, 1999; Porter, Wolf, & Miller, 1998). Melinda was able to present citations to support her claim that this baby was experiencing pain. This suggests that Melinda's previous empathic observation of other neonates had caused her to doubt the standard view that neonates do not experience pain; this doubt led her to do further research in the library. Research confirmed her own perceptions and further heightened her perception of pain indicators. Compassion thus focused her perception; it also generated a sympathetic response to this baby and disposed Melinda to act to alleviate his suffering.

Baby T's parents noticed a pattern in his behavior: signs of his withdrawal followed the dressing changes. Melinda listened to the parents and gave weight to their concerns. In doing so, she developed and confirmed the parents' trust in her benevolence and character. Her continued advocacy for their son further exhibited the fidelity to trust that patients and their families rightly expect of nurses.

SELF-CONFIDENCE AND MORAL COURAGE

This nurse clearly embodied an appropriate respect and positive regard for her own professional knowledge and for the central nursing role in human healing. The shift from physician loyalty as a nurse's primary duty to patient advocacy is a mere 30 years old. In the past, nurses generally did not express disagreement with a physician, let alone presume to enter into a discussion about a patient's care. Self-confidence as a nurse was essential in this case, providing a necessary foundation for Melinda's moral courage. Research confirms that nurses are, in fact, reliable interpreters of infant pain indicators (Maloni et al., 1986; Penticuff, 1989; Pigeon et al., 1989). Awareness of this fact should further bolster self-confidence for Melinda and other neonatal nurses.

Melinda was taking personal risks by refusing to assist the physician, by involving the parents, and by continuing to insist on the administering of pain medication. She persisted in her efforts to obtain the medication that she judged was necessary for her patient; she did not easily retreat. Melinda tried humor, presented physiological data and scientific research, refused to assist in the procedure without the medication, and finally involved the parents. There were risks in speaking frankly with the parents and in having them present for dressing changes. In this case, she suffered verbal abuse from the physician and perhaps a strained working relationship with him in the future. Greater penalties could have resulted.

INTEGRITY

In isolation, this one incident would not present a major challenge to integrity. But, although Baby T received the pain medication that he needed, the issue of pain relief for neonates will continue to be an issue in this, and other, NICUs. Repeated conflict between nurses' responsibilities to their extremely vulnerable patients, to the physicians with whom they share their work, and potentially to the hospital that employs them does threaten nurses' integrity. It becomes increasingly difficult to remain whole and balanced in the face of ongoing conflict.

✓ APPLY PRACTICAL REASONING TO MODIFY MORAL CONCEPTS

The virtue ethics decision process directs us to consider whether any modification of moral considerations is necessary to adequately address the practical moral issue being considered. How would we determine that such a modification is necessary? The process is essentially an argument from analogy. The virtue of practical reasoning enables us to interpret and adapt moral considerations to solve new practical moral problems. But some problems may actually require us to rethink and revise our moral considerations: The problem is so dissimilar to previous issues that we cannot simply apply or adapt the old concepts to the new setting.

The process of argument from analogy is summarized in the virtue ethics decision process. In the NICU case, the relevant moral considerations are the alleviation of suffering and the promotion of collaboration among health care professionals. If it were true that neonates are not physiologically capable of experiencing pain, then clearly the usual obligations to alleviate and control pain would not apply to these patients. But the evidence clearly supports the view that neonates do experience pain.

The other dissimilarity between neonatal patients and many other adult or pediatric patients is that neonatal patients cannot clearly express their pain. Recognizing and accurately interpreting pain indicators in neonates is a practical problem. It does not change the underlying moral consideration that physicians and nurses should do what they can to alleviate pain in their patients. The problem is a practical issue of how to respond effectively to this moral concern in this particular context.

The need for collaboration among health care professionals is not conceptually different in the NICU than it is in other areas of care. Because the status of seriously ill neonates can change so rapidly and frequently, it is especially important to have in place efficient processes for resolving disagreements about patient care in the NICU. This again does not require a change in the moral consideration regarding collaboration, but it may require some changes in organizational practices.

Box 5–3 provides another example of modifying a basic moral concept.

✓ REMOVE IMPEDIMENTS TO CHARACTER DEVELOPMENT

The goal of virtue ethics is to develop and sustain moral character in both individuals and in the organizations that shape their lives. Consequently, an important aspect of applying virtue ethics to particular issues is critically examining both individuals and organizations for impediments that undermine the development or embodiment of

---

Box 5–3   Modifying a Moral Concept

Unjustified Killing of Innocent Persons

The discussion of voluntary active euthanasia leads us to consider a modification in our concept of unjustified killing of innocent persons. The relevant moral consideration in the debate about voluntary active euthanasia is that it is wrong to kill a human being who is not threatening one's life or the life of another innocent person. A person who is dying and who asks a physician to end his or her life is clearly not a threat to the physician's life. This suggests that it would be morally wrong then for the physician to end this life. But advocates of voluntary active euthanasia argue that euthanasia cases are not analogous to the usual murder case. Murder is tragic because it unexpectedly takes away a person's life and all that he or she might have done in the future with that life (Brock, 1994).

But in the euthanasia case, the dying person has concluded that continuing a life filled with suffering is not a valuable future. In the usual murder case, death takes away a valued future. In euthanasia, the patient requesting to die does not value his or her future. Consequently, advocates of voluntary active euthanasia argue that the cases of murder and voluntary active euthanasia are so dissimilar that the same moral consideration cannot be applied to both. The dissimilarity in the cases forces us to consider a modification in our concept of unjustified killing of innocent persons.

the virtues of the relevant community. Examples of impediments in individuals might include having been socialized to follow orders, a defeatist attitude that believes that nothing can ever change, or a defensive attitude that responds to all new suggestions with "but we have always done it this way." Each person obviously brings an individual history and personality to his or her professional work. Excessive fear, cynicism, and anger may be the residue of personal responses to past experiences. These attitudes and emotions can undermine efforts by a community to embody its ideal virtues. Some may object that these are matters of psychology rather than ethics. Although we may outline rather clear disciplinary boundaries, in practice, psychology and ethics overlap. Virtue ethics does not merely decide what communities should do; it also critically assesses the responsibilities of communities and their members to promote and facilitate the process of consistently embodying their ideals.

In the NICU case, one impediment is the physician's lack of current education regarding neonatal experiences of pain. Recent surveys indicate that many physicians and nurses continue to be unaware of current research, suggesting that their professional organizations have educational work to do (Anand, 1995; Stang & Snellman, 1998). But this particular hospital can address the educational need through appropriate in-services.

Another impediment here is this physician's tendency to resort to verbal abuse of those in less powerful positions. Although physicians are surely not the only guilty parties, verbal abuse of nurses by physicians is a serious concern. Although verbal abuse does have personal psychological dimensions, it is primarily an issue about the abuse of power. Physicians who verbally abuse nurses do so because they can get away with it. They are much less likely to treat their peers in this way. It is the responsibility of organizations to have in place appropriate policies that clearly communicate that abusive behavior will not be tolerated. There also need to be clear and well-publicized procedures for reporting abuse, a well-defined process for investigating claims of abuse, and clear organizational sanctions that will be applied when necessary. Unless health care organizations are willing to impose sanctions to address substantiated cases of abusive behavior by physicians, they will continue to reinforce that behavior and communicate that professional groups are not equally valued.

✓ PROVIDE INSTITUTIONAL SUPPORT FOR CHARACTER DEVELOPMENT

Individuals and organizations have a responsibility to support the ongoing development of a community's virtues. In the case of Baby T, some steps could be taken to support the virtues of compassion, fidelity to trust, self-confidence, and integrity. These actions should decrease the need for repeated acts of moral courage to alleviate neonate suffering and also promote further development of collaborative work among the unit's doctors and nurses. Each organization should consider what policies or processes are most suited to its particular context. Three examples of organizational supports are considered here:

1. *Initiation of an ongoing dialogue between nurses and physicians regarding pain control in neonates*
2. *Development of a protocol to evaluate pain and to recommend interventions*
3. *Institution of a nurse–physician peer group to review conflict issues*

INITIATE DIALOGUE

This unit does not have a mission statement that interprets the hospital's mission in the NICU. Discussion and writing of such a statement could provide a useful context for dialogue about how pain control for neonates relates to the hospital's mission of compassion and the alleviation of suffering. The unit's physicians and nurses could agree to read and discuss together some of the current literature on neonatal experiences of pain. This literature would provide a shared database for further dialogue and consensus building. The dialogue and a written policy help to normalize physician–nurse discussions about the use of pain medication for particular neonates. Raising questions regarding pain treatment is less likely to require moral courage on the part of nurses and less likely to be perceived as a challenge to physician authority. As a result, discussion of pain issues could be incorporated in the daily rounds of the health care team.

DEVELOP A PAIN MANAGEMENT PROTOCOL

The unit should also develop a protocol to assess pain and recommend interventions. No standard tool presently exists to measure and rate the intensity of infant pain. A variety of physiological and behavioral signs have been documented as indicators of infant pain (Bildner, 1999; Howard & Thurber, 1998). With minimal use of equipment, neonatal nurses can observe most of these indicators. A pain management protocol should include a standardized method of documenting pain assessments. It should also include guidelines for the minimum standard for frequency of pain assessment and for starting and escalating therapy (Franck, 1997).

Resistance can be anticipated, especially from physicians who would object that this protocol would remove their control of care of their patients. This predictable response highlights the need for the protocol to be developed through a collaborative process that includes physicians, nurses, and administration. Drafts of the protocol could be taken to existing committees such as the hospital pediatric committee and the neonatal subcommittee, which have representatives of these three groups. Pain management should be a collaborative process. The pain management protocol should be used as an instrument that facilitates communication and discussion. The protocol is not a cookbook or rule that dictates pain treatment; it is a resource that guides the process of individualizing pain treatment.

ESTABLISH A CONFLICT RESOLUTION PEER GROUP

Conflicts regarding pain management will continue to occur even after a shared mission statement and clear protocol are in place. Clear methods for resolving these conflicts are essential. A nurse–physician peer group could be instituted to discuss difficult cases and resolve conflicts. Alternatively, difficult cases could be referred to the hospital ethics committee for consultation. The unit-level approach is preferable, however, insofar as it encourages further dialogue among health care providers who work together in this unit.

Establishing such a peer group may be difficult to implement. It requires that these two groups be recognized as peers and that they sit at the table as such. In spite of the dramatic changes that have occurred as nurses have defined their role more autonomously and developed their own knowledge base, many physicians, nurses, and administrators do not perceive these professionals as peer groups. On the other hand, there have been encouraging developments. Care conferences bring together a variety of professionals to discuss the direction of treatment in complex cases or to resolve conflicts regarding care. Such conferences have become commonplace in many practice settings. Although collaboration and equal respect for each professional perspective is not guaranteed, these are increasingly the expectation in such conferences. Nurses in NICUs often have specialized education and valuable years of experience that make them indispensable partners in a context where a patient's health status may change quickly and critical events are the norm. As a result, NICUs are often characterized by a higher degree of professional collaboration than in traditional medical–surgical units. Consequently, NICUs are a good venue for piloting nurse–physician peer groups. The rapid pace of technological development impacting care in NICUs makes the need for an open discussion of values and appropriate treatment absolutely essential.

Specific policies and practices such as these are necessary to support nurses as they strive to provide adequate care for their patients. Without this kind of institutional support, only the most courageous nurses will take the kind of steps that Melinda did in Baby T's case. In other cases, patients will continue to suffer unnecessary pain. In the absence of adequate institutional supports, long-term effects of ongoing stress, lack of trust, and poor communication will undermine this community's virtues.

Step 5. Implement and Evaluate the Plan

Each of the proposed solutions needs to be monitored and evaluated at regular intervals. Quality improvement principles can be used to evaluate the quality of pain management in the NICU (Friedrichs et al., 1995). It is especially important for the professionals of this NICU community to continue to review new information about pain control in neonates as well as new protocols for pain assessment and intervention that may be developed elsewhere.

Setting Professional Boundaries

Our second application of virtue ethics addresses a broad issue in home health nursing, rather than a specific case. Once again, we will follow the five steps of the framework for ethical analysis, including step 4, the virtue ethics decision process (see Box 5–2).

Step 1. Identify the Problem or Issue

The issue is where to draw professional nursing boundaries in the context of home health nursing. Caring relationships between home health care nurses and their patients and families are complex, professional, and primarily therapeutic, promoting the health needs of home-bound patients. Because the care occurs in the context of the home, professional boundaries that separate the health care professional from the patient and family can be difficult to define and maintain. In more traditional settings for nursing care, such as hospitals, clinics, or practitioner offices, a patient enters the professional's territory. Established norms of behavior prescribe how patients and nurses should interact in these contexts. Furthermore, though nurses in these traditional settings seek to make patients active partners in their care, the professional sets the ground rules for the interaction. In home health, the guest/host dynamic is reversed; thus, professional boundaries are more complicated and ambiguous.

Home health nurses need to take responsibility for defining, modeling, and maintaining appropriate boundaries. These professional boundaries are emotional or relational borders that separate the health care professional from the patient and family. Failure of nursing professionals to set these boundaries can be destructive and painful to both patient and nurse. Box 5–4 presents a number of boundary situations that are typical in home health nursing.

Box 5–4   Communities in Dialogue:

Setting Boundaries

Policies and guidelines aimed at helping home health nurses maintain appropriate professional boundaries should emerge from discussions among administrators, nurses, and other members of agency communities. These need to be reviewed regularly in light of changing contexts. Consideration of the following situations may assist home health care communities as they develop these policies and guidelines.

Which of the following activities violate appropriate home care nurse–patient boundaries?

- Giving one of your patients an attractive wall calendar
- Advocating for the services of a home health aide for longer than allowed for a patient you particularly like
- Picking up groceries for a patient
- Accepting ballet tickets from a patient
- Giving your home phone number to a patient
- Dating a current or former patient
- Having dinner with patient and family in their home
- Seeing a patient after hours to attend to spiritual needs
- Taking care of family members other than the assigned patient
- Changing storm windows for a patient
- Accepting a quilt made for you by a deceased patient's partner

Step 2. Analyze the Context

Cultural attitudes and policies regarding the ill and the elderly as well as the cultural expectations of caregivers are important aspects of the context of home care nursing. Both of these contextual factors shape and influence the values and expectations of home health nurses and their patients.

THE ILL AND DISABLED

Independence is valued in American culture. Many people with illnesses or worsening disabilities prefer to live in their own homes, maintaining as much independence as possible. Yet, policies and programs to support this independent living remain patchy and fragmented in the United States. Some services are available to deliver meals, to perform some basic household chores, and to provide health services for individuals at home. These services are provided by a variety of agencies and compensated through a variety of sources.

North American society is highly mobile, and families may be widely scattered, separated by many miles. As a result, home bound individuals may not have families that are available to offer physical and emotional support. Even when family members are geographically close, they frequently have jobs and their own children that keep them busy. Loneliness and social isolation are, consequently, common problems for homebound patients.

In spite of available services, many who are homebound due to illness or disabilities do not have an adequate level of support for either their physical or psychosocial needs. Not surprisingly, then, home health nurses will be asked to perform chores or run errands that may not fall within their job descriptions. Many homebound individuals and their families frequently form significant emotional bonds with caregivers.

CAREGIVER EXPECTATIONS

The nursing profession has emerged from a nineteenth century context in which nursing acts were carried out by female relatives as one part of their "natural" womanly duties (Reverby, 1987). Women were often brought from across the country to care for members of their extended families. Although their service was regarded as a "labor of love" (and therefore unpaid), it was not optional or voluntary: It was a duty derived from what was perceived to be women's compassionate, submissive, and dutiful nature. Self-sacrifice was taken for granted as a woman's duty. As nursing moved to the patriarchal, hierarchical hospital setting in the late 1800s, this concept of duty continued to serve as the foundation of nursing.

Contemporary American and Canadian nursing have rejected the Victorian ideals of submissiveness, self-sacrifice, and loyalty as defining nursing virtues. Nonetheless, residual effects from this nineteenth century ideal of the feminine caregiver remain both in the cultural consciousness and in the personal consciousness of nurses. Caregiving continues to be perceived as a "feminine" activity, in spite of increased focus on the joys and responsibilities of fatherhood or the entry of women into male-dominated professions and men into female-dominated ones. Women continue to do the majority of caregiving in homes (Hochschild, 1989), in grade schools, and in nursing. And though nineteenth century norms of self-sacrifice are no longer accepted, cultural norms of "feminine" behavior still include expectations of nurturing, caring, and solicitous behaviors (Basow, 1992; Bartky, 1990).

Friedman (1987) notes that even though many men and women's actual behavior does not conform to cultural gender stereotypes of masculinity and femininity, they nonetheless expect and evaluate behavior against these gender yardsticks. This dissonance between what we *say* we expect of caregivers and what we may *actually* expect at a deeper level of our psyches may create some conflicts for nurses as they try to articulate and maintain appropriate professional boundaries.

Step 3. Explore Options

One option for setting clear boundaries is for home health agencies to develop strict guidelines that proscribe specific behaviors for employees. A second option is to allow each nurse to make boundary decisions on a case-by-case basis. A third option is for organizations to develop guidelines that prohibit behaviors that are clearly unacceptable for home health nurses, while encouraging individual nurses to make their own judgments in other less clear cases. Agency guidelines would be developed collaboratively by employees and managers and reviewed regularly. In addition, opportunities for peer discussion of difficult cases and support for mentoring relationships would be priorities.

What is essential to all of these options are the criteria that will be used to develop guidelines or to make individual decisions. The process by which these are made, however, is also important. The following discussion shows that the third option, prohibiting clearly unacceptable behaviors while encouraging individual judgments in other cases, reflects the commitment of virtue ethics to community dialogue and reflection as well as to the ongoing development of character and moral judgment.

Step 4. Apply the Virtue Ethics Decision Process

✓ IDENTIFY RELEVANT COMMUNITIES

Following the virtue ethics decision process outlined in Box 5–2, we begin by identifying the relevant community in this case as the community of home health care nurses. This community is, of course, a part of the larger community of professional nurses. In addition to providing health care services for individuals and families at home, home health care nurses, like all health care professionals, assume responsibility to identify and respond to needs and priorities along the continuum of care as well as to educate and advocate. Consequently, although home health care nursing will have its own particular challenges and concerns, it shares with other areas of nursing a commitment to health restoration, promotion, and care.

✓ IDENTIFY RELEVANT MORAL CONSIDERATIONS

The essential moral consideration in this case is the need to maintain appropriate professional boundaries with patients. To be a professional is to enter into a special trust relationship with one's patients and the communities one serves. Patients and society entrust themselves to the care of health professionals; health care professionals commit themselves to act in the interests of those they serve. The ability of health care professionals to promote health and alleviate the suffering of their patients requires competence, trust, and an assurance of concern for their patients (Benner & Wrubel, 1989, p. 4). Professionals must balance the need to develop a caring personal relationship with the need to preserve the distance necessary for making objective professional judgments. They must also set professional limits that allow energy and time for essential self-care.

✓ IDENTIFY AND APPLY RELEVANT VIRTUES

Home health care nursing shares the set of nursing virtues outlined in Chapter 4 (pp. 103–104). This set of virtues must be interpreted, applied, and perhaps modified in the particular contexts of home health nursing. The three virtues that seem most relevant to the issue of professional boundaries are the virtues of justice, compassion, and fidelity to trust. Each of these is discussed below.

JUSTICE

Justice requires that we give what is due to each person including respect and promotion of well-being. It also requires that we distribute resources fairly. Parents teach their children this moral consideration of justice as fairness early on. For instance, a parent may ask a little girl to divide a candy bar and give her sibling the bigger piece. The issue of giving gifts to patients clearly raises the question of fairness. Would you give a wall calendar, or a birthday card, or homemade banana bread to all of your patients or only to a select few? Any behavior that sets one patient aside as special—other than special medical and nursing care needs—violates the professional responsibility to treat each patient with equal respect and care. This does not mean that nurses should treat patients impersonally any more than fairness in parenting rules out valuing the special uniqueness of each child.

Nursing students are similarly urged to tailor care to individual patients. Balancing the need for individualized care, on the one hand, and fairness, on the other, can complicate one's ability to define appropriate boundaries. A generally reliable guideline will be that if nurses give gifts, gifts should be given to all patients. For the home health nurse practicing in a more intimate environment, this rule may be more difficult and even more important to follow. Individual home health agencies may decide to adopt a uniform policy for all of their employees that would prohibit giving gifts entirely, an acceptable policy that promotes fairness.

Other examples also raise questions of fairness. Treating family members can be ruled out rather easily since they are not part of the approved plan of care. Treating them would unfairly use unapproved resources. A more difficult case involves the decision to provide special services for a special patient whom one especially enjoys. An example might be choosing to advocate for the support of a home health aide for longer than allowed. You believe that this patient's safety at home is jeopardized without the aide. This is a good reason for going out of your way to advocate for this patient. Nonetheless, you have other patients who also need similar extensions or other services, but you may choose not to advocate for them this way. Is your choice to do extra for one patient justified simply because you like that person?

Doing chores, such as buying groceries and changing storm windows, is a similarly difficult issue. One could ask whether these favors would be done for all patients or whether they are "special" favors done for only a select (favorite?) few. It may be tempting to note that not all patient situations are alike. Some patients clearly have family members or friends who can pick up groceries, change storm windows, or take the patient on an outing. Others do not. Or, if the neighbor who normally picks up groceries is ill or her car is in for repair, could the nurse pick up a few things just this once? Because patient situations vary, it may seem that certain special favors are justified in some cases.

This may, in fact, be true. But these examples raise further issues about how much of themselves home health care nurses should be willing to give to their patients. If home health nurses choose to treat particular patients differently, they should ask themselves what more they would be willing to do and what other special favors or chores patients may expect them to do? These questions lead us into the discussion of the appropriate boundaries of compassion.

COMPASSION

Of professional boundary issues, the majority that arise in home health nursing will be related to the issue of proportionate compassion. The duty to care is a moral imperative that is derived from the voluntary "profession to care" that all nurses make when they join the community of nursing. Effective nursing care includes competent performance of activities to meet patient needs and appropriate affective responses to patients. The virtue of compassion is related to both of these aspects of care.

Etymologically, *compassion* means "feeling with." Compassion, however, is more than simply having a feeling; it entails a desire and disposition to do something to improve someone else's situation. Compassion in caring for patients seems so clearly essential to effective nursing that one might assume a nurse could never have too much compassion. But care for others can become disproportionate relative to the individual needs of nurses and to the other commitments that define them as persons.

One reason that setting professional boundaries is difficult is that ultimately it requires maintaining a balance between one's own needs and identity and those of one's patients. Many of the situations in Box 5–4 challenge nurses to maintain this balance of needs and identity. Judgments about this balance cannot be easily summarized in rules, though some general guidelines for home health care professionals may be useful.

Compassion, like all virtues, integrates thinking, feeling, and acting. More specifically, as noted in Chapter 4 (p. 109), the thinking element in compassion is an empathic recognition of another's suffering; the feeling element includes an appropriate affective response; and the action required is the disposition to alleviate the suffering or to comfort. Clearly, compassion entails some vulnerability. Nurses risk being overwhelmed by patient suffering when they empathize and sympathize with their patients. Nurses must preserve some emotional distance in their practice for their own sake and for the sake of their patients. There are appropriate limits to compassion. More compassion will not always be better than less.

Aristotle maintained that all virtues involve balance. He defined a virtue as a mean relative to two extremes of character (*Nichomachean Ethics*, II, 6). For instance, courage is a mean relative to the extremes of cowardice on the one hand; and rashness or foolhardiness on the other. The mean, however, will not necessarily be "halfway between" the two extremes, but in between in a way that takes into account the relative strengths of our individual tendencies toward deficiency or excess. For many of us, courage will be a mean that directs us more toward rashness, because most of us are more inclined to be cowards than we are to be recklessly bold. For many teenagers who are filled with a sense of invincibility, courage will require more caution, and so the mean will lean away from boldness and toward caution.

A deficiency of compassion is readily identified as moral callousness or moral insensitivity, a failure to respond in feeling or action to the suffering of others. We do not as readily have a name for the opposite extreme of having too much compassion. But, if we keep in mind that virtues involve balance, we can see that compassionate responses can lead to distorted care when they lack appropriate proportionality.

The virtue of compassion requires nurses to strike a balance between the condition and demands of patients and their families, on the one hand, and the condition and demands of self, on the other. "Demands of self" does not refer to self-interested desires to be comfortable or to avoid inconvenience. Compassion is an altruistic virtue that assumes one is willing to make some effort, to risk some inconvenience, to invest some resources in helping others. But the costs of time, energy, and resources must be proportionate relative to other legitimate needs of the caregiver.

The cultural expectations of those in the "feminine" role of caregiver that we noted earlier can make it difficult for nurses to achieve and maintain this balance between their needs and their patients' needs. Patients may expect nurses—who are most often female and, in any case, performing what has been defined as a feminine role—to be especially giving, nurturing, and self-sacrificing. Similarly, nurses may have similar expectations of themselves or may evaluate their own behavior against their cultural feminine stereotype. The lack of an adequate social support system for many home bound individuals only adds to the pressures on home health nurses to "do extras."

Burnout, depression, or persistent emotional and physical fatigue can occur when disproportionate weight is given to the demands of those served relative to the interests of the nurse. Failure to set and maintain appropriate professional boundaries may be a symptom of this distorted compassion. If we look at particular instances, we may easily miss the pattern here. It could be reasonable to accommodate a patient's request to do a dressing change at 4 P.M. rather than as scheduled at 2 P.M. Or there might be individual occasions when actions outside of the nurse's professional role would be appropriate. One can easily imagine a situation, for instance, in which attending a Fourth of July barbecue at a patient's home might be mutually refreshing and enjoyable. Perhaps that date or occasion has special significance to the patient and the nurse may feel honored to share in the celebration. Over time, however, these special cases may collectively add up to giving disproportionate weight to patient needs and well-being and too little weight to self-care. Home health nurses will encounter numerous situations in which the desire to support patient efforts to live fulfilling lives can lead to a pattern of behavior that undermines boundaries.

FIDELITY TO TRUST

The third virtue affected by professional boundaries is fidelity to trust. This virtue requires that nurses act in ways that confirm the trust that patients have in them to consistently promote their patients' well-being. Patients entrust themselves to the care of their health care providers. Taking this step is an act of faith; it is faith in the benevolence and good character of these professionals. The cases of accepting ballet tickets, dating a patient, and accepting the homemade quilt represent conflicts of interest that potentially violate this covenant of trust. Conflicts of interest arise when a professional has a personal interest in the outcome of a transaction on behalf of a patient. When such transactions are sufficiently substantial that they do or reasonably might affect the independent judgment the professional is expected to exercise on the patient's behalf (or on behalf of the employing agency), then they must be avoided.

Dating one's patient is clearly a case of such a conflict of interest. The nurse's objectivity is obviously undermined. In addition, concerns about an imbalance of power in such dating relationships could also be raised. The propriety of accepting gifts is less clear-cut. Accepting ballet tickets is probably not alone sufficient to affect the nurse's judgment. Furthermore, it might be more difficult to decline gifts like the quilt that have personal meaning to patients or their families. But the covenant of trust between health care professionals and their patients is fragile but essential for effective health care. Avoiding even the appearance of conflict is important in this context.

✓ APPLY PRACTICAL REASONING TO MODIFY MORAL CONCEPTS

We have seen that justice, compassion, and fidelity to trust are the key moral concepts underlying the issue of setting professional boundaries. Although boundary issues may be more complicated and ambiguous in the home health setting, there is no essential disanalogy between the nurse–patient relationship in this setting and the traditional nurse–patient relationship in a hospital or a physician's office. Patient needs and nurses' needs must be balanced in all care settings. Consequently, there is no reason to think that situations in the home health setting will require any modification of the moral concepts related to maintaining professional boundaries.

✓ REMOVE IMPEDIMENTS TO CHARACTER DEVELOPMENT

Virtue ethics encourages both individuals and organizations to remove impediments to character development. The cultural stereotype of women and nurses as self-sacrificing is an impediment that may undermine the ability of nurses to maintain appropriate professional boundaries. Although this stereotype is often challenged today, women in most cultures are still expected to do a disproportionate share of the caregiving in relationships and families. This cultural expectation may carry over into nursing where patients, employers, and sometimes colleagues may expect nurses to sacrifice their time, energy, and emotional resources to give care to their patients. Individual nurses, professional nursing organizations, and home health care agencies can help to remove this impediment by educating nurses and the patients and communities they serve about the appropriate responsibilities for home health nurses.

✓ Provide Institutional Support for Character Development

Individuals and organizations also need to provide support for the ongoing development of character in their communities. Home health agencies can support efforts to maintain appropriate boundaries by sponsoring ongoing opportunities for nurses to share stories about their successes and failures as well as to discuss difficult cases—past and pending. Nurses in home health care often work in isolation from their peers. As a result, they have fewer opportunities to observe colleagues working and interacting with patients. This makes it even more essential that home health agencies and home health nursing organizations institutionalize conversations about boundary issues so that mentoring and co-mentoring can occur. Role-playing of cases can provide opportunities for experienced nurses to model practical responses to difficult situations.

Agencies also should draft policies that provide some guidelines in this area. Policies and guidelines should emerge from discussions with administrators, nurses, and other members of agency communities. The policies and guidelines should also be discussed and reviewed regularly. Some guidelines may prohibit behaviors such as seeing patients when not on duty or accepting money, gifts, and valuables from patients and families. Other guidelines may suggest that certain behaviors can be problematic and should generally be avoided. These behaviors might include sharing meals with patients or doing minor home repairs. Most judgments about professional boundaries are not black and white. As we have noted, the majority of cases concern creating a pattern of behaviors that collectively maintains an appropriate balance between patient care and self-care. The balance may not be the same for each nurse. Policies and guidelines must be flexible, while alerting nurses to common areas of difficulty.

Adequate funding of home health would reduce some areas of conflict for home health nurses. American health policy continues to favor acute care. The need for nursing and non-nursing support that enables people to stay at home remains a lower priority than acute care. As a result, home health nurses experience moral distress when services and nursing care vital to patient safety and health are inadequately funded. Because these situations are a constant fact in home health, compassionate nurses may frequently feel a need to provide "extra" services for their patients. Home health agencies and professional nursing associations must be actively involved in educating policy makers and the public about the needs of homebound patients.

Step 5. Implement the Plan and Evaluate the Results

Our analysis of the issue of setting professional boundaries in home health care leads to an action plan that includes education of nurses and their patients, opportunities for mentoring and dialogue among nursing peers, and the development of agency guidelines. Each of these components should be developed collaboratively by agency managers and nurse employees. In addition, each component should be monitored and evaluated at regular intervals to assess how adequate it is in meeting the needs of nurses and the patients they serve.

Further Connections

Numerous issues in health care ethics would benefit from the application of a virtue ethics perspective. Each of the nursing virtues deserves careful consideration, including consideration of how each virtue is supported or undermined by policies and practices within health care organizations and the nursing profession.

Among these nursing virtues, fidelity to patient and community trust presently faces some of the most serious threats. The increasing commercialization of health care promotes practices that undermine community trust. The increasing use of provider incentive packages in managed care is one practice that is eroding this essential virtue. Inappropriate and poorly designed managed care incentive systems can encourage undertreatment of patients as well as place providers in a position of conflicting loyalties to their patients and to their employing organizations. Two other practices represent a serious threat to community trust. In some communities, there is a lack of providers who will care for Medicaid- and Medicare-insured patients. Other practitioners are opting out of insurance programs altogether, shifting the responsibility of reimbursement entirely to their patients. These practices reflect the lack of adequate and coherent health care policy in the United States. Providers deserve fair compensation for their services. Nonetheless, health care professionals pledge themselves to promote their patients' interests rather than simply pursuing their own financial interests. Nurses and physicians must exercise their responsibilities as patient advocates, encouraging approaches to provider incentives and reimbursement for services that will promote appropriate care and ethical practice.

Fidelity to trust is also potentially undermined in the precarious role of nurse case managers (NCMs) in managed care organizations. The assumption has been that through care, communication, and coordination of care, NCMs can improve quality of patient care while reducing costs. Increasingly, however, NCMs are discovering that the interests of patients and the employing system may be fundamentally opposed in significant ways. In addition, balancing the needs of patients against the needs of the employing system is extremely difficult, if not impossible, at the individual case manager level in light of the imbalance of power between these parties.

In addition to the consideration of particular virtues, some issues demand careful application of the virtue of practical reasoning. Relevant moral considerations must be identified and then interpreted and adapted to resolve new practical moral problems. Decisions regarding the appropriate treatment of patients in persistent vegetative states, for instance, require us to reconsider the value of respect for human life and our understanding of when death occurs.

The issue of partner notification and epidemiological tracking of human immunodeficiency virus (HIV)-positive patients requires careful consideration of the goals of these practices and the moral values of confidentiality, nondiscrimination, and public health that have informed these practices in the context of other sexually transmitted diseases. Does the adaptation of these moral considerations to the aquired immune deficiency syndrome (AIDS) virus justify present policies that require neither reporting of HIV-positive persons to a health department nor notification of their sexual partners?

One final example of the need for reinterpretation and adaptation of moral considerations is the current debate regarding medically futile treatment. In recent years, some physicians and some hospitals have refused to provide treatments that they believed provided no medical benefit to particular patients, that is, medically futile treatments. Traditionally, the concept of medical futility has embodied the moral consideration that the precious resources of a community should not be wasted. Certainly, it is wasteful to initiate or continue treatment that cannot provide a health benefit to a patient.

Closer examination of this concept, however, reveals that what should count as a benefit and who should decide what counts are questions not easily answered. At stake in the controversy about futility are not only practical moral judgments about how to use community resources wisely but also practical moral judgments about how to balance professional integrity and patient autonomy. The nursing virtue of mediation may be particularly valuable here as nurses play a vital role in facilitating cooperation and communication among patients, families, and care providers (Taylor, 1995).

Chapter 3 (pp. 86–88) noted the profound impact that genetic technology will have on health care in the twenty-first century. Technology is an unavoidable aspect of human experience. Genetic technology can be used mindlessly to enforce socially prescribed blueprints of perfection or to enhance human lives. There are no shortcuts to achieving the latter goal: We must tackle the hard questions about what we want for ourselves and our children, what traits and capacities are desirable, and why. Our human identities are not determined by our genetic code. They are created through a complex interaction between our genetic structure and our physical/cultural environment. Ethical questions regarding the use of genetic technology cannot be answered solely through an abstract application of rules. They also require contextual communal conversations that are informed about the biology of genetics as well as the social realities of parenting, health and disabilities, and political and economic parameters. We must consider what advantages proposed genetic enhancements will offer future children, while recognizing the limits of our abilities to imagine the environment and fashions of the future. Choices must allow for individual development as well as environmental development (McGee, 1997). The challenges of these and many other contemporary ethical issues remind us that it is our capacity to reinterpret and adapt moral considerations to changing circumstances that makes communal living satisfying and fruitful.

Conclusion

Our examination of the issues of neonatal pain control and professional boundaries has clearly shown that virtue ethics can provide concrete guidance for both individuals and organizations. This chapter also revealed several strengths of the virtue ethics perspective: its emphasis on (1) the interdependence of individuals and their organizational environments, (2) critical examination of both individual character and organizations, (3) lived experience and contextual judgment, and (4) the benefits to our social nature as human beings through ongoing dialogue and mentoring.

KEY POINTS

- Nurses experience moral distress when they are unable to translate their moral choices into moral action or when they feel that nursing virtues are undermined.
- Virtue ethics provides critical tools for analysis of nursing community goals, adaptation of nursing virtues to changing contexts, and evaluation of individual and organizational contexts of ethical decision making.
- Individuals and organizations have a responsibility to support the ongoing development of community virtues. When repeated acts of moral courage are necessary in the workplace, impediments must be removed and organizational supports created to sustain nursing virtues.
- Feminine cultural stereotypes may contribute to expectations by both patients and nurses that nurses will sacrifice their own needs to provide extra services for their patients.
- The virtues of justice, compassion, and fidelity to trust enable nurses to maintain appropriate professional boundaries with their patients.

REFLECT AND DISCUSS

1. Select two of the nursing virtues from Box 4–1. Describe ways in which health care organizations can support these virtues.
2. In some situations, nurses understand what is the right action to pursue, but they conclude that it would be too costly in terms of time or personal risk. This conclusion may be personally and professionally painful, but are these necessarily instances of moral distress? Do these situations necessarily lead to a loss of integrity?
3. Review the opening scenario in Chapter 4 (pp. 93–94) concerning the home health nurse caring for a mother with postpartum depression. When the patient becomes frightened that depression is hindering her ability to care for her newborn, the nurse secures her permission to phone the physician to discuss treatment options. As a result, appropriate interventions were implemented. What should the nurse have done, however, if the patient had said "don't call my doctor"? To address this situation, with its conflict between patient autonomy and patient safety, what virtue(s) would be needed?
4. Have you recently disagreed with a physician about an order for pain medication? How did you respond to this situation? Are there adequate policies and procedures in your organization that support constructive resolution of these disagreements? If not, what recommendations would you make for developing or restructuring these policies and procedures?
5. Describe two other nursing situations in which you have experienced moral distress. What nursing virtues were undermined or impeded in these situations? What individ-

ual or organizational impediments restricted your ability to carry out the actions that you believed to be morally appropriate? What organizational policies would you recommend to support the relevant nursing virtues in these situations?

6. What challenges in preserving professional boundaries do you face in your nursing practice? How could you or your work organization support your efforts to preserve a healthy balance between meeting your patients' needs and meeting your own needs?

REFERENCES

Als, H. (1982). Toward a synactive theory of development: Promise for the assessment and support of infant individuality. *Infant Mental Health Journal, 3,* 229–243.

American Nurses Association (2000). *Code of ethics for nurses* (working draft #9). Available: http://www.ana.org/ethics/code9.htm [2000, November 17].

Anand, K. J. (1995). Pain in the neonatal intensive care unit. *IASP Newsletter,* November/December, 3–4.

Anand, K. J., & Hickey, P. R. (1987). Pain and its effects in the human neonate and fetus. *New England Journal of Medicine, 317,* 1321–1329.

Aroskar, M. A. (1995). Envisioning nursing as a moral community. *Nursing Outlook, 43,* 134–138.

Barr, P. (1992). Focus on ethics: The unknown fear—moral distress. *Nebraska Nurse, 25*(1), 13–14.

Bartky, S. L. (1990). Feeding egos and tending wounds: Deference and disaffection in women's emotional labor. In S. L. Bartky (Ed.), *Femininity and domination* (pp. 99–119). New York: Routledge.

Basow, S. A. (1992). *Gender stereotypes and roles.* Pacific Grove, CA: Brooks/Cole.

Benner, P. (1991). The role of experience, narrative, and community in skilled ethical comportment. *Advances in Nursing Science, 14*(2), 1–21.

Benner, P., Tanner, C., & Chesla, C. (1995). *Expertise in nursing practice: Caring, clinical judgment, & ethics.* New York: Springer.

Benner, P., & Wrubel, J. (1989). *The primacy of caring: Stress and coping in health and illness.* Menlo Park, CA: Addison-Wesley.

Bildner, J. (1999). Neonatal pain management. In J. Deacon & P. O'Neill (Eds.), *Core curriculum for neonatal intensive care nursing* (pp. 510–521). Philadelphia: W. B. Saunders.

Brock, D. (1994). Voluntary active euthanasia. In T. Beauchamp & L. Walters (Eds.), *Contemporary issues in bioethics* (pp. 490–499). Belmont, CA: Wadsworth.

Childress, J. F. (1994). Principles-oriented bioethics: An analysis and assessment from within. In E. R. DuBose, R. P. Hamel, & L. J. O'Connell (Eds.), *A matter of principles?: Ferment in U.S. bioethics* (pp. 72–98). Valley Forge, PA: Trinity Press International.

Chinn, P. L. (1990). Toward the 21st century: Nursing theory, research, and practice. Paper presented at the 1990 23rd Annual Communicating Nursing Research Conference, Western Institute of Nursing, Boulder, CO.

Clancy, G. T., Anand, K. J. S., & Lally, P. (1992). Neonatal pain management. *Critical Care Nursing Clinics of North America, 4*(3), 527–535.

Cooper, M. C. (1991). Principle-oriented ethics and the ethic of care: A creative tension. *Advances in Nursing Science, 14*(2), 22–31.

Davis, A. J., Aroskar, M. A., Liaschenko, J., & Drought, T. S. (1997). *Ethical dilemmas and nursing practice.* Stamford, CT: Appleton & Lange.

Franck, L. S. (1997). The ethical imperative to treat pain in infants: Are we doing the best we can? *Critical Care Nurse, 17*(5), 80–87.

Franck, L. S., & Gregory, G. A. (1993). Clinical evaluation and treatment of infant pain in the neonatal intensive care unit. In C. Berde, N. Schecter, & M. Yaster (Eds.), *Pain in infants, children, and adolescents* (pp. 519–537). Baltimore, MD: Williams & Wilkins.

Friedman, M. (1987). Beyond caring: The de-moralization of gender. In M. Hanen & K. Nielsen (Eds.), *Science, morality, and feminist theory* (pp. 87–100). Calgary, Alberta, Canada: University of Calgary Press.

Friedrichs, J. B., Young, S., Gallagher, D., Keller, C., & Kimura, R. E. (1995). Where does it hurt? An interdisciplinary approach to improving the quality of pain assessment and management in the neonatal intensive care unit. *Nursing Clinics of North America, 30,* 143–159.

Gilles, F. H., Shankle, W., & Dooling, E. C. (1983). Myelinated tracts: Growth patterns. In F. H. Gilles, A. Levington, & E. C. Dooling (Eds.), *The developing human brain* (pp. 117–183). Boston: Wright.

Grunau, R. V. E., Whitfield, M. F., Pretrie, J. H., & Fryer, E. L. (1994). Early pain experience, child and family factors, as precursors of somatization: A prospective study of extremely premature and fullterm children. *Pain, 56,* 353–359.

Hochschild, A. (1989). *The second shift.* New York: Avon Books.

Howard, V. A., & Thurber, F. W. (1998). The interpretation of infant pain: Physiological and behavioral indicators used by NICU nurses. *Journal of Pediatric Nursing, 13*(3), 165–174.

Johnston, C. C., & Stevens, B. J. (1990). Pain assessment in newborns. *Journal of Perinatal and Neonatal Nursing, 4*(1), 41–52.

Maloni, J. A., Stegman, C. E., Taylor, P. M., & Brownell, C. A. (1986). Validation of infant behavior identified by neonatal nurses. *Nursing Research, 35,* 133–138.

McGee, G. (1997). *The perfect baby: A pragmatic approach to gentics.* Lanham, MD: Rowman & Littlefield.

McGrath, P. J., & Craig, K. D. (1989). Developmental and psychological factors in children's pain. *Pediatric Clinics of North America, 36,* 823–836.

Meinhart, N. T., & McCaffery, M. (1983). *Pain: A nursing approach to assessment and analysis.* Norwalk, CT: Appleton-Century-Crofts.

Parker, R. S. (1990). Nurses' stories: The search for a relational ethic of care. *Advances in Nursing Science, 13*(1), 31–40.

Penticuff, J. H. (1989). Infant suffering and nurse advocacy in neonatal intensive care. *Nursing Clinics of North America, 24,* 987–997.

Pigeon, H. M., McGrath, P. J., Lawrence, J., & MacMurray, S. B. (1989). Nurses' perceptions of pain in the neonatal intensive care unit. *Journal of Pain and Symptom Management, 4,* 179–183.

Porter, F., Wolf, M., & Miller, J. (1998). The effect of handling and immobilization on the response to acute pain in newborn infants. *Pediatrics, 102*(6), 1383–1388.

Ray, M. A. (1994). Communal moral experience as the starting point for research in health care ethics. *Nursing Outlook, 42,* 104–109.

Reverby, S. (1987). A caring dilemma: Womanhood and nursing in historical perspective. *Nursing Research, 36,* 5–11.

Rodney, P., & Starzomski, R. (1993). Constraints on the moral agency of nurses. *The Canadian Nurse, 86*(8), 23–26.

Shapiro, C. (1998). Pain in the neonate: Assessment and intervention. *Neonatal Network, 8*(17), 7–21.

Stang, H. J., & Snellman, L. W. (1998). Circumcision practice patterns in the United States. *Pediatrics, 101*(6): E5.

Sundin-Huard, D., & Fahy, K. (1999). Moral distress, advocacy and burnout: Theorising the relationships. *International Journal of Nursing Practice, 5*(1), 8–13.

Taylor, C. (1995). Medical futility and nursing. *Image: Journal of Nursing Scholarship, 27*(4), 301–306.

Wilkinson, J. M. (1987/88). Moral distress in nursing practice: Experience and effect. *Nursing Forum, 23*(1), 16–29.

Yarling, R. R., & McElmurry, B. J. (1986). The moral foundations of nursing. *Advances in Nursing Science, 9*(2), 63–73.

Yeo, M., & Moorhouse, A. (1996). *Concepts and cases in nursing ethics* (2nd ed.). Peterborough, Ontario, Canada: Broadview Press.

6

Feminist Ethics: Reconstructing the Community

CHAPTER OUTLINE

EXPERIENTIAL ACCOUNT: Clinical Trial Ignores Mothers

Alison Colson, FNP, volunteers at Eleanor Roosevelt Health Services, a clinic in a major Midwestern city that charges sliding-scale fees to women without health insurance. At the clinic, Alison sees scores of women who are human immunodeficiency virus (HIV) infected. One of Alison's clinic patients, Serena, sought prenatal care six months earlier when she discovered she was pregnant. Although Serena works 36 hours per week for a local retailer, she has no health insurance. None-theless, Serena feels fortunate to be participating in one of the Centers for Disease Control and Prevention's (CDC's) AIDS Clinical Trials Groups (ACTGs). Protocol 076 is designed to study the vertical transmission of HIV from mother to infant. HIV-infected pregnant women who participate in the trial receive continuous oral zidovudine (AZT) treatment during pregnancy, intravenous AZT during childbirth, and oral AZT treatment for the newborn infant to determine whether this regimen will reduce the rate of HIV transmission through pregnancy and birth.

Serena and her baby would not receive AZT treatment apart from their partic-ipation in this clinical trial. Alison believes that Serena is benefiting from this treat-ment and hopes that Serena's baby will be born without the HIV infection as a result. Alison has witnessed many other infants whose chances for a healthy life have been severely compromised as a result of viral transmission during pregnancy and recognizes that benefits for future babies of HIV-infected women are enor-mous.

At the same time, Alison is distressed by the nearly exclusive focus of Protocol 076 on the prevention of pediatric AIDS. Although infants in the trial continue to receive AZT for 18 months after birth, their mothers receive it for only six weeks postpartum. Serena cannot afford to continue the AZT after the trial is completed. This saddens Alison, who is angry about the lost opportunity for monitoring the effect of AZT on disease progression in women. At its conclu-sion, the study may reveal much about effects of AZT during pregnancy on devel-oping fetuses, but it will reveal nothing about long-term effects of this treatment on the babies' mothers (Faden, Kass, & McGraw, 1996). Alison wonders why the CDC regards Serena's well-being and that of other women like her as any less important than the well-being of their newborns?

Concepts of Feminism and Feminist Ethics

Feminism can be defined as a world view that values women and confronts systematic injustices based on gender (Chinn & Wheeler, 1985). A feminist is a person who rejects the ways in which women and their experiences have been criticized, ignored, and devalued. A feminist also is someone who works to bring about the social changes necessary to promote more just relationships among women and men. Feminist ethics challenges perceived male biases in ethics, which have contributed to the devaluing of women's moral experience and to the subordination of women. While virtually all nurses today support the view that women and men are equal in value, they may be unaware of how traditional gender biases continue to affect ethi-cal theories, nursing practice, and health care.

The opening scenario provides one example of how traditional beliefs and values about women continue to harm them in health care. Traditionally, women have been valued primarily for their reproductive and nurturing capacities and as objects of sex-ual pleasure. A woman's highest calling has often been identified as the nurture and support of a man and his children so that he can engage in activities outside the home that benefit society.

It may seem that contemporary North American society rejects views of women's value as determined by the degree to which they support others. Many would insist that women are equal to men and should be valued in themselves and not merely for their supportive, nurturing roles in society. The clinical trial in the opening scenario suggests that women are still often valued only for their traditional, instrumental roles. Faden and colleagues (1996) persuasively demonstrate that, until recently, AIDS research focused on women only as transmitters of the virus to others, either through sexual activity or gestation. Researchers largely ignored the health interests of women themselves. Gender-biased expectations of women as care providers also are demonstrated in the unequal division of household and child care labor that persists in spite of women's increasing employment outside the home (Hochschild, 1997; Lennon & Rosenfield, 1994) and in the unequal expectations for male versus female children to care for elderly parents (Horowitz, 1985).

Proponents of rule and virtue ethics could argue that neglect of women's health interests and disproportionate focus in AIDS research on the health interests of men and infants is unjust to women. A feminist ethicist would agree, but would add that this injustice reflects the continuing systematic subordination and oppression of women. This commitment to eliminating the subordination of women (and the interrelated oppression of other groups) distinguishes feminist ethics from other ethical theories (Jaggar, 1992; Sherwin, 1992; Wolf, 1996). A range of feminist schools of thought have developed differing accounts of the causes of women's subordination and have proposed strategies for eliminating this oppression. Feminist ethics draws on and reflects these various feminist perspectives.

Women are oppressed when their interests are *systematically* subordinated to those of men. A system of male authority that oppresses women through its social, political, and economic institutions is referred to as a *patriarchy*. Many women (and men) do not recognize the oppression of women. If we look only at individual instances of women being treated unjustly, we can interpret them as isolated events and fail to perceive the deeper pattern of oppression. Frye (1983) highlights this point in her definition of *oppression* as an interlocking series of restrictions and barriers that reduce the options available to people on the basis of their membership in a group. Oppression is thus a pattern of discrimination against a collective group—not simply isolated acts of discrimination against individuals. Feminist ethics begins from the conviction that the subordination of women is morally wrong and works to uncover institutionalized practices that form the web of oppression. Freire's (1971) description of this critical process as the unveiling of the world of oppression is an apt one. If one routinely views the world through a veil, one's view is filtered through a fine mesh of interlocking threads. One becomes so accustomed to this view that one is unconscious of the veil's effect on perception: the view with the pattern of threads is simply the way one has learned to see the world. When women and men are socialized into a world in which men and what men do are valued over women and what women do, the norms and practices that institutionalize this bias become the largely unnoticed threads of the veil of oppression. It takes effort and sustained analysis to identify particular practices that form the veil. Feminist ethics is committed to this ongoing analytical process.

Feminist ethics is also committed to the constructive process of designing alternative ways to restructure relationships, social practices, and institutions. Social transformation is the ultimate goal of feminist ethics. It is, therefore, unavoidably political, a fact that makes some people uncomfortable. Since we tend to think of politics as the use of power to get whatever is in the best interest of one's own group, to say that feminist ethics is political suggests that women are fighting to reverse the oppression, to control men, and to have their own way whatever it takes. As Tong (1993) notes, however, feminist ethics is political in the classical sense of politics as designing political/social institutions so that they promote rather than impede human flourishing. Because individuals and communities are interdependent, individuals can be good persons only in a just society. Ethics and politics, therefore, are necessarily inseparable.

Sexism is a set of beliefs that asserts the inferiority of one sex (usually women) and thus justifies sexual inequality (Newman, 1995). Sexist ideology asserts that clear, unchangeable differences between men and women support the preferential treatment of men. Yet in a community in which women are systematically oppressed, neither women nor men can be free or flourish. While men are not oppressed as a subordinate group in a sexist society, they are harmed by sexism. They are alienated from their authentic self-development and deprived of the opportunity to develop skills and traits associated with those devalued as "feminine." Nonetheless, sexism supports men's overall interests (power, domestic and sexual service, preference and privileges) at the expense of women's (Sherwin, 1992). The system that supports women's oppression restrains men's self-development, but men (as a group) maintain a dominant position.

Feminist ethics strives for social transformation that will empower all people to live freer, fuller lives. The primary question of rule ethics is what actions are right or wrong, while virtue ethics asks us to consider what kind of people we should be. Feminist ethics again shifts our focus and poses distinct questions:

1. *How are women harmed by their subordination to men under patriarchy?*
2. *How are men harmed by patriarchy?*
3. *How can relationships, social practices, and institutions be restructured to empower women and men?*

Contexts in Philosophy and Nursing

Feminist ethics, like rule ethics and virtue ethics, is influenced and shaped by the social context from which it has emerged. As we have noted before, this does not mean that it is relevant only to this particular historical and cultural context. But awareness of this context will aid our understanding of concepts and perspective in feminist ethics.

Feminists Critique Ethics

Until the late 1960s, criticisms of women's subordination are largely absent from literature of Western ethics. Noteworthy exceptions include Mary Wollstonecraft's *A*

Vindication of the Rights of Woman (1792/1965), John Stuart Mill's *The Subjection of Women* (1869/1988), Frederick Engels' *The Origin of the Family, Private Property and the State* (1884/1942), and Simone de Beauvoir's *The Second Sex* (1949/1961). Consideration of feminist ethics in philosophy coincided with the resurgence of feminist activism and a renewed interest in practical ethics. In the late 1960s, feminists and mainstream philosophers began to debate practical issues of contemporary social life such as sexual morality, abortion, racism, war, animal rights, environmental issues, and behavior of multinational corporations. This practical focus in philosophy reflected in part the social upheaval and public critique of institutions occurring in Western societies. Feminist ethical debate emerged first from grassroots activism and moved quickly to academic settings. Early discussions focused on issues such as reproductive rights, equal opportunity in the workplace, women's unpaid labor in the home, media portrayals of women, and issues of sexuality including rape and the presumption of heterosexuality. The scope of ethical concern later broadened to include discussions of pornography, surrogate motherhood and in vitro fertilization, militarism, the environment, and the effects of third world development on women (Jaggar, 1992).

By the late 1970s and early 1980s, feminists were questioning whether traditional ethical theories provided adequate conceptual resources for analysis of these so-called women's issues. Some feminists began to look for a distinctively feminine approach to morality, while others called for a more radical rethinking of traditional moral concepts and the process of developing ethical theories.

Critical analysis and debate regarding the relevance of gender to ethics did not originate with contemporary feminism. A number of eighteenth and nineteenth century authors formulated positions on what was called "women's morality" (Tong, 1993). These can be grouped into three categories:

1. *Men and women have distinct but equal moral virtues; the uniqueness of each should be preserved.*
2. *Moral virtue is gender neutral.*
3. *Women's morality is distinct and either it is already superior to men's or it would be in a world free of sexual inequality.*

These authors disagreed about whether male and female morality are inherent in biology, the result of social conditioning, or due to both factors. Interestingly, activists in this first wave of feminism (roughly 1848 to 1920) used arguments from all of these positions to advocate for granting voting rights to women. Feminists continue to be inspired by their earlier counterparts, and echoes of these perspectives on gender and ethics can be heard in contemporary debates in feminist ethics.

Gender Bias in Traditional Ethics

Historically traditional ethics has valued attributes and interests that are culturally identified with men over those identified with women. A number of major moral theorists have denied women's moral agency, claiming that women were incapable of mature, moral reasoning. This view is not limited to early theorists such as Aristotle, Rousseau, and Kant. Using Kohlberg's (1958, 1981) instrument for assessing moral development, women as a group have consistently scored lower than men have. Kohlberg's model of moral development had been the virtually undisputed standard since its development in the 1950s until Gilligan's gender critique in 1982. Although Kohlberg does not claim that women are necessarily incapable of mature moral reasoning, it is remarkable that his conclusions about gender differences have been so readily accepted in contemporary research on moral development.

Women have continued to be excluded and marginalized in other ways in ethics. The Western moral tradition has frequently ignored and denigrated the private or domestic realm. Because women generally have been responsible for this domain, it has been associated with the feminine. Many ethical theories have focused on public venues associated with masculine work and roles. Until recently, this preference could be observed by scanning the index of introductory ethics texts. Major topics included issues in government and law (e.g., the death penalty, wars, terrorism), business (e.g., truth telling and honesty in advertising, bribes in international business), and medicine/health (e.g., euthanasia, famine in the third world). Absent were topics perceived as beyond public regulation such as friendship, parenting, division of household labor, and date rape.

Even in contemporary ethical discussions, women's interests are frequently ignored or devalued. One glaring example is the way in which philosophers have debated the issue of abortion as an abstract discussion about the moral status of a fetus and competing fetal and maternal rights. Regardless of the conclusion that an individual may draw about the morality of abortion, women are acutely aware that pregnancies occur within the bodies and lives of particular women. Being pregnant is not simply a matter of "carrying" a baby: it involves a developing relationship that occurs within a woman's body. The design of Protocol 076, focusing only on the vertical transmission of HIV from mother to infant, reflects this tendency to reduce pregnant women to fetal containers.

Feminists argue that another reflection of gender bias in Western ethics has been the tendency to emphasize masculine but not feminine values. Values that are associated with men, empirically, normatively, or symbolically, in a particular culture are considered "masculine." Independence, autonomy, reason, will, hierarchy, culture, and transcendence are frequently cited as examples of culturally defined masculine values that are embodied in Western ethical theories. Interdependence, community, connection, emotion, body/nature, and immanence are commonly cited examples of culturally defined feminine values that are absent or denigrated in the Western tradition (Jaggar, 1991).

Feminist claims of gender bias in Western ethics are summarized in Box 6–1. As Jaggar (1992) notes, not all feminists agree with all of these criticisms or their applicability to specific ethical theories or debates. Furthermore, even where there is general agreement that gender bias exists in traditional Western ethics, feminists propose a variety of strategies to revise ethical theory. There is consensus that problems of gender bias cannot be fixed simply by adding topics of special interest to women in ethics texts. Such a response assumes that issues can be neatly divided into men's and women's issues or that women as a group share the same "special interests." More significantly, this approach avoids asking why Western ethics has privileged certain interests and perspectives over others. Adding new topics is not enough; many feminists believe that new questions need to be raised and a different sort of critical analysis applied.

- Historically, major moral philosophers claimed that women were incapable of mature, moral reasoning or less capable of moral development than men.
- Western moral tradition frequently ignored and devalued the private or domestic realm, which has become symbolically associated with the feminine.
- Western ethical theories have tended to embody values that are culturally masculine, such as independence, autonomy, reason, hierarchy, culture, and transcendence.
- Values such as interdependence, community, connection, emotion, body/nature, and immanence, which are culturally feminine, have often been absent or denigrated in these theories.

Nursing in Transition

As we noted in Chapter 4 (pp. 105, 107), nursing has its roots in Victorian culture that assumed a natural hierarchy of men over women. This hierarchy was reflected in the structure of Victorian social organizations. While changes pioneered by Florence Nightingale were revolutionary, they did not seriously challenge the Victorian conception of the role and status of women in society. Her work was radical in that it transformed nursing from undisciplined and menial work performed primarily by women of reduced economic means into an honorable occupation for "better class" women. The reputation of the "new nurse" as a well-trained, highly disciplined, and devoted professional contrasted sharply with that of the illiterate, slovenly nurse of the previous era. As remarkable as this transformation was, Nightingale's conception of nursing did not question the Victorian view of women's role and character. Nursing was conceived as a natural extension of a woman's domestic role and the virtues of the new nurse were strikingly similar to the Victorian ideals of feminine submissiveness, self-sacrifice, and loyalty (Kuhse, 1997; Reverby, 1987).

Though Nightingale and other early nursing leaders did not expect blind obedience from nurses, their metaphors of subservient, loyal soldiers have enormously shaped both nursing self-perception and its perception by others (Kuhse, 1997). Nurses continued to perceive themselves primarily as instruments of physicians and medicine until the 1960s. The 1960 revision of the American Nurses Association (ANA) *Code for Nurses* reflects a significant shift in self-perception through the use of language of co-participation of nurses in the care of patients, rather than language of subordination. This shift does not appear in the *International Council of Nurses' Code for Nurses* until 1973. These revisions introduced the idea that patients rather than physicians are the nurse's primary responsibility. In addition, a previous reminder to nurses that they are obligated to carry out physician orders is replaced in the international code by one that encourages nurses to sustain cooperative relationships with co-workers in nursing and other fields.

As Kuhse (1997) notes, the change in metaphor from physician's helpmate to patient advocate is the result of several factors. Declining public confidence in medicine encouraged a new patient–nursing alliance. Nurses were also becoming better educated and more highly skilled. As a result, nurses developed a greater appreciation for their own knowledge and expertise. This also contributed to growing dissatisfaction with their traditional subservient role. Increasingly, nurses wanted to be recognized as professional members of a health care team whose judgments would be counted when significant decisions were made. Feminism was certainly another factor. Its critique of traditional sex-role stereotypes has obvious implications for the traditional concept of nurses as physicians' handmaidens. Many nurses were no longer willing to play the submissive role expected of them (Kuhse, 1997).

Nursing and Feminism

Despite considerable compatibility between the strengthened self-image of nurses and certain feminist ideals, nurses have not always perceived feminism's effects on their discipline in a positive light. While feminism provided impetus and resources for the critique of a subordinate nursing role, some nurses also felt disparaged by feminism's critique of traditional caregiving roles of women. Liberal American feminism in the 1960s and 1970s, represented by groups such as the National Organization for Women, focused on obtaining equal educational and occupational opportunities for women and men. From this feminist perspective women were oppressed largely by the cultural constraints that isolated them in the domestic sphere and excluded them from full participation in the public sphere. Political activism focused on opening up traditionally male-dominated fields and professions to women.

Success was counted by increased percentages of women entering law, medicine, managerial positions, and political office. Young girls were assured that they could do anything that men do; they were also encouraged to choose better-paying fields like engineering, construction work, or computer programming over lower paying ones like hairdressing and clerical work. In the past, educated women had been encouraged to choose either nursing or teaching (especially of young children). Now a new message suggested that women no longer had "to settle" for these roles. Competent female students interested in health care were encouraged to become a physician rather than "just a nurse." Feminists seemed as ignorant as physicians and hospital administrators of the special knowledge and expertise of nurses.

Many women felt deeply alienated by the feminist movement. Some who chose to be full-time parents felt dismissed as "just a mother." Others who worked outside the home because of economic necessity derived their primary identity through their roles as wife and mother. While increasing numbers of nurses pursued advanced degrees and perceived their jobs as careers, many left full-time nursing when they became mothers and valued their jobs for the flexibility of work hours and mobility that nursing provided. Feminism for many women seemed simply irrelevant or worse, as reflected in its caricature by some as a group of well-off, man-hating separatists who deprecated women's traditional gifts and roles.

As a result, many nurses felt doubly discounted by feminism's seeming disregard for motherhood, first as professionals who prided themselves on empathetic caring, and second as women who valued their roles as mothers. This explains to some degree the positive reception in nursing of one strand of feminist ethics known as *care ethics*.

Women's Health: Bridge Between Nursing and Feminism

Despite the problems many nurses experienced with feminist ideology, nurses have played a central role in the women's health movement from its beginning. Nursing work in this area has provided an important bridge between nursing and feminism. Women seek health information and care at greater rates than men do. They often also assume significant responsibility for their children's health and for the men with whom they share their lives.

When the Boston Women's Health Book Collective published its first edition of *Our Bodies, Ourselves* in 1969, there was little information easily available about women's health. There has been a virtual explosion of information and resources since that time. The women's health movement is a grassroots, consumer-driven effort to provide women with tools needed to take care of their health at home and in the workplace (Boston Women's Health Book Collective, 1992). Women have increasingly demanded self-determination in matters of health care, and nurses have responded. Nurses have been instrumental in expanding the purview of women's health from a traditional focus on reproductive matters to a concern with a wide range of factors that affect women's health (McBride, 1997). Theorists and practitioners in women's health have applied feminist concepts of symmetry of power in provider–patient relationships, shared decision making, and the goal of social change (Andrist, 1997; Sampselle, 1990). This work provides significant evidence of the relevance of feminist ethics to nursing practice.

It is clear that the relationship between feminism and nursing has been mixed. Without question, feminism provided essential support and analytical resources for redefining the nursing role. Furthermore, the application of feminist principles has redefined the scope and practices in women's health. But feminism's disparaging critique of traditional caregiving roles has alienated some nurses.

Understanding Patriarchy

Distinctively feminist health care ethics is just beginning to emerge. Like feminism itself, it is not one theory but a common project that unites a variety of theorists who share the view that patriarchal values are perpetuated and reflected in all major social institutions—including health care institutions. Patriarchy does *not*, however, refer to individual men or even a collection of men. It refers to the kind of society in which men *and* women participate. And this patriarchal society is, in Johnson's words, "*male-dominated, male-identified, and male-centered*" (1997).

A society is male-dominated when the positions of authority—in politics, business, government, health care, education, law, religion, and so on—are generally held by men. Consequently, even the status of men who may occupy subordinate social positions is enhanced by the male control of authority in a patriarchal society. Patriarchal societies are male-identified in that the culture's norms about what is good, normal, and desirable are associated with men or masculinity. Cultural ideas and values associated with women and femininity are correlatively devalued. Finally, a patriarchal society is male-centered in the sense that attention is focused primarily on men and what men do. It is important to note that in a male-dominated, male-identified, and male-centered society one will likely find some women in significant positions of authority and power. Dominant systems can allow some exceptions to the rule. This often deflects a deeper critique of the system.

Social systems, like patriarchy, have a profound impact on all of our lives. Johnson uses the metaphor of a tree to illustrate how our individual lives are part of the complex system of patriarchy. His patriarchal tree is presented in Figure 6–1. It shows how individuals are linked to a system with deep roots of core principles and values, a trunk composed of social institutions and branching into the multitude of groups, organizations, and communities in which we live our lives, and finally reaching out to the individual leaves representing each of us who participate in the system of patriarchy. This tree metaphor helps us to see that patriarchy is something much more than "men," either as individuals or as an entire group. When feminists critique patriarchy, they are analyzing a deeply rooted complex system (Johnson, 1997).

Patriarchy also, as Johnson (1997) observes, provides paths of least resistance that encourage men to accept gender privilege and perpetuate women's oppression and encourage women to accept and adapt to their oppressed position. Patriarchy has a profound ability to shape our sense of who we are and our perception of the options available to us. This awareness can engender a sense of powerlessness in us. But just as the tree produces the leaves, it is equally true that the tree depends on the leaves converting light into organic material in order to survive (Johnson, 1997).

We are shaped by partriarchy, but we can also resist and change it. We have power as individuals to learn about the roots of patriarchy and how they affect us. And we have power to imagine alternatives and to work with others to change our lives. This reminds us that feminist ethics is committed to the two tasks of (1) uncovering institutionalized practices that form the web of women's oppression due to patriarchy and (2) designing strategies for resisting this oppression and for restructuring society.

Care Ethics

Some authors have responded to the marginalization and neglect of women in traditional ethical theory by proposing an approach to morality that affirms values that have been characterized as feminine in Western cultures. Gilligan's widely publicized work has played a central role in the development of a distinctively feminine approach to morality. In her 1982 book, *In a Different Voice: Psychological Theory and Women's Development*, Gilligan (a former student of Kohlberg) argues that women typically

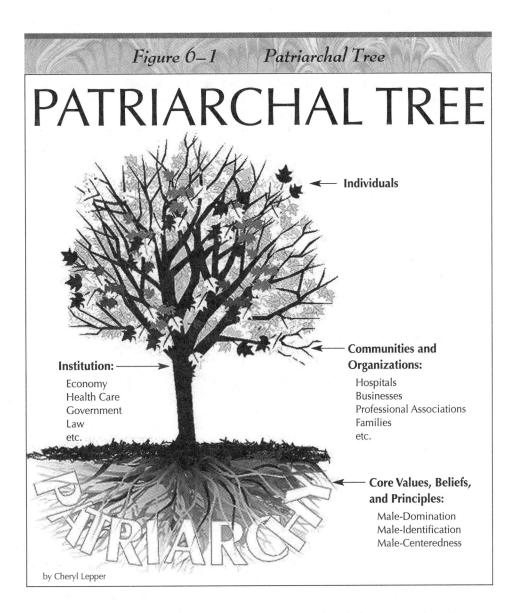

Figure 6–1   Patriarchal Tree

PATRIARCHAL TREE

← **Individuals**

← **Communities and Organizations:**
Hospitals
Businesses
Professional Associations
Families
etc.

Institution: →
Economy
Health Care
Government
Law
etc.

← **Core Values, Beliefs, and Principles:**
Male-Domination
Male-Identification
Male-Centeredness

by Cheryl Lepper

speak with a different moral voice than men do. She concludes from her research that women tend to espouse an ethics of care, while men tend to espouse an ethics of justice. An *ethics of care* perceives morality in terms of the responsibility to care for others and to preserve and foster connections between persons rather than in the terms of conflicting rights and duties that characterize an ethics of justice.

Some authors regard care ethics as one type of feminist ethics. Others, however, argue that though its development is linked with that of feminist ethics, care ethics lacks essential elements of a feminist ethic. Perhaps care ethics can best be regarded as an embryonic form of feminist ethics. Most feminists agree that a feminist approach to ethics will, at a minimum, begin with two convictions: (1) that the subordination and oppression of women is morally wrong, and (2) that the moral experience of women is as worthy of respect as that of men. Care ethics has focused on the second conviction while remaining relatively silent on the first. Care ethicists such as Gilligan, however, do criticize traditional Western ethics for assuming that masculine values are normative, and androcentrism (being male-identified) is one element of Johnson's definition of a patriarchal society. Thus, care ethics does incorporate to some degree a critique of patriarchy.

On the other hand, it should be acknowledged that this critique plays a minor role in the care ethics perspective. Nonetheless, the development of care ethics has played an important role in the evolution of feminist ethics, especially in feminist health care ethics.

Ethics in a Different Voice

The feminine moral perspective of care ethics sees humans as intrinsically relational and interdependent. As a result, morally mature persons seek to resolve conflicts in ways that preserve and strengthen relationships. A feminine ethics of care thus emphasizes values of connection, sharing, and community—values often overshadowed or discounted in male-biased ethics that emphasize independence, autonomy, and hierarchy. Box 6–2 contrasts the ethics of care and the ethics of justice.

Box 6–2   Contrasting Moral Voices

Ethics of Care	Ethics of Justice
• Traditionally associated with feminine perspective.	• Traditionally associated with masculine perspective.
• Human beings are intrinsically relational.	• Human beings are intrinsically separate individuals.
• Morality conceived in terms of responsibilities to care.	• Morality conceived in terms of conflicting rights and duties.
• Emphasizes connection, sharing, community.	• Emphasizes independence, autonomy, and hierarchy.
• Resolves conflicts in ways that preserve and strengthen webs of connections.	• Resolves conflicts by determining overriding rule.
• Moral decision making is attentive to the context of relationships.	• Moral decision making involves the logical application of universal rules.

Modern theories of ethics, which emerged from the Enlightenment period of 1750 to 1914, describe the negotiation of moral rules between self-interested strangers. Care ethics asserts, however, that moral development begins within the context of intimate family relations, which are personal connections with particular individuals. Caring for these persons requires complex skills of attending to the individual needs within each person's concrete contexts. This caring process, as mothers, nurses, and caregivers will attest, requires holistic perception and judgment that draws on intuition and emotion as well as linear, logical thinking. Emotionally engaged attention, care advocates claim, provides resources for ethical responses that surpass those provided by rule-bound moral frameworks. Perceptual engagement of this sort enables engaged practitioners to respond to others in their particularity and uniqueness. Ethical solutions will thus be more inclusive and more grounded in who people really are than is possible in a rule-based ethic.

The care ethics critique of Enlightenment ethics parallels those of virtue ethics, communitarianism, and postmodernism. The care ethics and feminist critique echo virtue ethics' criticism of rule ethics' preoccupation with rules, impartiality, and a restricted notion of reasoning that excludes any role for emotions in moral decision making. The prescriptions feminists propose for healing the abstract rationalism of Enlightenment ethical theories, however, are different than those outlined by non-feminist theorists.

Nursing Finds a Voice

The affinity of nursing to care ethics seems obvious. Nursing literature of the 1980s and 1990s is replete with claims that care is foundational to nursing (Benner, 1984; Bishop & Scudder, 1985; Cooper, 1991; Davis, 1985; Fry, 1992; Gastman, 1999; Leininger, 1984; Ray, 1987; Watson, 1985). Fry describes care as the foundational value on which any theory of nursing ethics must be built, Watson as the moral ideal of nursing, and Leininger as the essence of nursing.

In the 1960s and 1970s, nursing was deeply involved in efforts to establish itself as a profession separate from medicine with its own unique identity. Nonetheless, as Kuhse (1997) notes, justifications of the nurse's role as patient advocate and nursing discussions of other ethical issues in nursing continued to rely on traditional ethical theories and concepts (drawn primarily from rule ethics). The language of rights, autonomy, and duties dominated these discussions (Benjamin & Curtis, 1981; Curtin & Flaherty, 1982; Davis & Aroskar, 1983; Jameton, 1984; and Bandman & Bandman, 1985.)

The publication of Gilligan's *In a Different Voice* in 1982 and Noddings's *Caring: A Feminine Approach to Ethics and Moral Education* in 1984, seemed to many nursing theorists to provide a more adequate perspective for articulating an ethics appropriate to nurses. In doing so, nurses could define themselves as a different, though not inferior, profession than medicine (Kuhse, 1997). Gilligan and Noddings are widely regarded as the mothers of care ethics.

Gilligan (1982) asserts that the link between gender and moral orientation is not absolute and that both care and justice perspectives are open to women and men (p. 2). Although the ethic of care is more characteristic of women and the ethic of justice is more characteristic of men (Bebeau & Brabeck, 1989), women and men can and do use each other's moral language (Gilligan & Attanucci, 1988; Walker, deVries, & Trevethan, 1987). Gilligan proposes that a mature human being will be comfortably bilingual. A society that fails to recognize and value the voice of care as much as it has traditionally valued the voice of justice is one that is impoverished and handicapped.

Despite her disclaimer, Gilligan identifies the voice of care with women and the voice of justice with men throughout *In a Different Voice*. Furthermore, regardless of Gilligan's intentions, her work most often has been understood as advocating a distinctive moral voice for women (Friedman, 1987; Kuhse, 1997). Other writers have argued that women develop a distinct moral perspective as a result of experiences such as menstruation, pregnancy, and lactation (Alcoff, 1995; Almond, 1988; Whitbeck, 1984). Gilligan's work has spawned numerous empirical studies that attempted to test her gender hypothesis that women are more likely to use an ethic of care and men an ethic of justice (see Friedman, 1987, for a summary of this literature). The results of this research are inconclusive. Some studies suggest that correlations between gender and moral language may actually reflect educational and occupational differences (see Walker's summary, 1984). It seems clear, however, that men and women use both the care and justice perspectives to address moral dilemmas; no clear division by gender is demonstrable.

As noted earlier, the idea that men and women have different modes of moral thinking and different moral virtues is not the invention of contemporary feminism. A number of early feminists believed women possessed moral virtues that were not only complementary to men's virtues, but also superior and more "noble." In the nineteenth century, Mary Wollstonecraft disagreed with the valorization of feminine virtues and warned that their cultivation contributed directly to women's political and economic subordination. Many contemporary feminists share her concern about the dangers of gender essentialism.

Gender essentialism assumes that women and men have unique characteristics and dispositions that are determined by their biological differences. As Wollstonecraft notes, such a position may become a double-edged sword for women. Thus, while some feminists have extolled the superiority of women's more pacifist nature (versus men's supposedly aggressive nature), historically women were excluded from higher education and political participation due to their allegedly inferior intellectual nature.

Care ethics need not assume that feminine qualities of nurturing, cooperativeness, and responsiveness to others are "essentially" female. But care ethics authors have sometimes been perceived in this light, and it is important to note the risks involved in this interpretation. If women are more naturally disposed to compassion and self-giving, for instance, then shouldn't men and children accept and expect women's self-sacrifice on their behalf? And if their nature prepares them to be peacemakers and protectors of virtue, they will seem unsuited for the aggressively competitive world of business and politics. On the other hand, when young boys mistreat pets or bully smaller children, will these actions be dismissed as typical unempathetic male behavior? If a pregnant woman becomes addicted to cocaine, will she be written off as biologically defective?

Such deterministic thinking is unlikely to promote the feminist goal of ending women's subordination and transforming society. A care ethic based on biological essentialism is also problematic as a model for nursing ethics. Male nurses would be incapable of embodying the moral ideals of nursing if the theory assumes that empathetic caring is inherent in women and lacking in men. Furthermore, if medicine is based on an ethics whose characteristics are inherently male, then women would apparently never achieve the moral ideals of medicine. Both of these conclusions are unacceptable.

Some writers try to avoid an essentialist view of gender and moral perspective by focusing on women's experiences rather than on their biology. They argue that the experience of mothering encourages the development of certain moral sensibilities. Noddings (1984), Ruddick (1989), Whitbeck (1984), and Held (1993) argue that there is a link between the work women typically do in the "private sphere" and their distinctive moral voice. Thus, most (though not all) women develop what Ruddick calls "maternal practice." Like any human practice, it is a cooperative activity that has its own standards of excellence and requires special abilities and particular ways of thinking (Ruddick, 1989). More than expression of love or empathy, maternal practice is a form of learned thought. Held insists that child rearing is not a blind instinct but human activity that involves conscious choice and deliberate, thoughtful actions (Held, 1993). The moral sensibility and judgment characteristic of maternal thinking is developed through thoughtful performance of mothering roles. Experienced mothers combine intuition, "attentive love," and critical realism to make complex judgments to protect and nurture their children (Ruddick, 1989).

Noddings (1984) states that care ethics is "feminine in the deep classical sense, rooted in receptivity, relatedness, and responsiveness" (p. 2). Nonetheless, memories of being cared for are accessible to all human beings. "Care" is more foundational to ethics than justice since it is our longing to be in a special caring relationship that provides the motivation for us to be moral. Consequently, Noddings argues, this impulse to act in behalf of a particular other is latent in all of us, but our natural tendency to care must be enhanced through education. Society, in general, and traditional ethicists, in particular, have undervalued human caring. Because of their responsibilities for caring, women tend to remember and preserve the memory of caring and being cared for more than men (Noddings, 1984). As a result, they have an important educational role to play.

In most cultures and in most economic classes, women have had primary responsibilities not only for nurturing children, but also for tending and maintaining marriages, friendships, extended familial relationships, and general emotional housekeeping whether in the home or at work (Bartky, 1990). Young girls are socialized to assume these caregiving responsibilities. They may assume other roles as well, including typically masculine work roles, but they are nonetheless expected to be nurturers. Women's experiences in nurturing roles provide resources for relationship-based ethics that equal the richness of resources men derive from their experiences in the public sphere. From this perspective, socialization and social roles rather than biology account for the distinct feminine voice. Consequently, both women and men can assume public and private roles and benefit from the moral perspective and sensibilities these roles encourage.

The moral sensibility and contextual judgment that care ethics describes is strikingly similar to the contextual, embodied, and personal caregiving that Benner eloquently portrays in *From Novice to Expert* (1984). As we presented in Chapter 4, excellent nursing practice, including "skilled ethical comportment" (Benner, 1991) requires perceptual awareness and discretionary judgments that depend on responsiveness to the specificity and relational aspect of each nursing situation. Expert nurses develop an embodied practical knowledge, enabling them to approach complex situations from an experience-rich, holistic rather than a rule-governed basis. The sensitivity and judgment cultivated through care ethics will enrich nursing (Benner, 1984/2001; Benner & Wrubel, 1989; Gadow, 1985, 1988; Fry, 1992). Numerous applications are possible, including:

- The capacity to respond holistically to complex ethical situations
- The ability to respond to objective clinical concerns while preserving patient dignity and personal identity
- Supporting another person's meanings and values, often at times when those values are most threatened

Effects of Power Imbalance

Because women's moral experiences are as important as men's, they should be studied and mined for insights just as thoroughly as more characteristically male experiences have been. We need to recognize the moral significance of personal relationships with specific persons. Because personal feelings and emotions are ethically significant in moral deliberation, they must be examined as critically as ideas and beliefs. Ethical theories must recognize the necessity and value of specific contexts for moral judgments. It is not enough, however, to combine the best insights from men's and women's experiences in order to create an ideal ethical theory. We must also consider how social structures may have shaped those experiences.

Feminists support the efforts of care ethicists to make visible and value the moral perspective of women and those who perform the "feminine" work of caregiving. Feminists, however, are alert to the likelihood that in a sexist culture, women's adeptness at caring is related to their subordinate status.

Distortions of Feminine Caring

Gilligan observes that traditional ethics sees the male moral voice as representing all people. The normative voice, however, is not simply a male voice but the voice of the dominant group in society. It is a masculine voice insofar as those in power have tended to be men, but it is also a white, North American/European, upper-middle-class voice. It is hardly surprising then that not only do women as a group score lower on Kohlberg's measure of moral development, but African Americans and Hispanics score lower as well (Cortese, 1990).

Furthermore, attributes associated with the ethic of care (e.g., relationality, responsiveness to needs, intuition, and immanence) are characteristic of many non-Western, non-European cultures that were colonized by Western Europeans

(Harding, 1987). Consequently, feminists argue that though recovering and listening to the moral voices of the marginalized is vital, it is also important to be aware how subordinate voices may have been distorted by unjust power relations. Thus, the recovery by care ethics of characteristically feminine values plays an important role in the development of a feminist nursing ethics. These are values that have been critical to nursing's identity. But a feminist nursing ethics must also include a critical examination of how unequal power relations within health care systems may have distorted subordinate voices, including the subordinated voices of nurses.

Characteristic perceptions and dispositions of care may be necessary defensive strategies of subordinate groups. For those who live in close proximity to their oppressors, cultivating sensitivity to the emotional needs of others, responding efficiently to those needs, and striving to please (or at least to create the appearance of doing so) are important skills of self-protection (Goode, 1989). Although women may learn to excel at nurturing for other reasons as well, surviving in a patriarchal society is an important motivation.

Manipulation, Deceit, and Sabotage

Subordinate groups who lack direct power often learn how to use intimate knowledge of the dominant group to achieve their own ends. The finely honed ability to read and interpret the needs and emotions of others can be used to manipulate those in authority. These skills of perception also enable subordinates to be situational chameleons who change their tone, values, or loyalties to take advantage of each situation (Card, 1990).

In nursing this distortion of the attributes of care is described in Stein's (1968) classic essay on the "doctor–nurse game." Although communication between physicians and nurses has improved to some degree since Stein's 1968 study (Stein, 1990), this remains an area of primary concern for many nurses (Anderson et al., 1996). When nursing knowledge conflicts with physicians' medical claims, nurses believe that their expertise will frequently be discounted. Consequently, they may resort to hiding their expertise, feigning deference to medical authority, and manipulating physicians in order to get what they feel is necessary for their patients. Although nursing literature applauds courageous assertion of nursing knowledge, individual nurses must consider consequences of damaging their working relationships with physicians (Kuhse, 1997). Thus, manipulation and deceit become standard practice in many cases. Another frequent response is passive–aggressive behavior toward physicians. A nurse may appear to passively accept a physician order which she or he perceives as contrary to a patient's best interests, but then proceed to sabotage that treatment plan (Meyers, 1994).

Internal Conflict

A second symptom of the distortion of care in nursing is the evidence of a diminished ability of nurses to care for one another. As Roberts (1983) notes, self-hatred and low self-esteem result from the internalization by oppressed persons of the devaluing of their culture and values. "Horizontal violence" or conflict within the oppressed group, wherein members feel the need to reject their marginalized group identity, is a common outcome. Self-hatred and alienation may be expressed in unfair criticism and verbal abuse of other group members, as reflected in the common observation that "nurses eat their young" (attributed to L. Curtin in Bent, 1993). Rage and frustration about one's own abuse and powerlessness that cannot be expressed safely to the oppressors is instead communicated—often unconsciously—within the oppressed group (McCall, 1996; Roberts, 2000).

Lack of cohesion within nursing groups is another subtle manifestation of internalized self-hatred and low self-esteem. Limited participation in professional organizations suggests that nurses lack pride in their own group and are reluctant to associate with other powerless people (Roberts, 1983; Baldwin, 1995; Bowman, 1993). The ongoing debate over the appropriate education for entry-level nurses is another indicator of group division, as is resentment and disparagement of colleagues who pursue advanced degrees.

Self-Sacrifice

Gilligan and Noddings advocate the need for self-care as well as care for others. Neither author, however, adequately acknowledges how Western culture has expected women to care for others at the expense of their own health and well-being (Houston, 1989). This ideal of sacrificial giving of the self is an obvious way in which caring is distorted by the structures of patriarchy. As noted in Chapter 5 (pp. 149–150), the cultural expectations of those who fulfill the feminine role of caregiver can make it difficult for nurses to balance their needs with those of their clients. Nightingale appealed directly to the conventional association of a good (virtuous) woman with a good caregiver in order to present nursing as an acceptable, even noble, occupation for women in an era when "better class" women were expected to be at home (Kuhse, 1997). Hospitals quickly exploited this moralized association of nursing with selfless, devoted care of others in training programs that exchanged hard work, low pay, and perpetual moral scrutiny for little actual training.

That this exploitation did not end with the Victorian era is evident today when hospitals attempt to shame nurses who strike for better working conditions and a just wage. Management ad campaigns often portray striking nurses as "bad" people (i.e., bad "feminine" people) who are willing to sacrifice patient well-being to satisfy their own "selfish" needs (Growe, 1991).

Distortions of Masculine Virtues

Members of dominant groups are also harmed by oppressive systems. Some men suffer from oppression based on class, race, sexual orientation, or religious practice. In these cases, they are harmed by systems of dominance that are designed to oppress them. But men are also harmed by the patriarchal structures that are designed to oppress women. In this case, men are not oppressed by patriarchy since this system of restraints serves their overall material interests (power, domestic and sexual service, freedom from undesirable roles) at the expense of women's interests (Sherwin, 1992). But men, like other dominant groups, experience deformation of character as a result of living in a patriarchal system. These deforming effects include arrogance, moral blindness, defensiveness, and alienation from authentic self-development (Card, 1990).

Men, like other superordinates, take for granted the system that gives them their status. They are typically unaware of the incremental but cumulative advantages they garner from the social structure. As a result, they tend to assume that their greater accomplishments in society are the result of a natural superiority rather than systematic bias (Goode, 1989). Arrogance and moral blindness are predictable consequences. Because individual men are not responsible for creating the patriarchal system, they are often blind to the advantages it gives them and to the ways in which they perpetuate it. As a result, many men take offense at suggestions that they are to blame for women's oppression.

Sustaining an oppressive system (even if only by not resisting it) exacts a significant price from the oppressor group. Patriarchy is based on control as its core principle: Men are taught to be in control and to fear being controlled, especially by other men (Johnson, 1997). Relationships of intimacy and trust may be difficult as a result. Furthermore, the need to be in control (or at least to appear to be) also limits men's ability to explore their own emotional and spiritual selves. Alienation from oneself and others is a natural result for a person who values control above all else (Johnson, 1997; Sherwin, 1992).

Many men and women are unaware of the corrosive effects of the systematic oppression of women, which distort masculine and feminine roles and qualities. To promote awareness, feminists insist that moral experiences of women and men must be critically examined.

Institutional Constraints

As noted earlier, care ethicists have been motivated by a desire to recover a feminine moral voice that has frequently been disparaged by traditional Western ethics. In articulating rich descriptions of this unique voice, they have sought not only to illuminate the resources of this moral perspective but also to enhance the self-respect of those most identified with this voice. Benner (1984/2001), for instance, explicitly stated that her work was a response to the crisis in nursing in the 1980s: She hoped to combat the disillusionment, demoralization, and devaluation of clinical nursing in North America by uncovering the nature and significance of nursing care. The positive effect of Benner's work during this critical time cannot be overestimated. Yet, as Bowden (1997) makes clear in her thoughtful analysis of Benner's work, Benner's work may inadvertently contribute to a sense of personal failure and impotence on the part of nurses. Bowden states that while her critique is not limited to Benner, she focuses on Benner's work (and her later collaboration with Wrubel) because of its extraordinary perceptiveness. Bowden's critique is generally representative of many feminist analyses of care ethics.

Bowden describes *From Novice to Expert as* ". . . one of the richest descriptions available of the nature of clinical nursing practices and their distinctive ethical possibilities." She argues, however, that Benner's inattention to the disabling effects of the structural components of the nursing crisis actually undermines Benner's stated goal of nursing empowerment. Benner briefly acknowledges institutional and cultural barriers to excellent clinical care, but in her desire to avoid characterizing nurses as victims, she radically underestimates the effect of these barriers. She fails to give nursing practice the same insightful attention to personal and sociohistorical factors that she uses to analyze the phenomenology of illness. Nurses are encouraged to cope with disempowering institutional and societal barriers to caregiving through the same creative, holistic thinking that they bring to helping patients cope with illness. Without a critical analysis of the ways in which a hierarchical, gendered health care system devalues and disrupts nursing care, however, a nursing care ethic risks encouraging exploitation of nurses' capacities and holding them individually responsible for failures of nursing care (see also Bowman, 1993). It is implied that an excellent nurse should be able to "cope." But where are the external experts who will mediate, advocate, educate, and empower nurses in the way that they support patients faced with assaults to bodily and personal integrity?

Benner ignores the framework for institutional critique that is inherent in the virtue ethics perspective she articulates. Virtue ethics advocates the removal of impediments to a community's virtues and development of institutional supports for them. Individuals and communities are interdependent and co-responsible for character. Feminist ethics shares this concept of interdependence but also adds the need to critically assess the effects of power relations, including those related to gender, on the moral ideals and character of a community and its members.

Epilogue to Care Ethics

Gilligan's most important contribution to feminist ethics may be her unmasking of the tendency in Western ethics to define male experience as normative human experience. Through a critical review of traditional psychological theories of moral development, Gilligan reveals that the harm to women is not restricted to ignoring their moral experiences. The more fundamental harm is that men's moral experience has been represented as the *human* moral experience. Men's experience has been used to define a normative standard, and women have been judged to be deficient when evaluated against this norm. Gilligan observes that each of the major psychological theories of moral development were based on studies of men only. Some theorists, like Kohlberg, whose initial study followed 84 boys, included only male subjects in their models of moral development. Others, like Erickson, studied males and females but then ignored the different experiences of women when constructing their models of "human" development. Thus, men's experiences became the basis for models that prescribed the correct stages of moral development.

It is hardly remarkable then, Gilligan notes, that when men and women have been tested against these standardized models, women as a group have consistently been scored at a lower level of moral maturity than men as a group. This "evidence" thus confirmed the traditional claims of philosophers from Aristotle to Schopenhauer, who proposed that women lacked an adequate capacity to conceptualize and apply abstract moral principles. The unmasking of this tendency to make male experience normative is a fundamental element of feminist work in all disciplines. Gilligan has helped thousands to recognize this misrepresentation of male experience as universal human experience in the area of ethics.

Care ethics is a feminist ethics insofar as it recognizes that this tendency of traditional theories to make male experience normative has contributed to women's subordination. Feminist ethics continues Gilligan's process by seeking to uncover the roots and effects of unjust power relations, particularly those based on gender. Feminists recognize that all women do not experience sexism in the same way. Gender oppression is interwoven with many other identifying factors such as race, ethnicity, sexual orientation, class, and religious affiliation. A feminist approach to nursing ethics and bioethics will explore the effects of power relations in the areas of health and health care. The goal is ultimately the transformation of attitudes and health care institutions by finding ways to link the concerns, visions, and perspectives of diverse networks of people. Feminists share with many nurses the desire to avoid victimization and the paralysis of feeling impotent. Their goal is not simply to rage against oppression, but to create spaces for reflection and action (Rinehart, 1998).

Creating a Feminist Nursing Ethics

Health care systems, organizations, and concepts are embedded within the specific social contexts of particular societies. Patriarchy is a significant feature of most societies, though it is uniquely embodied in each society (Sanday, 1981). Feminists want to understand how health care is shaped by its roots in patriarchy and how patriarchal values have shaped health care systems. They do not all share the same analysis nor the same conclusions. But there are some shared themes. We will examine four:

1. *How health care perpetuates hierarchies of power*
2. *A relational account of justice*
3. *Health care's role in the social construction of reality*
4. *Contributions of feminist epistemology to health care ethics*

Perpetuating Hierarchies of Power

Given the larger social context of patriarchy, it is not surprising to find that health care helps to perpetuate the hierarchies of power found in this social system. Patriarchy is a system of control that grants privileges not only to men, but also to whites and those with greater economic resources. Health care systems perpetuate the oppression of women, especially women of color, that is part of the larger patriarchal society.

THE HEALTH CARE SYSTEM

The organization of health care systems is itself a reflection of male-identified values of control and hierarchy. Furthermore, health care in North America reflects the male-dominated character of these societies. Power remains concentrated in the hands of a mostly white male elite; yet the current system relies on the dedication of a large body of subordinate, almost entirely female and mostly white nursing staff. Nurses, in turn, retain authority over an even larger, mostly minority, nonprofessional support staff (Hine, 1989). While nursing began with Nightingale's vision of separate but equal spheres of responsibility for medicine and nursing, economic interests rapidly led to the subordination of nursing (Ehrenreich & English, 1978; Reverby, 1987). In the enormous expansion of health care institutions in North America after World War II, nursing's ability to articulate and institute its own vision of caring has been constrained by the interlocking interests of academic medical empires, financiers, and hospital suppliers and drug companies.

Contemporary applications of budgetary management reflect this continuing subordination and control of nursing. An example is the rationing of patient care by means of predetermined "target hours" and "patient classification systems," using formulas determined by hospital experts and medical diagnoses. As patient–nurse ratios grow, nurses must provide fewer services to more patients more quickly (Bowden, 1997). Campbell further explains how documentary procedures in Canadian nursing are used to transform nurses' professional, experiential knowledge into quantifiable data, which is used to control, regulate, and order nursing practice according to costing formulas. Nurses become increasingly alienated from their caring potential as judgments about patient care are removed further and further from the bedside. The professional and ethical authority of nursing is undermined as judgments about nursing care are controlled by economic and professional interests of others (cited in Bowden, 1997). The scenario in Box 6–3 further demonstrates nursing's subordinate position in the health care system. Because nurse practitioners now bill for their services, invoices itemize charges for nursing care. Previously, costs of nursing care were invisible to patients because they were included but not itemized in charges for a hospital room or physician services in the clinic setting.

Box 6–3 Nursing Care: Contradictions in Patient Perceptions

Emma, a 76-year-old female, is referred for management of congestive heart failure and atrial fibrillation to a chronic care clinic managed by nurses. Emma has been taking Coreg, spiroaldactone, and warfarin. The providers in the clinic are nurse practitioners who monitor and treat Emma's heart disease to maximize her functional status so that she can remain in her assisted living apartment. The program stipulates visits on at least a monthly basis, because Emma needs to have her International Normalized Ratio level evaluated regularly.

The initial clinic visit requires approximately one hour for a detailed history and physical, functional assessment, an analysis of baseline lab and radiologic data, determination of community resources needed, and education about the disease process, its treatment, and the care that would be provided. Follow-up visits usually take about 20 minutes and include a focused history and physical, analysis of INR, adjustments to treatment if needed, education, and evaluation for needed community resources.

Box 6–3   Nursing Care: Contradictions
in Patient Perceptions (cont.)

During her first visit, Emma remarked that she was very pleased to be able to get this care. On her third visit, she brought in her Medicare bill, which itemized charges of $140 for the initial visit and $68 for the second visit, as well as charges for lab work or other diagnostic procedures. Emma carries supplemental insurance and thus incurs no out-of-pocket cost for the care. She commented that she could not believe that it cost so much to have a nurse see her. When asked how she would characterize the quality of her care, she said it was great and provided more detail and time than her physician spends with her. Part of Emma's concern arose from the fact that the billing indicated the name of a physician she had never seen. Rather than obtain provider numbers for the nurse practitioners, the clinic had chosen to bill under the physician's name. Emma stated that this must be why the bill was so high: The clinic was charging her physician rates since nursing care certainly couldn't be this expensive. When asked if she would like to stop coming to the clinic and return to physician follow-up, she quickly declined. She explained she believed that the care provided was really helping her but repeated that the cost for "just a nurse" seemed high.

Questions

1. What conflicting beliefs are evident in Emma's response to receiving this bill for nursing services?
2. What might this nurse practitioner and all nurse practitioners do to educate patients about the value of the services that they provide?

GENDER-BIASED MEDICAL RESEARCH AND TREATMENT

Health care perpetuates gender oppression in a number of ways. Medical research is one area where gender bias has been clearly documented. It has frequently relied on male research subjects, while generalizing the results to women without sufficient evidence of their applicability to women. This research bias likely contributes to gender discrimination in medical treatment.

The Council on Ethical and Judicial Affairs (CEJA) of the American Medical Association concluded that "medical treatments for women are based on a male model, regardless of the fact that women may react differently to treatments than men or that some diseases manifest themselves differently in women" (1991, p. 559). A clear example is the research on taking aspirin to reduce the risk of heart disease. The primary study in this area, published in 1988, examined the effects on 22,071 men, demonstrating that one aspirin every other day reduces the risk by over 50 percent for men over 50. The National Institutes of Health (NIH) declined to fund a similar study on women until 1991, despite repeated requests by one of the primary investigators of the original study.

Many drugs routinely prescribed for and taken by women have never been tested in women. Women—and their health care providers—are left with the undesirable choice between taking a drug without reliable data on its effect on women or forgoing the possible benefits of the drug. The most common justification for omission of women as research subjects is the assertion that cyclical hormone changes make them more difficult to study and that these changes cause effects that would pollute the "clean" data generated by the study of male subjects. The male body is uncritically accepted as the norm for "human biological function," despite uncontroversial evidence that drug metabolism, dose-response reaction, and other significant markers of clinical effect are different in women. Furthermore, the fact that their body chemistry may make research more difficult hardly justifies excluding women from drug research. The point of such research is to generate knowledge that aids in the treatment of people, half of whom are women and many of whom do have menstrual cycles (Merton, 1996).

Recent studies have revealed disturbing inequalities in the treatment of the same health problems in men and women. Among women and men who experience renal failure, women between the ages of 46 and 60 are only half as likely to receive a kidney transplant as men in the same age group. Cardiac disease, the leading killer of both men and women, takes the lives of nearly equal numbers of men and women. Nonetheless, men receive better care for heart attacks and are more likely to recover from them. Women are far less likely to be given angiograms, are 50 percent as likely to receive balloon angioplasty and clot-dissolving drugs, and are referred for cardiac catheterization less than 20 percent as often as men (Merton, 1996; Nelson & Nelson, 1996).

The lack of adequate data may be one reason for this discriminatory treatment. Research in cardiovascular disease has concentrated almost exclusively on men. Although women constitute two thirds of the elderly, a major federal study on health and aging studied only men in its first 20 years. Only men were included in a research study on the effectiveness of aspirin in preventing migraine headaches, in spite of the fact that there are three times more female than male migraine sufferers. Perhaps the most absurd example of gender bias and lack of adequate data is an NIH-funded project using only male subjects that drew conclusions regarding the impact of obesity on breast and uterine cancer (Nelson & Nelson, 1996).

Research related to the HIV epidemic provides a poignant illustration of the male-centeredness of medical research and the devaluing of women. Researchers have tended to treat HIV-positive women primarily as "vessels" and "vectors" (Faden, Kass, & McGraw, 1996). In a 1987 report, the CDC reported four ongoing studies involving women; three focused on vertical transmission from mother to infants (including Protocol 076), and the fourth studied possible intervention strategies to prevent the spread of HIV from prostitutes to their male partners. Despite a dramatic increase in the rate of infection in women, no natural history study of nonpregnant women was begun until April 1993. In 1983, when the CDC launched its first full-scale natural history study of HIV and AIDS to follow 5,000 homosexual and bisexual men, the absolute number of infected men was dramatically larger than the number of women. But between the first report of a case of AIDS in a woman in 1981 and 1991, the number of cases of AIDS in women had increased 1,000 times—nearly 10 times faster than in men. As Faden and colleagues note, lack of information about HIV development in women has likely compromised the ability of practitioners to diagnose and treat the infection in women (Faden, Kass, & McGraw, 1996).

AIDS research has not only been male-centered, but also male-identified insofar as it has assumed that the manifestations of the infection in men are equally applicable to women. Until 1993, the CDC case definition of AIDS did not include any "woman-specific" conditions. In spite of growing evidence by 1987 that HIV-infected women suffered from a variety of recurrent gynecologic problems, the CDC steadfastly refused to revise its definition until 1993. The CDC stated that if these gynecologic conditions were included, some women with these conditions but without HIV disease would be counted in the AIDS statistics. A confirming HIV serology, however, already required for other AIDS-defining conditions, could have avoided this problem (Faden, Kass, & McGraw, 1996).

Women were harmed in several ways through the CDC's decision. First, some women could have been diagnosed earlier if physicians had known to associate recurrent gynecologic conditions with HIV. Second, since persons diagnosed with AIDS are eligible to receive Social Security and medical benefits, many women with AIDS were unable to secure desperately needed assistance. Third, both HIV-infected and HIV-negative women were harmed when their communities did not receive intervention and education dollars allocated by the federal government based on the proportion of AIDS cases in those communities (Faden, Kass, & McGraw, 1996).

Women are harmed when research questions appropriate to women are not studied and when researchers assume that differences between men and women are irrelevant in medical research. Women are treated unjustly when their health interests are ignored or their health is considered less important than men's. Examples cited here are not isolated or accidental instances of the exclusion and underrepresentation of women in medical research. They are the reflection of a systematic diffusion throughout the "tree of patriarchy" into the many branches of social groups and organizations. There is no reason to expect scientists and physicians to be exempt from this influence or to assume that they intentionally discriminate against women. Many are likely unaware of this pattern of discrimination. Oppression, as Young (1990) notes, is structural and systemic: It is not a matter of one group consciously trying to keep another group down. Medical researchers have been educated and socialized into a system of gender oppression. Their work will reflect this system's core values, attitudes, and beliefs *unless* they persistently resist them (Sherwin, 1994).

TREATMENT OF WOMEN OF COLOR

The critique of paternalism in medicine has been one of the most significant achievements of traditional health care ethics. Since the 1960s, ethics have emphasized the need to respect and to promote the autonomy of individual patients in light of the inherent and historical power imbalance between an ill patient who is dependent on the expert knowledge and beneficence of physicians. While feminists join in this opposition to paternalism, their critique of the physician–patient relationship widens the scope of analysis. Public political forces, including sexism and racism structure the physician–patient relation. Thus, paternalism cannot adequately be addressed simply by encouraging physicians to respect their patients' autonomy, to seek informed consent, and to improve their communication skills. Physicians do not encounter their patients merely as individuals nor in isolation from the larger society. As Roberts (1996) observes, ". . . moral dilemmas between doctor and patient are interpreted and resolved according to power arrangements outside the doctor's office" (p. 121). Since women of color experience the intersections of gender and racial oppression, critical examination of their experiences reveals yet another way that medicine perpetuates hierarchies of power.

There is clear evidence that race and class differences affect the quality of care patients receive (CEJA, 1990; Wennecker & Epstein, 1989; Whittle et al., 1993; and Todd, 1989). African American patients, for instance, are less likely than white patients to receive lifesaving treatments such as bypass surgery, intensive care for pneumonia, long-term dialysis, and kidney transplants (CEJA, 1990). The effects are felt in the context of routine physician–patient interactions as well. Todd (1989) concluded from her study of these interactions that "the darker a woman's skin and/or the lower her place on the economic scale, the poorer the care and efforts at explanation she got" (p. 77).

The experiences of women of color in the health care system are shaped by the complex and unique history of each minority group's interaction with this system in a racist society. For African American women, for instance, this history includes the use of slave women as guinea pigs to develop gynecological surgery for white women, forced sterilizations that continued into the 1970s, segregated hospitals, and the legacy of distrust created by the Tuskegee syphilis study (Roberts, 1996; Beardsley, 1990; Townes, 1998).

Roberts (1996) explores how physician decisions to report drug abuse in pregnant women are shaped by racial stereotypes and assumptions. One study found that in spite of similar rates of substance abuse across racial and socioeconomic lines, African American women are reported to public health authorities for substance abuse during pregnancy 10 times more frequently than are white women (Roberts, 1996). Between 1991 and 1996, of almost 200 women arrested and charged with criminal offenses after their newborns tested positive for drugs, most were poor and African American. Because most states have no laws that require testing and reporting, many hospitals have no formal testing protocols. Thus, testing is generally left to the discretion of individual health care professionals. It is entirely appropriate for health care professionals to be concerned about the effects of substance abuse on newborns. The pattern of disproportionate reporting of African American women is, however, unfair (Young, 1994).

How should we understand the greater incidence of reporting pregnant African American women for substance abuse? So pervasive a pattern of discrimination cannot be explained adequately in terms of racial prejudice and bias on the part of individual health care professionals. Roberts (1996) argues that physicians are more willing to report African American women because these physicians are "part of a society that considers these women to be less deserving of motherhood and in greater need of state control of their reproductive decisions" (p. 128). She supports this position by pointing to the history of systematic, institutionalized limitation of African American women's reproductive freedom. This history includes the brutal coercion of their reproduction during slavery; publicly funded birth control clinics, established in the South in the 1930s, which attempted to reduce fertility among black women; and forced sterilizations (Roberts, 1996).

Roberts's analysis underscores the need for health care ethics to move beyond the traditional view of the physician–patient dyad as a private relationship between two persons. Physicians and other health care professionals do not encounter patients in isolation from larger public forces that shape these encounters. Feminist health care ethics reminds us of the tendency of health care professionals and organizations to perpetuate hierarchies of power that exist in the larger society. Unless we recognize this tendency, we will miss opportunities to resist these forces and to empower patients, their communities, and health care professionals.

Relational Account of Justice

Recognizing how the health care system tends to oppress social groups already marginalized in the larger society points to the need for a relational account of justice. A relational account is an approach that asserts that justice requires not only the respect for persons as unique individuals, but also an understanding of people as members of social groups (Wilkerson, 1998; Young, 1990). People's lives are defined and affected in many ways by their relation to social groups. Members of oppressed groups may have a greater need for health care due to the effects of their oppression, the obstacles that complicate their access to care, and their experience of care as linked to stigma and control. Furthermore, as with women, care for other oppressed groups may be based on insufficient research and medical education that tends to focus on the white male as the norm (Wilkerson, 1998).

As Young (1990) notes, mainstream moral and political theories of justice focus on issues of distribution and access to health care resources. Adopting the Enlightenment perspective of rationality and objectivity, both conservative and liberal accounts of justice share medicine's stance of detachment. The proper perspective for public policy is, consequently, assumed to be one of "objective" distance and neutrality. The goal is then construed as developing policies that give all individuals equal standing, equal access, and equal resources.

From this perspective, mainstream theorists in health care ethics condemn as unjust instances of overt discrimination or unequal access to care. But this "objective" concept of justice does not motivate deeper analysis of disparities of power and influence that may create different health care needs, different barriers to care, and different experiences of health care for oppressed groups. Some harms achieve the status of an injustice only when one considers groups. For instance, an individual woman may have no right to participate in an experimental drug protocol. But drug protocols that systematically exclude a group based on gender or race may constitute a significant moral wrong (Merton, 1996; Wolf, 1996).

Some aspects of injustice cannot be described adequately in terms of unjust allocation and distribution of goods (Wilkerson, 1998; Young, 1990). The perception of African American women as inherently unfit mothers is but one example. To understand this injustice, feminists assert that we must include oppression as a central aspect of injustice in health care. Then, as Wilkerson (1998) proposes, we will recognize that "treating people with respect entails not merely granting them respect as *individuals* but actually transforming social relations so that oppressed *groups* can occupy places of respect in the social structure" (p. 109).

Health Care and the Social Construction of Reality

Feminists have long been concerned with how gender and sexuality are socially constructed. They have been critical of positions that assume that a woman's or a man's biological sex should determine personality traits, characteristic behaviors, or social roles. *Gender is a social role.* Like other social roles, gender carries with it a set of social expectations that include rights, obligations, behaviors, and duties. Gender stereotypes reflect cultural expectations about maleness and femaleness. These conceptions of masculinity and femininity are socially constructed (Newman, 1995).

Berger and Luckmann (1966) define the *social construction of reality* as the process through which facts, knowledge, truth, and so on are discovered, made known, reaffirmed, and altered by the members of a society. This process can be understood in terms of three stages. The first of these is *externalization*, wherein people develop knowledge about some aspect of the world by creating theories or explanations that they then "externalize" by publicizing them in a variety of ways. For example, physicians, psychiatrists, and scholars developed and publicized compelling theories about the nature of chronic drunkenness to persuade most people in our society to understand alcoholism as a disease.

The second stage of social construction, the process of *objectivation*, occurs when ideas, theories, and explanations become accepted as "self-evident" facts. In the third stage these facts (what "everyone knows") are *internalized* through socialization; children are taught these facts as the way the world is (Newman, 1995).

Social institutions and the people who control them play a significant role in shaping and sustaining perceptions of reality. In some cases, socially accepted facts are supported by widely confirmed evidence, as with the now established fact that the sun is the center of the universe. But in other cases, "experts" have interpreted data to support theories that serve their interests, as when Nazi scientists provided data to support theories of Aryan biological and intellectual superiority. Many "facts" about human beings and the social forces that shape them are not clearly demonstrable as true or false. Reality is complex, and more than one theory or explanation is possible much of the time. But some accounts of reality, such as the position of Aryan superiority, cannot be succesfully defended and must be critically analyzed.

In any society, there is a struggle for the power to influence or control society's conceptions of reality. This does not necessarily imply that persons in positions of power intentionally manipulate perceptions for their own malevolent or selfish ends. Feminists suggest, however, that it does mean we should be aware of the power that people, groups, organizations, and institutions have to define values, create visions, and influence society's conception of reality. Consequently, feminists encourage us to ask whose interests are served by a particular conception of reality and whose interests are harmed or ignored by it (Sherwin, 1992). Because health care institutions, especially medicine, play a significant role in defining women's health and sexuality, health care ethics must consider these questions.

SOCIAL CONSTRUCTION OF WOMEN'S HEALTH

The power of those in medical authority to define illness is one of the important ways that medicine constructs social reality. Women's health advocates have been critical of the tendency to medicalize normal events in women's lives. Menstruation, birth control, weight reduction, childbirth, parenting, exercise, menopause, and aging are defined as medical problems that "require" physician care. In some sense, medicine has defined women as inherently defective or pathological throughout much of their lives (The Boston Women's Health Collective, 1992; Sherwin, 1992). The authority to label something as unhealthy, diseased, or ill is a powerful position that has often been used to justify treating women differently than men and to authorize extensive medical management of women's lives.

As Sherwin (1992) observes, menstruation has always been recognized as a distinguishing feature of women's bodies, but its perception as an illness is relatively recent. Early theorists regarded menstruation as a healthy means of cleansing and purifying the body. Throughout the eighteenth century, menstruation was commonly regarded as natural and healthy. Women were encouraged to maintain regular activities during menses (Martin, 1987; Sherwin, 1992). By the mid-nineteenth century, however, the medical community had reconstructed menstruation as a disability that warranted rest and withdrawal from normal activities, especially any that required mental effort. Feminist analysts agree that the change in approach reflects a major political and social shift rather than any development in medical knowledge (Clarke, 1990; Ehrenreich & English, 1978; Sherwin, 1992; Wilkerson, 1998). As Enlightenment theorists championed the right of rational persons to participate in the political and economic life of their communities, new justifications were needed to explain the exclusion of women from universities, paid work, and political participation. Medicine obliged by providing "scientific evidence" for the "zero-sum energy" theory. This theory asserted that the womb and the brain are in competition for blood and energy. Consequently, if a woman's energies were "drawn away" from her reproductive organs through mental effort, her organs would suffer developmental deformities with perpetual negative effects. Obviously then, academic study, political activity, and any other serious mental work was harmful to menstruating women. By the end of the century, physicians were leaders in the campaign to exclude women from universities and to undermine their participation in the women's suffrage movement (Clarke, 1990; Sherwin, 1992).

Apparently, working class women did not face the same risks to their health for they were not discouraged from continuing to work during menstruation. Medical authorities, in fact, suggested that working-class women were protected through the masculinizing effect of their labors and by the fact that they were unlikely to engage in any significant mental work anyway. The masculinizing effect of work was considered undesirable, of course, and women with other economic choices were expected to avoid it. Nonetheless, Carol Tavris (1992) demonstrates that the view of menstruation has repeatedly been constructed and reconstructed to suit the economic demand for women in the labor market. During World War II, when women were desperately needed in the workforce, medical researchers reversed their opinion that menstruation was incapacitating. Yet in the 1930s and again in the 1950s, researchers found significant evidence that menstruation disrupted women's work and employment. When the number of women in paid employment dramatically increased again in the 1970s, research supporting the disruptive view of menstruation dramatically increased as well (Tavris, 1992).

Although contemporary medical texts discuss menstruation as a normal, healthy physiological function, it is still often described in language that suggests pathology and decay. One well-known text describes the two main phases of the endometrium as the "proliferative" and the "secretory." The first phase is identified with growth and regeneration, while the second with "rapid loss," "degeneration," and "destruction" (Jones, Wentz, &Burnett, 1988, cited in Wilkerson, 1998). Such language still reflects a patriarchal definition of women as mothers, existing for the sake of others. Menstruation is perceived as failed production (and menopause as the loss of productive capacity), rather than as a functional process in its own right. Other organic processes involving production and secretion of tissue, such as the regular shedding and replacement of the stomach lining or the process by which seminal fluid picks up cast off cellular material as it goes through male ducts, are not similarly described as "failed production" or waste (Martin, 1987).

Recent feminist analyses of the medicalization of premenstrual symptoms and menopause reflect similar concerns about the representation of these uniquely feminine experiences as illnesses or biological failures. From a woman's perspective, Wilkerson (1998) notes, ". . . neither menstruation nor menopause—as opposed to certain *symptoms* that some women experience—is problematic or unhealthy (or somehow less healthy than pregnancy) in and of itself. Their definition as unhealthy reflects once again the male-identified and male-centered nature of patriarchy. The relatively noncyclic nature of male physiology is treated as the normative measure of health, beside which female cyclicity is considered deviant (Wilkerson, 1998).

Feminists present numerous examples of the social construction of women's health that serves the interests of men and children to the detriment of women themselves. Chapter 7 explores medical attitudes toward women's body size and the role these attitudes play in eating disorders.

MEDICAL CONSTRUCTIONS OF SEXUALITY

Is it a boy or a girl? This is often the first question asked at the birth of a new child. It is not intended to be a trick question, but in the case of an estimated 1.7 percent of newborns, the answer is extremely difficult to determine (Fausto-Sterling, 2000). Born with a range of anatomical conditions in which male and female attributes are combined, these children often, but not always, present with ambiguous genitals. The standard medical and nursing response to the birth of intersexed children is to attempt to "disambiguate" the newborn's identity (Dreger, 1998). After physical and genetic testing of an intersexed newborn, physicians are directed to assign either a male or female identity, to surgically modify the child's genitalia to conform believably to this identity, and later to provide medical treatment such as hormones to reinforce the assigned gender. The birth of an intersexed infant is regarded as a medical and psychosocial emergency—decisions must be made within 48 to 72 hours. Teams of specialists, including geneticists, pediatric endocrinologists, and pediatric urologists, are immediately assembled to decide the sex/gender of the intersexed infant (Chase, 1999; Parker, 1998).

The assignment of sexual identity is guided by two criteria: (1) preservation of potential female reproductive capabilities—thus, genetic females (babies lacking a Y chromosome) are declared girls no matter how masculine their genitalia appear; and (2) ensuring that genetic males (babies with Y chromosomes) have "adequate" penises if they are to be assigned the male gender. An adequate penis is one that will allow the individual to urinate standing up and to engage in sexual intercourse through vaginal penetration. A genetic male with an "inadequate" penis will be assigned the female gender and reconstructed to look female (Chase, 1999; Dreger, 1998; Fausto-Sterling, 2000). Reconstruction often requires multiple surgeries.

Constructions of Sex and Gender Are Intertwined

As noted earlier, feminists have challenged the assumption that gender differences emerge naturally from biological differences between the sexes. That differences in men's and women's behaviors and experiences are largely the result of cultural socialization is now more commonly accepted. Masculinity and femininity are thus social constructions. But though gender roles and behavior may vary across time and culture, human beings everywhere are either biologically male or female. Or at least most people perceive this to be the case, assuming that two biological sex categories are universal, exhaustive (there is no third sex), and mutually exclusive (a person must be one or the other). The male–female dichotomy is so entrenched within our social structure that those who challenge it are likely to be regarded as crazy (or as foolish academics out of touch with reality) (Lorber, 1989; Newman, 1997).

"Sex" is not a purely physical category. The ways in which we experience our bodies—including awareness of our sexuality—are influenced by our development within particular cultures and historical periods. In other words, sex is also socially constructed. Examining the medical model for the *treatment* of intersexed infants reveals how social theories of sex and gender are intertwined and influence medical response. Because incidence is low, few nurses may be called on to provide care for intersexed infants and their parents. Still, this issue is foundational for all, because it illuminates how medicine helps to construct sexuality for everyone and not solely for intersexed individuals.

The Psychosexual Neutrality Thesis

The traditional model of intervention and treatment of intersexed infants, developed in the 1950s, is based largely on the work of John Hopkins sexologist, John Money (1955; Money and Ehrhardt, 1972) and is endorsed by the American Academy of Pediatrics (1996). The foundational postulate of this model is the belief that individuals are psychosexually neutral at birth. Consequently, Money and associates have for decades assured physicians that they could create either gender within any child as long as necessary cosmetic alterations are performed early and the medical team and parents consistently relate to the child according to the chosen gender designation.

Because parents play a key role in the child's psychosocial health, the medical and nursing team must make every effort to instill the parental conviction that what has been assigned is the child's true sex. As soon after birth as possible, health care providers explain basic embryological facts to parents, namely that all fetuses initially have identical genitalia and the potential to develop into either sex. Building on this information, they explain that the infant's genitalia are incompletely developed and further diagnostic tests are needed to determine whether their child is a boy or a girl. Physicians and nurses are cautioned never to suggest that the child has two genders or is "half boy–half girl." Instead, parents should be assured that physicians will be able to identify the "true" sex, and that once this "true identity" is determined, surgical and hormonal treatments will complete nature's intention (Elliott, 1998; Fausto-Sterling, 2000; Parker, 1998).

Although Money's model was developed almost entirely from his experience with one well-publicized case, this treatment approach until recently was largely unquestioned. Controversy currently surrounds this model, however, spurred by the revelation in 1997 that the key case supporting it was a medical failure (Colapinto, 2000; Diamond & Sigmundson, 1997). Box 6–4 summarizes this case.

Box 6–4   Assigning a Sex

"John" was born in 1965 as a typical XY male with a twin brother, but at eight months his penis was accidentally destroyed during a circumcision. A team of specialists headed by John Money decided that life for John without a penis would be intolerable and that he should be medically reconstructed and raised as a girl. Although it did not arise from congenital intersexuality, this case was regarded as the ideal test of the theory that individuals are born psychosexually neutral. John's twin provided a perfectly matched control. Money monitored "Joan's" development and repeatedly published reports of Joan's successful development of female identity. Reality, however, challenged these reports.

The story of David Reimer, the person behind the "John/Joan" pseudonym is told with insight and compassion in Colapinto's *As Nature Made Him* (2000). Despite his parents' commitment to follow prescribed treatment, David's Joan years were filled with struggle. David endured nearly universal rejection and ridicule by peers who perceived him as a highly masculine girl who frequently resorted to fist-fighting. Joan was never comfortable with her female identity and resisted medical treatments as well as her parents' "feminizing" socialization. After learning the truth at age 14 from his father, David chose to make the transition to a male identity. Trying to come to terms with what had happened, he experienced profound depression and twice attempted suicide. After several surgeries, David, who continued with testosterone treatment, is now married and has adopted his wife's children (Colapinto, 2000).

Significant numbers of intersexed adults have begun to speak out about medicine's attempts to "normalize" their sexuality. The Intersex Society of North America (ISNA) is an advocacy group of former patients who are speaking against the present model. They report that despite the good intentions of physicians and parents to spare them discomfort and shame, their medical treatments and genital surgeries have left them with precisely these feelings. They deplore the secrecy and deception that are an intrinsic part of the current treatment model and the lack of long-term follow-up to determine treatment efficacy. Many intersexed adults report that genital surgery has damaged their sexual function (Chase, 1996; Kessler, 1998). Furthermore, some studies of intersexed individuals who were not surgically altered indicate that a majority have lived well-adjusted lives (Colapinto, 2000). It is remarkable that the Money model has enjoyed nearly unquestioned dominance in the light of the slim data researchers have produced to support it (Colapinto, 2000; Fausto-Sterling, 2000; Dreger, 1998).

Cultural Relativity of Sexual Codes

Labeling someone as male or female is a social decision as are identifying criteria used to determine sex and choosing to make a determination at all. Choices about criteria and sex made in the medical management of intersexuality reinforce and help to further construct certain assumptions about sex and gender. Fausto-Sterling (2000) suggests that medical practice of sex conversion rests on three unexamined assumptions: "First, that there should be only two sexes; second, that only heterosexuality was normal; and third, that particular gender roles defined the psychologically healthy man and woman" (p. 44).

The first assumption may seem to be common sense. Yet various cultures have responded to intersexuals in different ways. Navajo culture recognizes a third-sex/third-gender called the *nadleeh*, regarded as holy and sacred; the birth of a *nadleeh* is a happy event since a *nadleeh* ensures wealth and success. They are considered leaders and are entrusted with family property (Elliott, 1998; Newman, 1997). In the Dominican Republic, there is a higher-than-usual incidence of 5-alpha-reductase deficiency syndrome. Children with this condition are genetically XY but are born sexually ambiguous. Typically raised as girls, at puberty they undergo significant masculinizing changes. Most change to a male gender role, and many go on to marry women. Despite this transition, they maintain their identity as a third sexual category called *guevedoce* ("penis at twelve"). People of this culture maintain a triadic sexual code, dividing their world into male, female, and *guevedoce*. The *guevedoce* are perceived not as men who are mistakenly raised as girls but as a third gender whose development is perfectly normal for individuals in their category (Elliott, 1988).

Fausto-Sterling (2000) notes that in premodern Europe, sex and gender were conceived as falling along a continuum rather than into the discrete categories commonly used today. Intersexed individuals (known as *hermaphrodites*) were merely variations on the sexual continuum. Practical issues of inheritance, marriage, dress, voting status, and so on required resolution; different societies applied their legal and religious codes in a variety of ways. While societal attitudes varied considerably, the intersexed were rarely condemned. Secular and religious lawyers and judges were the primary arbiters of intersexual status until the early nineteenth century. But with the emergence in the nineteenth century of biology as a discipline, intersexed bodies were redefined as a pathology that required a medical cure. By the twentieth century, physicians had become the chief regulators of intersexuality (Fausto-Sterling, 2000).

There is nothing inevitable about the current medical view of intersexuality. Occurring in an estimated 1.7 percent of all babies, intersexuality is much more common than the familiar trait of albinism, which occurs in .005 percent of all births (Fausto-Sterling, 2000). Whatever the exact statistical frequency of intersexuality, it is clear that many bodies combine anatomical components conventionally attributed to males or females. Contemporary Western medicine defines these as incorrectly developed male or female bodies; physicians and nurses describe them (inaccurately) to parents as incompletely developed male or female bodies. But they could also be described simply as *differently* developed bodies.

Genital "normalcy" has been considered a necessity for parental and social acceptance of an intersexed child and for the child's happiness. But as Chase (1999) observes, whether or not surgery is performed, the intersexed person's genitals differ from those of other people. The intersexed person's sexual orientation and sense of gender may differ as well. Stories shared by intersexed individuals suggest that their physicians' obsessive focus on their anatomy may actually promote feelings of freakishness (Colapinto, 2000; Dreger, 1998). It is not self-evident that the birth of an intersexed child should be handled medically or surgically. "Ambiguous" genitals do not constitute a disease. Congenital adrenal hyperplasia is the only intersex condition that poses a medical emergency. Its associated salt imbalance and cortisone insufficiency are life threatening for newborns. "Ambiguous" genitals themselves, however, are not.

A variety of authors within and outside of health care advocate drastic changes in the care of intersexed infants, proposing that care for these children and their parents should emphasize counseling, peer support, and education. Surgery would be performed only for physical emergencies. Children would receive age-appropriate information and, when old enough, could choose cosmetic surgery or a change of sex role if desired. The nurse would play a key role in this more holistic model as patient advocate and educator. By focusing on patient autonomy, mental health, and community-based peer support, health care providers could help intersexed individuals grow up to be socially and sexually functional adults with healthy self-esteem (Chase, 1999; Dreger, 1998; Kessler, 1998).

Perpetuating Sex and Gender Stereotypes

Although physicians and other health care professionals may be guilty of misleading parents and deceiving their intersexed children through the charade of "finding the child's 'true' sex," there is no health care conspiracy to preserve and protect the established cultural system of sex and gender. As Elliott (1998) notes, physicians treat intersexed children the way they do because they see the world as divided into boys and girls, men and women. They hope to spare these children ridicule, shame, and misery as they grow up in a culture that accepts sexual dimorphism as fact. Yet though physicians are motivated by benevolence rather than an ideological crusade to save our culture from sexual chaos, the traditional treatment nonetheless reflects gender stereotypes, fear of homosexuality, and professional arrogance.

Preserving female fertility is considered more essential that preserving sexual sensitivity in women. A clitoris that is longer than one centimeter in length is considered "cosmetically offensive" in girls and is generally surgically reduced with a resulting loss of sexual sensitivity. On the other hand, genetic males whose stretched penile length is less than 2.5 centimeters are usually reconstructed as females, including the removal of fertile testes. A great deal is expected of a "functional" penis, including the capacity for erection, penetration of a vagina, and ejaculation. An adequate vagina, on the other hand, is defined simply in terms of a receptive space. Not surprisingly, feminists and many intersexed adults object to the presumption that there is a "right" way to be female or male and that everyone must be made to fit these categories (Dreger, 1998). It is surprising that so few long-term studies have been done to determine the real life experiences of surgically altered intersexed adults and that physician groups have actively refused efforts by intersexed adults to share their experiences (Chase, 1999; Dreger, 1998). Whether they consciously choose to or not, health care providers wield tremendous power to shape our social reality. It is critically important that they and all members of society consider whose interests are served and whose are harmed or ignored by the social construction of sex and gender through the treatment of intersexed children (Sherwin, 1992).

Contributions of Feminist Epistemology

Epistemology is the study of knowledge—what we can know and how we can know it. Feminists have developed a number of theories about practices that produce knowledge. These theories go beyond Gilligan's claim that women tend to see moral problems differently in two ways (Wolf, 1996). First, feminists do not group all females under the category of "woman," nor do they suggest that all women experience the world in the same way. Second, feminists are concerned with investigating the broader relationship between power, gender, and the means of generating authoritative knowledge. These relationships and the practices that produce knowledge will vary in different circumstances and contexts. The process of knowing is always contextual and it is critical to attend to these differences.

Clearly, feminist epistemologies diverge from the view that ethics must begin from an impersonal, universal, and objective perspective. Many philosophers assume, as noted in Chapter 1 (pp. 14–15), that ethical judgments are valid only if derived from universal truths. Feminists reject this claim as infeasible, because the process of knowing is shaped by many aspects, including gender, race, class, personal history, family of origin, and so on. Knowing is more than an expression of individual feelings. Feminists are pluralists who insist that knowledge claims must be justified through a careful process of reasoned reflection and accept that these claims may conflict with those of other persons or groups. But critical reflection and empathetic dialogue create the possibility for links among the various communal conversations or what Haraway calls "webs of connection" (cited in Mahowald, 1996).

Given the oppression in our societies, some perspectives will be more privileged and thus more normative than others. As we have seen, the more privileged perspectives have an authoritative role in the social construction of reality, including what counts as illness or health. Health care ethics has championed "the patient," but feminists ask whose voice has not been heard. These voices and their perspectives offer insights into what is wrong and what needs to be changed in the current health care system. The goal is "the expansion of democracy in the production of knowledge" (Alcoff & Potter cited in Wolf, 1996). It is not simply an expansion to include more diverse experts, however. Health care ethics has largely been limited to discussion among bioethicists, medical and scientific experts, and governmental authorities. Yet Wolf (1996) is surely right when she argues that communal dialogue should include lay people and especially those most affected and potentially disadvantaged (such as women and intersexed individuals) by the outcome of ethical deliberations.

Health care ethics has tended to focus on what physicians or medical researchers should do. Feminist epistemology would require an equally vigorous analysis of health care issues from the standpoint of diverse patients, subordinate health care professionals and workers, research subjects, and community members (Wolf, 1996). New issues would be raised as a result of expanding the epistemological community, including how patients access the health care system, how and where care is delivered, what alternatives to Western medicine may be preferable, and how health care providers, researchers, and insurers can be held more accountable. More responsiveness to the distinct health needs of oppressed groups would be required. Inclusion of oppressed groups would surely also inspire more intensive discussion about how health care services should be defined. Issues of poor nutrition, lack of shelter, unsafe working and living conditions, abuse, addictions, and deficient prenatal services would become more prominent (Sherwin, 1994; Wolf, 1996).

Feminists insist that social and organizational structures shape the means of generating knowledge and that these means in turn shape these structures. Thus, expanding the epistemological community would also mandate a restructuring of health care practices. As patients and subordinate health care professionals/workers become more engaged in deliberations that shape their lives, they can develop and investigate new models for restructuring power relations that are associated with healing. The final section of this chapter will explore some possibilities for expanding the health care dialogue and restructuring power relations.

Models for Restructuring

Feminist health care ethics seeks not only to analyze hierarchies of power in health care but also to develop strategies to eliminate oppression. Those in positions of power and privilege rarely invite the less privileged to share the tasks of defining goals, shaping organizations, and determining operating procedures. A feminist health care ethics will be committed to empower marginalized groups to develop their voices and to assume leadership roles. Leaders generally acknowledge the importance of listening to constituents. But empowering marginalized groups involves much more than gathering input from focus groups. The point is not to merely "add on" new insights to the existing health care system but to extend to *all* who work within health care and those who are served by it the opportunity to shape the health care structures that so significantly affect their lives.

The Women and Children with AIDS Program at Chicago's Cook County Hospital exemplifies the process of empowering marginalized persons. In the late 1980s, when AIDS was considered a disease that primarily affected men, staff at Cook County Hospital realized that though services for gay men and male intravenous drug users were readily available in Chicago, no services existed for women and children with AIDS. A group of Cook County physicians, nurses, and social workers set out to address this urgent need.

Through dialogue with female patients, the staff came to understand that medical and social needs were inseparable. From the beginning, the program incorporated peer support groups within the standard of care, which benefited women who were isolated and neglected by their communities (Corea, 1992). The group setting also provided an opportunity for the women to identify for themselves their needs and concerns and then to educate the "experts" at Cook County about their experiences with HIV (Wilkerson, 1998).

As the Cook County team learned, "nonmedical" concerns profoundly impacted the progression of HIV in these women and their children. Their roles as women, mothers, and members of poor urban communities had to be addressed in order to develop an effective treatment program, placing their medical needs within a broader psychosocial context. Comprehensive support services were developed and provided at the same site where the women and children received medical care. Services included child care, professional counseling (especially for the alcohol and drug abuse that frequently accompany AIDS), health education, case managers to help women secure the medical and financial assistance they were entitled to, and legal advice (McClory, 1991). Support groups continued to provide feedback about medical and social issues the women were facing. Services were developed, modified, and discontinued as a result of this feedback.

Nurturing community leadership begins with cultivation of self-esteem and group pride. The Women and Children with AIDS program nurtured what its facilitators referred to as "the evolution of dignity." In their peer groups, women began to model for each other assertive behavior and strategies needed to secure assistance from large, unresponsive institutions. They developed strategies for negotiating condom use by their partners. Interested group members were further empowered through training as paid peer HIV-prevention educators for their communities (Corea, 1992). As the women learned to articulate their needs, advocate for themselves, and reach out to their communities, the response of their peers and the Cook County health team reflected their strengths and successes.

The Women and Children with AIDS program is one example of the feminist project of empowering marginalized groups to participate in shaping health care structures and the larger communities that affect their lives. These projects will vary widely based on their diverse contexts but programs that succeed in empowering marginalized groups can be characterized by several elements described in Box 6–5 (Belenky, Bond, & Weinstock, 1991; Staples, 1999; Wilkerson, 1998). Nurses who are committed to educating and empowering their patients are well positioned to support this process of development.

Whether in clinic, hospital, community health, or extended care facilities, opportunities abound for nurses to initiate efforts to restructure power relations that oppress and marginalize women and others in health care institutions. Nurses can begin by acknowledging the insights and strengths of women patients and then invite them to participate in designing alternative structures and practices within health care.

Box 6–6 explores issues related to the ongoing process of empowering nursing within the hierarchical health care structure. Changes have occurred in nursing, but more remains to be done as nurses strive to transcend their traditional position as an oppressed group. Nurses can learn from other marginalized groups who have found creative ways to resist oppressive practices and to restructure the power relationships that oppress them.

Box 6–5   Elements of Successful Empowerment Programs in Health Care

- **Create dialogue** aimed at developing a community–professional partnership. Leaders should invite people to tell their personal stories and draw out their thinking by asking good questions. Attention should be given to minimizing status differences between professionals and community members. Cultural differences should be recognized and incorporated into meeting conduct.
- **Conduct a community assessment** of resources and needs, an ongoing, cyclical process of generating and implementing ideas.
- **Nurture community leadership.** Professionals should apprentice themselves to community leaders who can teach them what they need to know about a given community. They should also assume that all community members offer insights and strengths, refrain from criticizing their ideas, and strive to understand why community members think a certain way.
- **Develop interventions** for health improvement by helping both community members and professionals understand how their communities could and should be organized. Encourage communities to consider health problems within the larger context of broader social forces.
- **Implement, monitor, and evaluate interventions.** Mirror strengths and successes to provide encouragement as projects develop.

Box 6–6   Communities in Dialogue:

Liberating Nursing from Its Oppression

Nurses continue to feel devalued as a result of managerial and medical dominance in health care. Empowerment of nursing requires understanding the cycle
of internalized self-hatred and the development of a more positive self-image.
Roberts proposes a model of identity development for nursing based on models
of other oppressed groups, including women and African Americans (Roberts,
2000). She proposes five steps toward nursing's liberation: (1) understanding
and talking about the dynamics that have perpetuated the system; (2) developing personal and professional pride through the celebration of their history,
developing a new positive voice, and taking it public; (3) developing a cohesive
nursing group through the reidentification of nursing leaders with staff nurses
and supporting leadership roles for nurses outside of administrative and education roles; (4) a synthetic stage in which the nurse becomes more able to work
in interdisciplinary groups and regains an ability to evaluate coworkers as individuals rather than as members of a group; and (5) involvement in activities
aimed at changing the hierarchical structure of health care as well as addressing
broader issues of social justice.

Questions

1. How can nurses apply the resources of a nursing health care ethics to this
   process of liberation?
2. Where do you anticipate the most resistance to this process within nursing
   and why?
3. When nurses return to school for a bachelor's degree or for graduate study,
   they often feel unsettled and disconnected from their co-workers. How can
   these nurses use the new insights of their education to facilitate the process
   of empowering nurses and developing group cohesion?
4. What obstacles impede the involvement of staff nurses in professional leadership roles? How can these impediments be removed?

Conclusion

Sexism permeates our culture. It limits the options available to women simply
because they are women. This sexism has shaped nursing's history and identity. It
continues to be a fact in the power imbalances within health care today that affect not
only nurses but the communities they serve. Committed as they are to holistic care,
nurses must not overlook the moral and health costs of this oppression. They can
advocate for themselves and for their communities, empowering themselves and others to resist and transform the oppressive practices within health care. Feminist ethics

Box 6–7   Feminist Ethics Summary

Primary Questions

♦ How are women harmed by their subordination to men under patriarchy? How are men harmed by patriarchy?

♦ How can relationships, social practices, and institutions be restructured to empower women and men?

Key Features

♦ The subordination of women (and other groups) is morally wrong and harms both women and men.

♦ Traditional theories of ethics have denigrated women as moral agents and devalued their moral experience. Feminists assert that the moral experiences of women are as worthy of respect as that of men, though both must be critically assessed.

♦ Committed to identifying and eliminating oppressive imbalances of power, especially those based on gender.

♦ Other moral questions and judgments are considered only if the act or practice in question is not itself one of a set of interlocking practices that maintains oppressive structures.

♦ Critique of oppression must be contextual: Particular practices must be critically examined in their actual context and circumstances.

♦ Feminist ethics seeks to design alternative ways to restructure relationships, social practices, and institutions in ways that will empower women and men.

♦ Feminist ethics also explores justifiable ways to resist oppressive practices.

provides nurses and others with resources they need for understanding, critiquing, and restructuring the relationships, practices, and institutions that are part of patriarchy. Box 6–7 highlights key features of feminist ethics.

KEY POINTS

• The commitment to eliminating the subordination of women (and other oppressed groups) distinguishes feminist ethics from other ethical theories.

• Although feminism provided resources for the critique of a subordinate nursing role, nursing's relation to feminism has been ambivalent.

• The history of Western ethics reveals a number of ways in which traditional ethics has privileged the interests of men over those of women and a culturally masculine perspective over a feminine one.

- Care ethics develops a distinctively feminine approach to morality that revalues the moral perspective of women and those, including nurses, who perform the "feminine" work of caregiving.
- Care ethics is a feminist ethics, insofar as it recognizes that the tendency of traditional theories to make male experience normative has contributed to women's subordination. Feminists, however, also note the tendency of a sexist culture to distort and deform the process of caring.
- Feminist health care ethicists seek to understand how health care perpetuates hierarchies of power and contributes to the social construction of reality.
- Respect for persons includes understanding people as members of social groups and recognizing that some harms achieve the status of injustice only when one considers group identity.
- Feminist epistemology calls for the inclusion of voices from the margins of health care whose perspectives offer special insights into what is wrong with and what needs to be changed in the current health care system.
- Nurses can play a critical role in the feminist project of transforming health care institutions through coalition building, partnerships, advocacy, and community empowerment.

REFLECT AND DISCUSS

1. Explain how feminist ethics includes both critical and constructive tasks.
2. How do feminists support their claim that women are oppressed by patriarchy, while men are harmed but not oppressed by it? How does this distinction influence the experience of male nurses and female physicians?
3. If the oppression of women is so pervasive inside and outside of health care, why are women (including many nurses) reluctant to acknowledge it? Since nurses are by far the largest group of health care professionals and women outnumber men as health consumers, how is patriarchy "enforced" or maintained in the health care system?
4. Care ethics may be described as an embryonic feminist ethic. How does care ethics promote the goals of feminist ethics, particularly in nursing? How might an emphasis on nurses' caring abilities without a critical analysis of gender-based power imbalances in health care encourage continued oppression of nurses?
5. Reconsider the case in Chapter 4, Box 4–6, regarding the use of quality improvement instruments. What insights does a feminist ethics perspective add to your assessment of this case? How might the nurses in this case redesign their policies for peer evaluation in light of feminist principles?
6. Some critics of feminist ethics argue that there should be no "men's ethic" or "women's ethic" but instead a humanistic ethic that applies to all. Some even argue that feminist ethics creates a new version of sexist ethics. Is feminist ethics sexist? Should the goal of ethical theory be to create a gender-free, humanistic ethics?
7. What do feminists mean when they say that gender and sex are socially constructed? How are they constructed and by whom? Give some examples. What implications does the medical treatment of intersexed individuals have for all of us?

8. If basic concepts such as sex and gender are socially constructed, then certainly ethical concepts such as right, wrong, good, bad, just, and unjust are as well. So are ethical beliefs simply a matter of preference or arbitrary choice? How do the approaches of feminist epistemology and ethical pluralism help us to answer this question?

REFERENCES

Alcoff, L. (1995). Cultural feminism versus post-structuralism: Identity crisis in feminist theory. In N. Tuana, & R. Tong (Eds.), *Feminism and philosophy: Essential readings in theory, reinterpretation, and application* (pp. 434–456). Boulder, CO: Westview Press.

Almond, B. (1988). Women's right: Reflections on ethics and gender. In M. Griffiths & M. Whitford (Eds.), *Feminist perspectives in philosophy* (pp. 42–57). Bloomington, IN: Indiana University Press.

American Academy of Pediatrics (1996). Timing of elective surgery on the genitals of male children with particular reference to the risks, benefits, and psychological effects of surgery and anesthesia. *Pediatrics, 97*(4), 590–594.

Anderson, F., Maloney, J., Oliver, D., Brown, D., & Hardy, M. (1996). Nurse–physician communication: Perceptions of nurses at an army medical center. *Military Medicine, 161,* 411–415.

Andrist, L. (1997). A feminist model for women's health care. *Nursing Inquiry, 4,* 268–274.

Baldwin, D. (1995). Territoriality and power in the health professions. In Final Report of the Council on Graduate Medical Education, National Advisory Council on Nurse Education and Practice, *Report on primary care workforce projections* (pp. 1–36). Washington, DC: U.S. Department of Health and Human Services.

Bandman, E. E., & Bandman, B. (1985). *Nursing ethics in the life span.* Norwalk, CT: Appleton-Century-Crofts.

Bartky, S. (1990). Feeding egos and tending wounds: Deference and disaffection in women's emotional labor. In S. Bartky (Ed.), *Femininity and domination* (pp. 98–119). New York: Routledge.

Beardsley, E. H. (1990). Race as a factor in health. In R. D. Apple (Ed.), *Women, Health, and Medicine in America* (pp. 121–140). New Brunswick, NJ: Rutgers University Press.

Bebeau, M. J., & Brabeck, M. (1989). Ethical sensitivity and moral reasoning among men and women in the professions. In M. Brabeck (Ed.), *Who cares?* New York: Praeger.

Belenky, M. F., Bond, L. A., & Weinstock, J. S. (1997). *A tradition that has no name: Nurturing the development of people, families, and communities.* New York: Basic Books.

Benjamin, M., & Curtis, J. (1981). *Ethics in nursing.* New York: Oxford University Press.

Benner, P. (1984/2001). *From novice to expert: Excellence and power in clinical nursing practice.* Menlo Park, CA: Addison-Wesley.

_____. (1991). The role of experience, narrative, and community in skilled ethical comportment. *Advances in Nursing Science, 14,* 1–21.

Benner, P., & Wrubel, J. (1989). *The primacy of caring: Stress and coping in clinical nursing practice.* Menlo Park, CA: Addison-Wesley.

Bent, K. (1993). Perspectives on critical and feminist theory in developing nursing praxis. *Journal of Professional Nursing, 9*(5), 296–303.

Berger, P. L., & Luckmann, T. (1966). *The social construction of reality.* Garden City, NY: Anchor.

Bishop, A., & Scudder, J. R. Jr. (1985). *Caring, curing, coping.* Birmingham, AL: University of Alabama Press.

Boston Women's Health Book Collective (1992). *The new our bodies, ourselves.* New York: Simon & Schuster.

Bowden, P. (1997). *Caring: Gender-sensitive ethics.* London: Routledge.

Bowman, A. M. (1993). Victim blaming in nursing. *Nursing Outlook, 41*(6), 268–273.

Card, C. (1990). Gender and moral luck. In V. Held (Ed.), *Justice and care: Essential readings in feminist ethics* (1995) (pp. 79–98). Boulder, CO: Westview Press.

Chase, C. (1996). Re: Measurement of evoked potentials during feminizing genitoplasty: Techniques and applications (letter). *Journal of Urology, 156*(3), 1139–1140.

_____. (1999). Rethinking treatment for ambiguous genitalia. *Pediatric Nursing, 25*(4), 451–455.

Chinn, P. L., & Wheeler, C. E. (1985). Feminism and nursing: Can nursing afford to remain aloof from the women's movement? *Nursing Outlook, 33*(2), 74–77.

Colapinto, J. (2000). *As nature made him: The boy who was raised as a girl.* New York: HarperCollins.

Corea, G. (1992). *The invisible epidemic: The story of women and AIDS.* New York: HarperCollins.

Clarke, A. E. (1990). Women's health: Life-cycle issues. In R.A. Apple (Ed.), *Women, health, and medicine in America.* New Brunswick, NJ: Rutgers University Press.

Cooper, M. C. (1991). Principle-oriented ethics and the ethic of care. A creative tension. *Advances in Nursing Science, 14*(2), 22–31.

Cortese, A. J. (1990). *Ethnic ethics: The restructuring of moral theory.* Albany, NY: State University of New York Press.

Council on Ethical and Judicial Affairs. (1990). Black-white disparities in health care. *Journal of the American Medical Association, 263,* 2344–2346.

_____. (1991). Gender disparities in clinical decision making. *Journal of the American Medical Association, 266*(4), 559–562.

Curtin, L., & Flaherty, J. (1982). *Nursing ethics: Theories and pragmatics.* Bowie, MD: Brade.

Davis, A. J., & Aroskar, M. A. (1983). *Ethical dilemmas in nursing practice.* Norwalk, CT: Appleton-Century, Crofts.

Davis, D. (1985). Nursing: An ethic of caring. *Humane Medicine Journal, 2*(1), 19–25.

De Beauvoir, S. (1961). *The second sex.* New York: Bantam (original work published 1949).

Diamond, M., & Sigmundson, H. K. (1997). Sex reassignment at birth: A long term review and clinical implications. *Archives of Pediatric and Adolescent Medicine, 150,* 298–304.

Dreger, A. D. (1998). "Ambiguous sex"-or ambivalent medicine? Ethical issues in the treatment of intersexuality. *Hastings Center Report, 28*(3), 24–35.

Ehrenreich, B., & English, D. (1978). *For her own good: 150 years of the experts' advice to women.* Garden City, NY: Anchor Books.

Elliott, C. (1998). Why can't we go on as three? *Hastings Center Report, 28*(3), 36–39.

Engels, F. (1942). *The origin of the faimly, private property and the state.* New York: International Publishers (original work published 1884).

Faden, R., Kass, N., & McGraw, D. (1996). In S. M. Wolf (Ed). *Feminism & bioethics: Beyond reproduction* (pp. 252–281). New York: Oxford University Press.

Fausto-Sterling, A. (2000). *Sexing the body: Gender politics and the construction of sexuality.* New York: Basic Books.

Freire, P. (1971). *Pedagogy of the Oppressed.* New York: Herder & Herder.

Friedman, M. (1987). Beyond caring: The de-moralization of gender. In M. Hanen & K. Nielsen (Eds.), *Science, morality, & feminist theory* (pp. 87–110). Calgary, Alberta, Canada: University of Calgary Press.

Fry, S. (1992). The role of caring in a theory of nursing ethics. In H. B. Holmes & L. M. Purdy (Eds.), *Feminist Perspectives in Medical Ethics* (pp. 93–106). Bloomington, IN: Indiana University Press.

Frye, M. (1983). *The politics of reality: Essays in feminist theory.* Freedom Press, CA: Crossing Press.

Gadow, S. (1985). Nurse and patient: The caring relationship. In A. Bishop & J. Scudder (Eds.), *Caring, curing, coping: Nurse, physician, patient relationships.* Birmingham, AL: University of Alabama Press.

Gadow, S. (1988). Covenant without cure: Letting go and holding on in chronic illness. In J. Watson & M. Ray (Eds.), *The ethics of care and the ethics of cure: Synthesis in Chronicity* (pp. 31–43). New York: National League of Nursing.

Gastman, C. (1999). Care as a moral attitude in nursing. *Nursing Ethics: An International Journal for Health Care Professionals, 6*(3), 214–223.

Gilligan, C. (1982). *In a different voice: Psychological theory and women's development.* Cambridge, MA: Harvard University Press.

Gilligan, C., & Attanucci, J. (1988). Two moral orientations: Gender differences and similarities. *Merrill-Palmer Quarterly, 34,* 223–237.

Goode, W. J. (1989). Why men resist. In S. Skolnick & J. Skolnick (Eds.), *Family in transition* (pp. 163–179). Glenview, IL: Scott, Freeman, and Co.

Growe, S. (1991). *Who Cares? The crisis in Canadian nursing.* Toronto, Ontario: McClelland & Stewart.

Harding, S. (1987). The curious coincidence of feminine and African moralities. In E. F. Kittay & D.T. Meyers (Eds.), *Women and moral theory* (pp. 296–315). Totowa, NJ: Rowman & Littlefield.

Held, V. (1993). *Feminist morality: Transforming culture, society, and politics.* Chicago:University of Chicago Press.

Hine, D. C. (1989). *Black women in white: Racial conflict and cooperation in the nursing profession, 1890–1950.* Bloomington, IN: Indiana University Press.

Hochschild, A. (1997). *The time bind: When work becomes home & home becomes work.* New York: Henry Holt & Company.

Horowitz, A. (1985). Sons and daughters as caregivers to older parents: Differences in role performances. *The Gerontologist, 25,* (6), 612–617.

Houston, B. (1989). Prolegomena to future caring. In M. M. Brabeck (Ed), *Who cares? Theory, research, and educational implications of the ethic of care* (pp. 84–100). New York: Praeger Publishers.

Jaggar, A. M. (1991). Feminist ethics: Projects, problems, prospects. In C. Card (Ed.), *Feminist ethics* (pp. 78–104). Lawrence, KS: University of Kansas Press.

Jaggar, A. (1992). Feminist ethics. In L. Becker & C. Becker (Eds.), *Encyclopedia of ethics* (pp. 361–370). New York: Garland.

Jameton, A. (1984). *Nursing practice: The ethical issues.* Upper Saddle River, NJ: Prentice Hall.

Johnson, A. G. (1997). *The gender knot: Unraveling our patriarchal legacy.* Philadelphia: Temple University Press.

Jones, H. W. III, Wentz, A. C., & Burnett, L. S. (1988). *Novak's textbook of gynecology* (11th ed.). Baltimore: Williams & Wilkins.

Kessler, S. (1998). *Lessons from the intersexed.* New Brunswick, NJ: Rutgers University Press.

Kohlberg, L. (1958). *The development of modes of thinking and choices in years 10 to 16.* Doctoral dissertation, University of Chicago.

_____. (1981). *The philosophy of moral development.* San Francisco: Harper & Row.

Kuhse, H. (1997). *Caring: Nurses, women and ethics.* Oxford: Blackwell.

Leininger, M. (Ed.). (1984). *Care: The essence of nursing and health.* Thorofare, NJ: Slack.

Lennon, M. C., & Rosenfield, S. (1994). Relative fairness and the division of housework. *American Journal of Sociology 100,* 506–531.

Lorber, J. (1989). Dismantling Noah's ark. In B. J. Risman & P. Schwartz (Eds.), *Gender in intimate relationships: A microstructural approach* (pp. 53–67). Belmont, CA: Wadsworth.

Mahowald, M. B. (1996). On treatment of myopia: Feminist standpoint theory and bioethics. In S. M. Wolf (Ed.), *Feminism & bioethics: Beyond reproduction* (pp. 99–115). New York: Oxford University Press.

Martin, E. (1987). *The woman in the body: A cultural analysis of reproduction.* Boston: Beacon Press.

McBride, A. B. (1997). Nursing and the women's movement. *Reflections 23*(3), 38–41.

McCall, E. (1996). Horizontal violence in nursing. *The Lamp, 53*(3):28–29, 31.

McClory, R. (1991, February 1). HIV's neglected victims: Women and children last. *Chicago Reader.*

Merton, V. (1996). Ethical obstacles to the participation of women in biomedical research. In S. M. Wolf (Ed.), *Feminism & bioethics: Beyond reproduction* (pp. 216–251). New York: Oxford University Press.

Meyers, J. (1994). Working in the Grey Zone: The Moral Suffering of Critical Care Nurses. Unpublished masters thesis, Gonzaga University, Spokane,WA.

Mill, J. S. (1988). *The subjection of women.* Indianapolis: Hackett Publishing (original work published in 1869).

Money, J. (1955). Hermaphroditism, gender and precocity in hyperadrenocorticism: Psycological findings. *John Hopkins Medical Journal, 96,* 253–264.

Money, J., & Ehrhardt, A. A. (1972). *Man and woman, boy and girl.* Baltimore: John Hopkins University Press.

Nelson, H. L., & Nelson, J. L. (1996). Justice in the allocation of health care resources. In S. M. Wolf (Ed.), *Feminism & Bioethics: Beyond reproduction* (pp. 351–370). New York: Oxford University Press.

Newman, D. M. (1995). *Sociology: Exploring the architecture of everyday life.* Thousand Oaks, CA: Pine Forge Press.

Noddings, N. (1984). *Caring: A feminine approach to ethics and moral education.* Berkeley, CA: University of California Press.

Parker, L. A. (1998). Ambiguous genitalia: Etiology, treatment, and nursing implications. *Journal of Obstetric, Gynecologic, and Neonatal Nursing, 27,* 15–22.

Ray, M. (1987). Technological caring: A new model in critical care. *Dimensions of Critical Care Nursing 6*(3), 166–173.

Reverby, S. (1987). *Ordered to care: The dilemma of American nursing, 1850–1945.* Cambridge: Cambridge University Press.

Rinehart, J. A. (1998). It may be a polar night of icy darkness, but feminists are building a fire. In M. Alfino, J. S. Caputo, & R. Wynyard (Eds.), *McDonaldization revisited: Critical essays on consumer culture* (pp. 19–38). Westport, CT: Praeger Publishers.

Roberts, D. E. (1996). Reconstructing the patient: Starting with women of color. In S. M. Wolf (Ed.), *Feminism & bioethics: Beyond reproduction* (pp. 116–143). New York: Oxford Univeristy Press.

Roberts, S. J. (1983). Oppressed group behavior: Implications for nursing. *Advances in Nursing Science, 5*(3), 21–30.

_____. (2000). Development of a positive professional identity: Liberating oneself from the oppressor within. *Advanced Nursing Science, 22*(4), 71–82.

Ruddick, S. (1989). *Maternal thinking: Toward a politics of peace.* Boston: Beacon Press.

Sampselle, C. M. (1990). The influence of feminist philosophy in nursing practice. *IMAGE: Journal of Nursing Scholarship, 22*(4), 243–247.

Sanday, P. R. (1981). The socio-cultural context of rape: A cross-cultural study. *Journal of Social Issues, 37,* 5–27.

Sherwin, S. (1992). *No longer patient: Feminist ethics and health care.* Philadelphia: Temple University Press.

_____. (1994). Women in clinical studies: A feminist view. In Institute of Medicine, *Report of the committee on the legal and ethical issues relating to the inclusion of women in clinical research* (pp. 11–17). Washington, DC: National Academy Press.

Stein, L. I. (1968). The doctor–nurse game. *American Journal of Nursing, 68,* 101–105.

_____. (1990). The doctor–nurse game. *American Journal of Nursing, 20,* 159–164.

Tavris, C. (1992). *The mismeasure of woman.* New York: Simon & Schuster.

Todd, A. D. (1989). *Intimate adversaries: Cultural conflict between physicians and women patients.* Philadelphia, PA: University of Pennsylvania Press.

Tong, R. (1993). *Feminine and feminist ethics.* Belmont, CA: Wadsworth.

Townes, E. M. (1998). *Breaking the fine rain of death: African American health care and a womanist ethic of care.* New York: Continuum Publishing Group.

Walker, L. J. (1984). Sex differences in the development of moral reasoning. *Child Development, 55,* 677–691.

Walker, L. J., deVries, B., & Trevethan, S. D. (1987). Moral stages and moral orientations in real life and hypothetical dilemmas. *Child Development, 58*(3), 842–858.

Watson, J. (1985). *Nursing: Human science and human care.* Norwalk, CT: Appleton-Century-Crofts.

Wennecker, M. B., & Epstein, A. M. (1989). Racial inequalities in the use of procedures for patients with ischemic heart disease in Massachusetts. *Journal of the American Medical Association, 261,* 253–257.

Whitbeck, C. (1984). The maternal instinct. In J. Treblicot (Ed.), *Mothering: Essays in feminist theory* (pp. 185–198). Totowa, NJ: Rowman & Allanfield, 1984.

Whittle, J., Congligliaro, J., Good, C. B., & Lofgren, R. P. (1993). Racial differences in the use of invasive cardiovascular procedures in the Department of Veterans Affairs Medical System. *New England Journal of Medicine, 329,* 621–627.

Wilkerson, A. L. (1998). *Diagnosis: Difference.* Ithaca, NY: Cornell University Press.

Wolf, S. M. (1996). Introduction: Gender and feminism in bioethics. In S. M. Wolf (Ed.), *Feminism & bioethics: Beyond reproduction* (pp. 3–43). New York: Oxford University Press.

Wollstonecraft, M. (1965). *A vindication of the rights of woman.* London: Dent (original work published 1792).

Young, I. M. (1990). *Justice and the politics of difference.* Princeton, NJ: Princeton University Press.

_____. (1994). Punishment, treatment, empowerment: Three applications to policy for pregnant addicts. *Feminist Studies, 20*(1), 33–57.

7

Applying Feminist Ethics

*F*eminists do not seek to develop a single, comprehensive, and universal theory that can be applied to every ethical issue. Rather than a single theory, feminist ethics is a common project to which a number of theorists are committed, a project distinguished by the commitment to eliminate the subordination of women (and the interrelated oppression of other groups). Feminists do not argue that issues of oppression are the only important ethical issues or that all other ethical issues can somehow be subsumed under the issue of oppression. They do not believe that a feminist ethical perspective is the only useful viewpoint from which to critically assess and resolve ethical issues. But insofar as oppression permeates relationships, organizations, and social institutions, feminists insist that considerations of oppressive power imbalances must be central to our ethical analysis of any issue. Ethical analysis of oppression and constructive alternatives must be combined with other considerations to address the multitude of moral dilemmas that confront human communities.

1. Identify the problem or issue.
2. Analyze context.
3. Explore options.
4. Apply the decision process.
5. Implement the plan and evaluate results.

Within the context of feminist ethics, this chapter considers eating disorders, especially among children and adolescents. Eating disorders are clearly a health problem, with physiological and psychosocial dimensions. But as this chapter will explore, these disorders emerge as well from significant gender-related influences. The chapter will demonstrate the application of the framework for ethical analysis introduced in Chapter 1 and reviewed here in Box 7–1. In step 4, a feminist ethics decision process is applied to the issue of eating disorders. The chapter concludes with a discussion of additional issues in nursing that would benefit from a feminist ethical analysis.

Eating Disorders

Step 1. Identify the Problem or Issue

Eating disorders are chronic syndromes affecting more than eight million people in the United States. The most common eating disorders—anorexia nervosa, bulimia nervosa, and binge eating—are on the rise in the United States and around the world. More than 90 percent of those with eating disorders are women, though the incidence among males is increasing (American Anorexia Bulimia Association, 2000; Department of Health and Human Services [DHHS], 2000). Eating disorders are widespread among all groups of women. Males with eating disorders, on the other hand, are most commonly found within specific subgroups such as wrestlers, dancers, and homosexuals (DHHS; Strong, Williamson, Netemeyer, & Geer, 2000). Because eating disorders are not widespread among men and often appear to be linked to particular male subgroups and activities, we will examine the issue of eating disorders primarily as it affects women.

Eating disorders are clearly an important health issue, especially for young women. Feminists believe that eating disorders and their treatment are also an ethical issue. Although eating disorders are complex, with multiple contributing factors, feminists believe that they result to a significant degree from the oppression of women in Western cultures. Causal explanations of eating disorders are controversial, however, and consequently, so are treatment approaches.

Although those in mainstream health care sometimes acknowledge feminist positions on eating disorders, they generally dismiss the feminist perspective as simply "theoretical" (see Grothaus, 1998, for example). Primary medical models for treatment of eating disorders not only ignore this perspective but often prescribe treatments that are contraindicated from a feminist viewpoint. *Ethical issues to be explored in this chapter include how women are harmed by exclusion of a feminist perspective on eating disorders and how inclusion of this perspective might alter treatment approaches.*

An overview of eating disorders will help to focus our examination of the applications of feminist ethics. Eighty-six percent of those with eating disorders develop the condition before age 21, with the majority of eating disorders developing between ages 12 and 18 (Chally, 1998; Grothaus, 1998). Eating disorders are one of the major health problems affecting children and adolescent females in the United States and other Western countries. The U.S. Department of Health and Human Services' Office on Women's Health estimates that 1 to 4 percent of all young women in the United States are currently affected by eating disorders (DHHS, 2000; National Institute of Mental Health, 2000). Although most prevalent among adolescents and young adults, they may continue for decades (Tiggemann & Steven, 1999; White, 2000).

Anorexia and bulimia are most common among middle- and upper-class Caucasian girls and young women. Nevertheless, increasing numbers of cases are being seen across all different ethnic and cultural groups. Variations may exist in the specific nature of eating problems as well as risk and protective factors, but no population is exempt (DHHS, 2000; Hesse-Biber, Marino, & Watts-Roy, 1999; Miller et al., 2000).

TYPES OF EATING DISORDERS

Several researchers suggest that rather than viewing eating disorders as a discrete category, anorexia nervosa and bulimia should be understood as the extreme end of a spectrum of eating disturbances (Hesse-Biber, 1989; Hsu, 1990; Shisslak, Crago, & Estes, 1995). Figure 7–1 represents this continuum of eating patterns. Normal eating and bodily satisfaction appear at one end of the continuum, while eating disorders appear at the other end. Between the continuum's two ends, we find a wide range of attitudes and behaviors related to food and body image. *Disordered eating* is a term

---

Figure 7–1 Continuum of Eating Patterns

Normal eating and bodily satisfaction	Development of risk factors	Disordered eating	Eating disorders

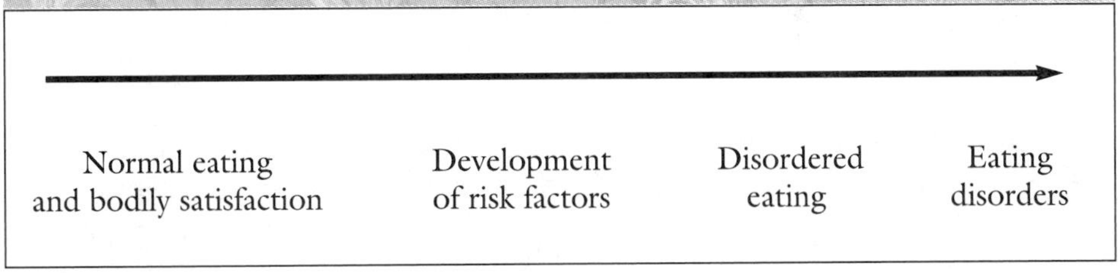

used to refer to problematic eating patterns, such as purging and binge eating, that are not sufficiently severe or don't occur often enough to be classified as clinical eating disorders (DHHS, 2000; Hesse-Biber et al., 1999).

Box 7–2 summarizes key eating disorders: anorexia nervosa, bulimia nervosa, and binge eating disorder. Presently, no universally accepted standard treatment for eating disorders exists, and relapse rates are high (DHHS, 2000). Experts agree, however, that treatment is most successful when eating disorders are diagnosed early.

Box 7–2   Summary of Eating Disorders

	Binge Eating Disorder (BED)	Anorexia Nervosa	Bulimia Nervosa
U.S. women affected	60–80% of college women engage in regular binge eating 15–50% of those in weight control programs, mostly women	1% of teenage and college women	2–3% of women 5–8% of teenage and college women 50% of anorectics develop bulimia nervosa
Typical onset	Late adolescence or early adulthood	Mid- to late adolescence	Late adolescence or early adulthood
Charac- teristics	Primarily identified by repeated episodes of uncontrolled eating Not associated with vomiting or excessive exercise to rid body of excess food Often feel out of control; experience guilt, depression, or disgust	Intense fear of fat and weight gain Weight loss is >15% of normal body weight Food/weight obsessions may include strange eating rituals, fixation on calorie/fat content, or overly rigorous exercise routines Perfectionistic and overachieving but lack self-esteem Intense need to control surroundings and emotions	Binge eating nearly always followed by purging; binges range from 1 to 2 times per day to several times per day Purging by self-induced vomiting, abuse of laxatives /diuretics, compulsive exercise, and/or fasting Many maintain normal or above body weight; bingeing /purging often done in secret; often do not seek treatment until 30s and 40s Often have difficulty with impulse control, stress, and anxiety

Box 7-2   Summary of Eating Disorders

	Binge Eating Disorder (BED)	Anorexia Nervosa	Bulimia Nervosa
Symptoms and medical complications	Often overweight due to high-calorie diet; medical problems similar to those found with obesity: high blood pressure, diabetes, high cholesterol, increased risk of gallbladder disease, heart disease, and some cancers	Starvation-related symptoms such as emaciation; dry, yellow skin with lanugo; brittle hair/nails; lowered pulse rate; loss of menstrual cycle; cold hands/feet; constipation; shortness of breath; weakness; reduced muscle mass; and swollen joints Irregular heart rhythms and heart failure; increased risk of osteoporosis Depression/anxiety; many at risk for suicide 6–7% mortality rate after 10 years and 18–20% after 20–30 years	Complications result from electrolyte imbalance and repeated purging: may include irregular heartbeat and/or cardiac arrest, heart muscle damage due to low potassium, dental problems, inflammation of esophagus, dehydration and damage to bowels, liver, and kidney Many suffer from clinical depression, obsessive–compulsive disorder, anxiety, and other psychiatric illnesses with an increased risk of suicide 0–19% mortality rate

TREATMENT PROGRAMS

Adolescents with eating disorders are treated in many types of programs and settings with a range of individual, group, and family therapy options. Most are treated in outpatient programs that employ a cognitive-behavioral treatment mode or selectively combine cognitive-behavioral principles with other approaches. Treatment usually involves a team of health care professionals that typically includes a pediatrician or internist, nutritionist, psychotherapist, and psychiatrist. Pharmacological therapies, particularly the use of antidepressants, are often utilized, but there is no definitive pharmacological approach to either anorexia nervosa or bulimia nervosa (Grothaus, 1998; Raymond, Mitchell, Fallon, & Katzman, 1994). Pressures from health insurers, however, have promoted a movement away from "the talking cure" and an increasing reliance on psychopharmaceutical management of many psychiatric disorders (Lester, 1997).

Step 2. Analyze the Context

In this section, we will explore several aspects of the context of eating disorders in Western (particularly U.S.) societies. These include psychosexual factors, cultural influences, and the impact of race, ethnicity, and sexual orientation.

PSYCHOSOCIAL FACTORS

Self-esteem is a measure of how much individuals approve of or respect themselves. Research suggests that women who have low self-esteem often have problematic eating patterns and distorted body images (Hesse-Biber et al., 1999). A significant amount of research has attempted to understand and explain the influence of families of origin on the development of self-esteem.

Family Dynamics

Hilde Bruch is perhaps the most admired and respected expert on anorexia nervosa in American medicine. She gained international notoriety for her works *Eating Disorders* (1973) and *The Golden Cage* (1979). Her work champions what has been the dominant psychotherapeutic view for the past two decades. Bruch argues that the heart of anorexia nervosa is a struggle for control by a girl who feels that although she is highly valued by her parents, she is unable to live up to what is expected of her in return. One of her patients described her predicament as that of a sparrow who feels too plain and simple for its gilded golden cage, but also restrained and limited by this cage. Bruch observed that her anorectic patients feel that they are expected by their parents to be exceptional children intellectually, athletically, and/or artistically. They also feel that somehow it is their responsibility to make their parents themselves feel successful, superior, and happy (Bruch, 1979).

The majority of Bruch's patients were from upper-middle-class and upper-class homes; a few were from upwardly mobile, success-oriented lower-middle-class and lower-class families. The families typically present themselves as well functioning, the parents expressing pride in their above-average parenting. Parents often express great surprise at their daughters' illness, noting that these young women have never been any trouble before this illness.

Below the surface of these apparently happy, harmonious families, Bruch found significant stresses. Fathers are frequently described as benevolent but removed both physically and emotionally from the lives of their daughters and absorbed in their pursuit of social and financial success. Mothers, often well-educated, intelligent women who sacrifice careers for the benefit of their families, tend to be submissive to their husbands and yet seem not to genuinely respect them. Daughters may feel a special responsibility for the well-being of their mothers or may express frustration with their mothers' submissiveness (Bruch, 1979).

In any case, young women with anorexia nervosa are excessively concerned with pleasing their parents and avoid disagreeing with their parents' choices and plans on their behalf. In these families, politeness and good behavior are absolute expectations. Feelings, particularly negative ones, are not expressed. As a result, the daughters expend enormous energy attempting to fulfill parental expectations even when what their parents want is not clearly expressed. Appearances are extremely important: The girls and their parents are preoccupied with what an action will look like, with what people will think, and with maintaining an image of success and happiness.

Bruch concludes that overprotective parents with rigid rules create an environment wherein the anorectic girl, like the sparrow trapped in the gilded cage, feels powerless and ineffective in conducting her own life and thus becomes a perfectionist who turns to control of food intake as an area in which to assert independence (Bruch, 1979, 1985). As one of Bruch's patients describes this quest for control: "You make of your own body your very own kingdom where you are the tyrant, the absolute dictator" (Bruch, 1979, p. 65).

The research literature on the families of anorectics is voluminous, and some recent analyses suggest that Bruch's description of these dysfunctional family patterns may be too simplistic (White, 2000). But there is significant agreement among psychodynamic theorists that anorectics suffer from a lack of individuation within their families of origin, overprotectiveness of parents, and rigidity in the family value system. These result in problems of autonomy, which in turn lead to a reduction of self-esteem (Frederick & Grow, 1996; Grothaus, 1998).

Less has been published about the families of bulimic patients than those of anorectic ones. Vanderlinden and colleagues (1992) report that families of bulimic patients often belong to higher social classes; control and emotional dependence are characteristic of family interactions, and strong tensions or conflicts are not directly expressed (cited in Grothaus, 1998). Other researchers have found that bulimic clients perceive their families as more distressed, less cohesive, less encouraging of independent behavior, and more controlling than women who do not experience an eating disorder (Grothaus).

There are conflicting views in the literature on the actual nature of the families of bulimic patients. Some find families that are disengaged, disorganized, and conflicted, while others find families in which individuals lack an independent sense of self (Levy & Hadley, 1998). In both cases, it is suggested that bulimic children fail to develop adequate personal authority or the ability to identify their uniqueness. This lack of individual identity contributes to lower self-esteem and the inability to form mature relationships with others. These factors are believed to contribute to the tendency of bulimics to be excessive people pleasers who lack self-control (Levy & Hadley; Brownell & Foreyt, 1986).

Negotiating Autonomy and Relationships

Psychological theorists note that self-concept is greatly influenced by how well someone is able to balance a sense of autonomy with a sense of relationship with others. Psychodynamic theorists like Bruch stress that the conflict between independence and dependence can be resolved only by a striving for increased separation and autonomy (Bruch, 1979). Psychoanalytic feminists propose, on the other hand, that a healthy self-concept is based on the development of relationships and connections to others (Chodorow, 1978; Gilligan, 1982). Steiner-Adair (1986) links the prevalence of eating disorders in adolescent girls to the cultural stress on separation and individuation at the expense of relationships. More recently, feminists Hesse-Biber and colleagues followed a group of college women with partial-syndrome eating disorders from their sophomore year to two years postcollege. Persons with partial-syndrome disorders engage in behaviors associated with eating disorders, such as bingeing, purging, use of diet pills, or fasting, but in less extreme ways than those with clinical eating disorders. Hesse-Biber and colleagues (1999) found that women in their study who got better were able to negotiate the tension between autonomy and relationship by nurturing both.

Hesse-Biber and colleagues also found that familial messages regarding weight and body satisfaction significantly influenced a woman's ability to balance autonomy and relationship. The women in their study who continued to exhibit problematic eating patterns were much more likely to grow up in families that overemphasized physical appearance and especially thinness than the women whose eating behaviors improved. Fathers, mothers, and siblings reportedly made frequent comments to the still-at-risk women about being too fat, needing to "thin down," looking chunky, or having fat bellies.

These findings are consistent with other research that shows that parental attitudes significantly affect body dissatisfaction and weight concerns, especially for girls (White, 2000). Particularly noteworthy is the finding by Streigel-Moore and Kearney-Cooke (1994, cited in White, 2000) that even when sons had higher body mass indexes (BMIs), both parents perceived their daughters as heavier relative to their height than their sons. Also worthy of note is one study's conclusion that children, especially girls, are influenced more by parental comments about their weight than by parental modeling of weight concerns and behaviors (White, 2000).

Impact of Sexual Abuse

Childhood sexual abuse has been related to eating disorders, especially bulimia nervosa. Documenting the extent of sexual abuse among those with eating disorders is fraught with difficulty because silencing of victims is a prerequisite for occurrence of such abuse. In her review of relevant research, Wooley (1994) cites reports of abuse among up to 60 percent of patients in reputable eating disorder treatment centers. The relationship between childhood sexual abuse and eating disorders is, however, a matter of intense debate in research and treatment communities.

Abuse is most frequently disclosed by female patients to female rather than male therapists. The findings of these female clinicians have largely been discounted as scientifically unreliable or simply ignored altogether. A primary reason given for this response is the unreliability of patients' self-reports without confirming controlled studies (Fairburn, 1992; Pope & Hudson, 1992, cited in Wooley, 1994). Although the process of self-reporting raises some legitimate concerns, it was via this process that researchers learned about most of the key phenomena of eating disorders, such as the drive for thinness, the denial of hunger, secret rituals of bingeing and purging, and compulsive exercising.

Although many studies based on self-reports were eventually followed up with controlled research, the earlier studies were granted provisional acceptance by the research and therapeutic community. Therapies were developed and rigorously advocated well before controlled studies became available. And reports based on clinical observations and patient descriptions were well accepted by clinicians because of their consistency. But extraordinary resistance to including sexual abuse among eating disorder risk factors (or according it importance in other ways) continues, despite more than 10 years of very consistent reports of cases and patient series (e.g., see Kearney-Cooke, 1988; Root & Fallon, 1988; Waller, 1992; Wooley, 1994). This pattern lends credibility to Wooley's assertion that "the relentless questioning of the veracity of abuse reports reflects an unwillingness to see male behavior as the cause of female illness" (1994, p. 189).

Ultimately, it is far more important for therapists and researchers to determine how to treat women with eating disorders who have a history of abuse than it is to determine the precise rates of abuse or their exact contribution to eating disorders. But achieving consensus on treatment approaches will require a greater willingness of male and female practitioners to work together to address this issue.

SOCIOCULTURAL INFLUENCES

Research has explored the influence of various sociocultural factors on disordered eating. We will focus on the post–World War II obsession with thinness, the impact of contemporary media, and the significance of class, race, and ethnicity.

Historical Perspective

Seid (1994) demonstrates the novelty and arbitrariness of current cultural beliefs about beauty, health, and eating by comparing them with the beliefs of other historical periods in Western civilization. Never before have men or women desired a body so "close to the bone." Slenderness has been admired in other eras. Fifteenth-century Gothics and sixteenth-century Mannerists painted elongated nudes, while women in the Romantic period (1830s–1850s) were encouraged to strive for tiny waists. Nonetheless, while admiring long limbs and tiny waists, the ideal woman's body of these eras was fully fleshed. Thinness was regarded as ugly and misfortunate.

In the mid- to late nineteenth century, fat was seen as a "silken layer" of elegant ladies. Dimpled flesh (cellulite!) was so desirable that thin women purchased inflatable rubber undergarments to enhance their backs, calves, shoulders, and hips. Plumpness was considered an indication of emotional well-being, a clean conscience, a good temperament, and especially, robust health. Fat was equated with a healthy reserve of energy and strength.

"Fatphobia" emerged in American society after World War II, linked to a moral concern that postwar plenty and leisure would make Americans physically and morally soft. Americans perceived themselves as flabby and unhealthy in spite of increasing life expectancy. A new ideology concerning weight was disseminated and perpetuated by insurance companies, the health industry, and the fashion industry. Insurance companies adopted the concept of "ideal weight" determined by height and bone structure. Health care providers promoted the identification of health and thinness and the belief that ideal weight is attainable by anyone through willpower and exercise. Late-twentieth-century fashions exposed to public view women's legs, thighs, and upper bodies. Women were now expected to achieve body ideals without the benefit of corsets, girdles, and other body-shaping undergarments. As Seid (1994) puts it, "the undressed body—the bare bones of being . . . had become the focus of fashion" (p. 10).

Seid notes that twentieth-century obsession with thinness has become a moralistic creed: "I eat right, watch my weight, and exercise." Virtue is quantified by numbers on the scale, BMIs, and body measurements. Thin persons are perceived as more competent, sexy, and exciting than the fat and flabby who are perceived as slothful, shameful, and disgusting. Although fashion standards of past eras were sometimes also harmful, our era is unique in its focus on the bare bones of the human body itself (Seid, 1994). A mere 5 to 10 percent of American women are physiologically capable of achieving the ideal female weight represented by many of today's actresses and models. As a result, 90 to 95 percent of American women are set up for failure.

Media Impact

American culture is a culture of "looksism" in which attractive appearance has important consequences at work, in relationships, and in the ability to generate income and influence others (Lennon, Lillethun, & Buckland, 1999; Pipher, 1994). TV, magazines, and movies reinforce the belief that women, in particular, should be more concerned with their appearance than with their ideas, achievements, or values. The American Association of University Women (1991) found that adolescent girls believe their self-esteem depends heavily on physical appearance and that their sense of self is significantly shaped by their body image.

The $130 billion advertising industry is a powerful educational force in America. The average American is exposed to over 1,500 ads every day. Cumulatively, this amounts to a year and a half of one's life watching commercials. Images in the mass media help to create and reinforce the latest ideals of body type and fashion. Women are disproportionately targeted by this advertising: Anderson and DiDomenico (1992) found that women's magazines contained 10.5 times more advertisements dealing with diet and weight loss than did men's magazines. Many people dismiss the effect of advertising and TV, noting that individual ads or TV programs are silly and mere fantasy. Research demonstrates, however, that the cumulative impact of media messages is significant (Solomon, 1992; Stephens, Hill, & Hanson, 1994). We may reject a particular product, clothing style, or personal style portrayed in the media, but we are less likely to reject the overall message about what is acceptable and what is not.

Kilbourne (1994) argues that the cumulative effect of media images on women is to make them feel inferior, anxious, and insecure: Women are taught to hate their bodies and thus learn to hate themselves. By normalizing the body type of a very small minority of women, advertising creates a huge market for products that promise to "fix" women's multiple deficiencies—their drooping breasts, disgusting cellulite, and so on.

Advertising cashes in on women's fear of fat, helping to perpetuate distorted visions of female beauty. Even the tall, thin bodies of models are further "stretched" through computer and camera tricks. Advertising also encourages food consumption. Ads portray rich, sensuous meals as a well-deserved reward for hard work or an essential aspect of socializing.

The obsessive diet-consciousness of most major women's magazines contrasts sharply with this hedonistic attitude toward food (Stephens et al., 1994). A yogurt ad, for instance, suggests "How to go from seeing yourself like this . . . to seeing yourself like this," where the "before" image is a pear. But, of course, most women are in fact pear-shaped (Kilbourne, 1994).

Advertising also reinforces the Western belief that women's bodies must be controlled. Women are, on the one hand, offered diet products that promise to make them powerful and energized. One brand of cottage cheese is touted as "Snacks for the Power Hungry," while a pantyhose ad exhorts women to "put on the power." On the other hand, the ability to control voracious appetites for food (and for power, sex, and equality) is extolled. Women are promised salvation from the temptations of sinful foods and freedom from guilt via low-fat ice cream and pizza. The message seems to be "Be independent and successful, but be feminine and non-threatening." This translates into the beauty ideal of the slim, lean, hard-bodied waif (Kilbourne, 1994).

Should a woman's self-control fail her, advertising sensationalizes self-indulgence with ads that seem to invite bingeing. Kilbourne (1994) notes this copy from an ice cream ad:

Maybe I'm a bit of a perfectionist. My CDs are in alphabetical order . . . Yet every time I have Häagen-Dasz I seem to lose control. Today, it was chocolate ice cream. I lost myself completely. Each creamy spoonful was a moment suspended in time. I would have stopped before I finished the whole pint. Only problem was, I couldn't find the lid (p. 412).

Do women really pay attention to these images and messages? Research suggests that they do. Taylor and colleagues (1998, cited in White, 2000) found that among elementary girls, the most significant predictor of weight concerns (thought to be the earliest onset symptom of eating disorders) was the importance placed on their weight and eating by their peers. The second predictor was the desire to look like girls on television, and for middle school girls it was the desire to look like models in magazines. Another study by Tiggemann and Pickening (1996, cited in White) found significant correlations between media consumption and two major traits of eating disorders. The amount of time spent by 15-year-old girls watching soaps and movies predicted body dissatisfaction, and the amount of time watching music videos related to a drive for thinness.

The pervasiveness of the "dieting mentality" in this society is truly frightening. Dieting is widely practiced regardless of weight status. Koff and Rierdan (1991) found that a large proportion of girls in their survey of 206 sixth graders were practicing weight loss behaviors, even though they did not perceive themselves as overweight. Another study found that two thirds of the black high school females and three quarters of the white females in one school district were dieting. The majority were not overweight and some were underweight (Emmons, 1996). Some estimate that on any given day in the United States, 50 percent of teenage girls are dieting (Pipher, 1994).

These facts do not necessarily imply that there is a conscious conspiracy among media producers to undermine women's health or to control their activities. Advertisers clearly do *create* and *exploit* women's anxiety about weight because it is so profitable to do so. On a deeper level, however, the media *reflects* cultural beliefs and values about women's bodies and their roles in society (Kilbourne, 1994; Faludi, 1991; Wolf, 1991).

Western Dualism and Self-Control

Bordo (1993b) notes that the philosophical history of dualism in Western culture is one of several cultural streams that converge in the anorectic syndrome. Human bodies, like all other aspects of human life, are constituted by culture. Bordo traces a dualistic heritage that comes to us from Plato, through Augustine, and then Descartes. The basic imagery of dualism remains fairly constant through this history. Human existence is bifurcated into the bodily or material realm and the mental or spiritual realm. There are central features of this dualism that turn out, Bordo observes, to comprise the basic body imagery of the anorectic.

First, the body is experienced as *alien*, something other than "me." This alien substance is "fastened and glued" to me, Plato suggests. For Descartes, it is an inanimate machine-like thing, entirely distinct from the true inner essential self—the soul or the thinking self. Second, the body is experienced as *a prison and a limitation*. All three philosophers describe the body as a prison or a cage from which the soul or mind tries to escape. Unable to escape, the soul/mind is alternately "dragged" by the body or is dragging itself about burdened by the ponderous weight of the body (Bordo, 1993b).

Clearly, the body is *the enemy*. It obscures our view, sabotages our willpower, and impedes our pursuit of truth. As a result, the body becomes the locus of *all that threatens our attempts at control*. As Bordo (1993b) puts it, "it overtakes, it overwhelms, it erupts, and disrupts" (p. 144). This enemy is so dangerous that all three philosophers instruct us in how not only to control the body, but ultimately how to kill off its desires and hungers.

Many anorectics share this same ultimate goal—to cease to experience hunger and desire. Anorectic women are as obsessed with hunger as they are with being thin. They describe their fear of being overcome by hunger, of giving in to their runaway desire for food. They experience hunger as an alien invader, an opportunistic marauder whose arrival is unpredictable (Bordo, 1993b). In fact, persons with eating disorders have difficulty identifying not only hunger, but cold, heat, and emotions as originating within themselves (Bruch, 1979).

Anorectics also echo dualism's theme of confinement in the body. Bordo (1993b) quotes one woman saying, "Please dear God, help me . . . I want to get out of my body, I want to get out!" Another woman, reflecting on her experience with anorexia, recognizes that self-starvation was an attempt to achieve her ideal of being thin by being without a body.

Bordo (1993b) does not suggest that anorectics are Platonists or Augustinians. She does argue that the images and ideals that these women articulate reflect the themes of dualism that run deeply in Western culture. Thinness represents a triumph of the will over the body; the ultrathin body—a sort of nonbody—is identified with an absolute purity and transcendence of the flesh. Fat is associated with pollution, mental decay, and evil (Bordo, 1993b).

Obviously, this dualistic view of the self is not new to contemporary Western culture. Bordo proposes, however, that contemporary culture is more obsessed than previous eras with the control of the body. Most anorectics do not begin with a conscious desire to become as thin as possible. They often start out to simply lose a few pounds, frequently in response to a parent's suggestion. But then they get hooked on the intoxicating feeling of achievement and of being in control (Bordo, 1993b). Seid (1994) describes this obsession with self-denial and control as a new American religion, which is practiced with varying degrees of devotion by a variety of people. This religion has its rituals of vigorous exercise, daily weigh-ins, and strict dietary guidelines. Pain and deprivation are signs of virtue; rewards of beauty, energy, and health are the promised salvation.

Bordo notes, however, that whether it is the female body-builders relentlessly chiseling their bodies, compulsive exercisers running beyond the remembrance of pain, or anorectics whittling down their frames, all pursue self-denial as an end in itself. Devoid of any pleasure in embodiment, they find pleasure in control and independence. But why are Americans in this era so concerned with control? Bordo (1993b) suggests multiple reasons. First, she notes that these acts of self-mastery are responses to the increasing sense of unmanageability in the culture. Much of life is simply not within our control—what we eat or how far we run, however, can be. In addition, Americans are deeply invested in the scientific fantasy of immortality and invulnerability. These rituals of self-control perpetuate the belief that deterioration and death can be held at bay indefinitely. Finally, Bordo shares Seid's belief that the self-control expressed in anorexia and compulsive exercising is also a moral rebellion against the abundance of the late twentieth century in North America (Bordo, 1993b; Seid, 1994).

RACE, ETHNICITY, AND SEXUAL ORIENTATION

Gender differences regarding body satisfaction are relatively consistent across racial/ethnic groups, but some notable differences do appear among women in different racial/ethnic groups. Those who emphasize the influence of culture in the development of eating disorders frequently assume that women of color are less exposed to this culture than white women, and thus less likely to suffer from disordered eating. From a review of available research literature, Crago, Shisslak, and Estes (1996) concluded that compared to Caucasian females, eating disorders are equally common among Hispanic females, more frequently among Native Americans, and less frequently among African American and Asian American females. It must be noted, however, that research on the prevalence of eating disorders among minority racial and ethnic groups is limited, and the results of this research have sometimes been equivocal. The latter seems to be particularly true for the research on Hispanic females with several studies finding similar incidence rates as Caucasian females and others finding Hispanics to be heavier, but less concerned with weight (see Jane, Hunter, & Lozzi, 1999).

Variations in the findings with regard to Hispanic females may be due in part to the fact that this category includes significant ethnic, racial, and socioeconomic heterogeneity. Furthermore, some research demonstrates that particular aspects of the body (such as skin texture and color and hair texture, thickness, and color) are weighted differently among different race/ethnic groups (Miller et al., 2000; Thompson, 1994). This suggests the need for more multidimensional assessments of body image in research comparing race/ethnic groups.

People of color in the United States are bicultural, influenced by often conflicting messages from within their race/ethnic groups and from the dominant culture

(Miller et al., 2000). Furthermore, the extent of acculturation varies widely within race/ethnic groups. Jane, Hunter, and Lozzi (1999), for instance, found that among Cuban American women ages 18 to 25, continued exclusive or primary use of Spanish language in the home and frequent consumption of Cuban meals were associated with less problematic beliefs and attitudes regarding eating behaviors. Thompson (1994) found that changes in a family's economic class and geographic location, reflecting the pressures of assimilation, were significant factors influencing parents' attitudes about thinness among African American and Hispanic women. In addition, although ethnic identity may in some ways mitigate the culture-of-thinness messages from the dominant society, internalized racism may also contribute to the development of eating disorders. Thompson found that some women of color coped with discrimination by minimizing the ways they felt different from others, including their body size.

Like race and ethnicity, there has been limited research on the significance of sexual orientation for prevalence of eating disorders. A recent study by Strong and colleagues (2000) concludes that sexual orientation is a significant factor for men, but much less for women. Heterosexual females reported the highest level of eating disorder symptoms as measured by the Eating Attitudes Test (EAT-26), heterosexual males reported the lowest level, and lesbians and gay males reported levels that were intermediate to the heterosexual groups. Overconcern about body size and shape was the strongest psychosocial correlate for eating disorders; heterosexual females, lesbians, and gay men all scored significantly higher than heterosexual men did on this variable.

Males account for only 10 percent of diagnosed cases of eating disorders, but of these cases, homosexual males account for 30 percent (Anderson, 1992; Carlat, Camargo, & Herzog, 1997). Strong and colleagues (2000) found that gay men were more concerned about body size and physical appearance than were heterosexual men. They were equally concerned about their physical appearance as heterosexual women but less concerned about body size than heterosexual women.

Consistent with other studies, Strong and colleagues (2000) found that lesbians were less concerned with physical appearance than heterosexual women or gay males. Lesbians also reported less influence from the media regarding internalization of the thinness body shape ideal. Nonetheless, lesbians reported only slightly lower levels of eating disorder symptoms than heterosexual women did, perhaps due to the fact that they still showed significant concern for body shape and size. Strong and colleagues conclude that only heterosexual males were found to be at low risk for eating disorders.

Step 3. Explore Options

The previous discussion reveals that eating disorders are complex syndromes with multiple contributing factors. While racial and ethnic differences exist, eating disorders are increasing in North America and Western European countries among Caucasian and minority groups. Responding to this challenge is a formidable task requiring collaboration from a variety of disciplines.

The ethical issue we are considering in this chapter is whether and how women are harmed by the exclusion of a feminist perspective on eating disorders, and how the inclusion of this perspective might alter treatment approaches. Consequently, we will focus on two options: (1) treatment approaches should integrate the findings from feminist analyses of eating disorders or (2) treatment approaches need not integrate findings from this perspective. We will see that, in practice, feminist analyses are sometimes incorporated, but in limited ways. Feminists argue that this limited incorporation still harms women because it does not recognize the most fundamental implications of the feminist perspective. Thus, a third option, the partial integration of feminist analyses, will also be considered.

Step 4. Apply the Feminist Ethics Decision Process

Box 7–3 outlines key aspects of a feminist ethics decision process in a useful checklist format. This decision process includes an emphasis on the feminist commitment to eliminate the oppression of women. Feminists also recognize that there are complex interconnections between sexism, racism, and class exploitation (Ferguson, 1991; Lugones & Spelman, 1986; Hooks, 1995). Consequently, their commitment incorporates a responsibility to address these interrelated forms of oppression.

Framework for Ethical Analysis

1. Identify the problem or issue.
2. Analyze context.
3. Explore options.
4. **Apply the Feminist Ethics Decision Process**
5. Implement the plan and evaluate results.

Box 7–3 Feminist Ethics Decision Process

4. Apply the Feminist Ethics Decision Process

- Identify social practices that underlie and contribute to the problem identified in Step 1.
- Evaluate how these social practices may contribute to the oppression of women:
  - By perpetuating patriarchal imbalances of power
  - By supporting the social construction of reality within patriarchy
- Consider how a relational account of justice reveals the harm done to women as an oppressed group.
- Consider special insights that those marginalized by these social practices provide to guide its restructuring.
- Design ways to restructure or resist the oppressive pratices.

✓ IDENTIFY SOCIAL PRACTICES THAT UNDERLIE AND CONTRIBUTE TO THE PROBLEM IDENTIFIED IN STEP 1

Feminists believe that the increase of eating disorders in the late twentieth century and their prevalence in women cannot be adequately explained without a feminist analysis. Social practices that contribute to the problem of eating disorders include (1) the cultural obsession with women's appearance, (2) the media's promotion of the thinness ideal, and (3) the treatment of eating disorders as primarily an individual psycho-physiologic problem.

Early treatment programs for eating disorders emphasized developmental issues, family problems, and perceptual/cognitive "dysfunction." The role played by the social construction of gender and other social factors was largely ignored. Today, treatment programs are much more diverse and multidimensional. The feminist/cultural contribution to the study and treatment of eating disorders has altered clinical perspectives and practice. Many programs now acknowledge a sociocultural context to the development of eating disorders. This may include the recognition of the cultural pressure on women for thinness, the effects of media imagery on vulnerable women, and the pressures on women due to changing and conflicting role expectations for women. But what is often missing in research and programs is a deeper analysis that asks *why* the culture/media promotes the thinness ideal, *why* women are more vulnerable to these messages, and *why* the ideal of thinness for women has become such a dominant ideal in the twentieth century. To address these questions requires us to understand how the social practices identified above perpetuate the patriarchal oppression of women.

✓ EVALUATE HOW THESE SOCIAL PRACTICES MAY CONTRIBUTE TO THE OPPRESSION OF WOMEN

Perpetuating Patriarchal Imbalances of Power

Wolf (1994) argues that cultural fixation on female thinness is related to female obedience rather than beauty. She notes that female fat is the subject of public passion, discussed in emotive language that exceeds that found in discussions of alcohol and tobacco use. Fat is portrayed as bulk waste, ugly and disgusting, and to be kept out of sight. But most importantly, female fat is a moral issue. When women eat "too much," they feel guilt. *Guilt* is a moral word, like "bad" or "wrong." Obesity (or even "normal" female fullness) is regarded with the scorn and moral commentary once reserved for sexually promiscuous women: "She has no self-respect," "she ought to be ashamed of herself," or "she has no self-control" (Steiner-Adair, 1994).

Feminists argue that the relentless focus on the size and shape of women's bodies and the pressures for women to conform to unrealistic weight norms is a direct response to the dangers posed by the women's movement in the twentieth century. Western women's preoccupation with dieting and thinness began when they received the vote around 1920. In the postwar years of the 1950s, fashion briefly celebrated women's natural fullness again as women were occupied with domestic nesting. But as women began to move in large numbers into male spheres in the 1960s and 1970s, "that pleasure had to be overridden by an urgent social expedient that would make women's bodies into the prisons that their homes no longer were" (Wolf, 1994, p. 96). Thus, a linear form rapidly replaced the more curvaceous forms that had characterized women's bodies and fashions for centuries (Seid, 1994). Big, ripe bellies; plump faces and shoulders; and dimpled buttocks and thighs disappeared from the artistic nude and fashion, replaced by an emaciated state that contradicts women's natural amplitude (Hollander, 1978).

The cultural obsession with women's appearance is a new form of social control. Beauty norms, which affect women's behavior as much as their appearance, are linked historically and politically to practices that include foot binding and corsets, which effectively restricted women's movement, as well as chastity belts and female genital mutilation, which restricted women's sexual expression. Yet the restrictions of the current beauty ideal are unique in that they are internal rather than external forms of control. Thus, while women are free to move into universities, law firms, construction crews, and legislatures, they carry the restrictions of their womanhood with them (Faludi, 1991; Rothblum, 1994; Wolf, 1994). Today's culture tells women they have the same opportunities as men of comparable abilities but then adds that they must obtain a body shape that is impossible for the vast majority of women. It is not incidental that anorexia initially occurred among white upper- and middle-class women who were best prepared educationally and economically to compete with men for positions of power and status (Bordo, 1993a; Steiner-Adair, 1994).

Pressure to control weight and eliminate fat is debilitating for many women, not only physiologically and psychologically but also politically. The women's movement had begun to empower women, increasing their self-esteem, efficacy, confidence, and courage. Chronic dieting and the inevitable cycles of failure, on the other hand, create passive, anxious women who feel defeated and powerless (Rothblum, 1994; Wolf, 1994). Women invest money, energy, attention, and concern into the process of achieving an impossible ideal of slenderness—resources that could be directed toward social and political transformation. Instead, women are encouraged to dismember themselves individually through unhealthy methods of bodily reduction and through ". . . their obsessive internal dissection of their bodies" (Steiner-Adair, 1994).

The culture of looksism and thinness also encourages women to dismember their collective body. Cultural beauty norms are enforced not only by the culture and by men but also by women themselves. Women allow one another less latitude with their bodies than they allow men (Bordo, 1993b). The generation of young women who would naturally constitute the next wave of feminism often are anxious to distance themselves from feminism. Twenty years of propaganda have taught many of them to identify feminists with unfeminine women who do not shave their legs and wear ugly shoes (Wolf, 1994). Others in this generation resent that society's expectations for them have increased as a result of the women's movement—they must be both ambitious and glamorous to be considered desirable. And they must work outside the home to support their family and continue to do most of the traditional work of the housewife.

Supporting the Social Construction of Reality Within Patriarchy

A feminist/cultural model describes the social construction of gender and of eating disorders as pathology. It seeks to understand the *meaning* of the ideal of thinness by analyzing what this ideal reveals about being a woman in our society. The feminine in

Western cultures is symbolically identified with the imprisoning and unruly body that Plato, Augustine, and Descartes excoriated.

We previously discussed how the Western cultural history of dualism and the need for self-control provide important contextual clues to the explosion of eating disorders in the twentieth century. These cultural influences, however, are unable to explain why 90 percent of those with eating disorders are women. Feminists insist that this fact can be explained only when we consider how Western culture's construction of gender intersects with the dualist and control axes (Bordo, 1993b). Box 7–4 shows contrasting pairs of terms within the historical mind/body dualism. Mind characteristics have been symbolically associated with males and body characteristics with females. Although many in our culture may know little of Plato or Augustine, these dualistic associations are alive. Most people in Western cultures identify slenderness with competence, self-control, and intelligence, while feminine curvaceousness is identified with "wide-eyed, giggly vapidity" (Bordo, 1993a, p. 55).

Is it any wonder that the onset of eating disorders, particularly anorexia, occurs at puberty as these young women unconsciously seek to avoid the development of a womanly body? Is it surprising that anorectics fight to transcend their fleshiness, striving to achieve the ideals of rationality, purity, and control represented by thinness or that bulimics wrestle with warring forces of insatiable hunger and the desperate need to eliminate polluting, flesh-making substances?

Feminists assert that eating disorders such as anorexia and bulimia are an extreme on a continuum of a sense of dis-ease with the body, a feeling shared by most women in Western cultures. The pervasiveness of the dieting mentality and the relentless self-critique of women's bodies support this view. Consequently, feminists contest the conception of eating disorders as a pathology with clear boundaries separating them from a "healthy" and "normal" condition. Rather, they see eating disorders as an extreme expression of a cultural disorder that affects all women to varying degrees.

Box 7–4 Mind/Body Dualism	
Mind (Masculine)	**Body (Feminine)**
rational	emotional, fickle
mature	childish
competent	incompetent
intelligent	mindless
self-controlled	unruly, turbulent
transcendent	cyclical, immanent
pure, virtuous	lustful, whoring
disciplined	soft, yielding
enduring	temporal, decaying

Although some women cope in ways that are more functional than others, the well-being of all women is undermined by the social construction of femininity in Western cultures (Bordo, 1993a; Orbach, 1986; Steiner-Adair, 1994).

Feminists submit that this cultural construct of gender helps to shape many other contributory factors of eating disorders, including the ideology presented in the media, the organization of the family, the construction of individual personality, and the training of perception (Bordo, 1993a). It is not accidental that media and fashion industries promote an unrealistic ideal of thinnness in this particular historical era and culture. As Bordo notes, the mythology of the devouring, insatiable female waxes and wanes. But it flourishes in periods when women become independent and assert themselves politically and socially (Bordo, 1993b). Eating disorders have become epidemic in the United States and elsewhere at a time when traditional boundaries for women's place in society have been challenged.

Accepting this cultural construct does not require belief in a conspiracy among powerful men orchestrating a campaign to control women politically and socially. We need only recognize that in periods of social instability and transformation, human beings often rely on comfortable formulas and may grasp for antiquated symbols of femininity and masculinity that define clear and definitive boundaries and roles. Thus, Madison Avenue and Hollywood do not arbitrarily create ideological images designed to torture and prey on vulnerable young women. Rather, as astute readers of the cultural psyche, they create images designed to respond to the palpable anxieties of this era.

One criticism of the feminist perspective on eating disorders is the argument that though cultural pressures may make women vulnerable to eating disorders, they cannot be the primary cause because all women in Western culture do not develop eating disorders (Storber, 1986). Feminists do not postulate an *identical* cultural situation for all women. We are all exposed to the homogenizing and normalizing ideology and images of femininity and beauty in the dominant culture. But unique combinations of environmental and biological influences shape individual identities. Thus, the dominant ideology of femininity is mediated by individual ethnicity, social class, age, sexual orientation, religion, genetics, education, family, and so forth (Bordo, 1993a). The interaction of these factors is complex and individualized, suggesting the need to resist overgeneralizations such as "women of color" are less susceptible to eating disorders.

Another criticism of the feminist perspective is that the feminist politicizing of eating disorders romanticizes anorectics as "heroic freedom fighters" and sacrifices seriously ill individuals for a political agenda (Brumberg, 1988; "Anorexia Nervosa," 1984). This criticism suggests that by positing a continuum of bodily dis-ease, feminists deny that those with eating disorders are genuinely sick and need medical treatment. Critics assert that these are diseases rather than a target for political protest. Feminists reject this either/or dichotomy (Bordo, 1993a). Eating disorders are debilitating, self-destructive disorders that tragically affect real, individual women. At the same time, the anorectic may resist the move into womanhood, maintaining a boyish figure and defeating the cyclic rhythms of her feminine body. The anorectic need not embrace a conscious political position, just as no conscious collusion among media and corporate leaders is necessary.

✓ Consider How a Relational Account of Justice Reveals the Harm Done to Women as an Oppressed Group

Women with eating disorders and women in general are harmed when researchers and health care practitioners fail to recognize how eating disorders are related to women's oppression as a collective group. As discussed in Chapter 6, a relational account of justice asserts that justice requires not only respect for persons as unique individuals but also an understanding of people as social groups. Some harms achieve the status of an injustice only when one considers how people's lives are defined by their membership in subordinate social groups. The relational account of justice reminds us that we must respect and respond with compassion to eating disorder patients as individuals, but also seek to transform social relations so that all women can occupy places of respect in society.

The feminist perspective points to two applications of this relational account of justice to the treatment of eating disorders. First, by isolating eating disorders from cultural ideology, mainstream medical treatment severely limits the ability of women to genuinely recover (Hutchinson, 1994; Sesan, 1994: Shisslak & Crago, 1994; Steiner-Adair, 1994). A woman who is ill deserves individualized treatment. But insofar as the disorder is rooted in a cultural ideology that devalues all women, treatment that fails to give significant weight to cultural oppression cannot hope to effect a thorough recovery.

The second application of the relational account of justice reminds us that all women are harmed by the cultural ideology that devalues feminine qualities and seeks to limit women's place in society. Eating disorders, Bordo suggests, provide "windows" opening onto problems in the social world (1993a) or "crystallizations" of much that is wrong with our culture's construction of womanhood (1993b). Without a systemic social analysis of how pressure to be thin perpetuates the oppression of women, the harm done to the vast majority of women will be missed.

✓ Consider What Special Insights Those Marginalized by These Social Practices Provide for Its Restructuring

Feminist ethics is committed to serious though not uncritical consideration of women's perceptions. The dominant treatment mode for eating disorders in the United States, a cognitive-behavioral approach, seems to discount women's experiences. The majority of treatment programs focus on weight gain, weight stabilization, and normalization of eating behaviors (Sesan, 1994; Lester, 1997). Cognitive therapists assert that eating disorders arise from "distorted attitudes," "disordered cognition," or "flawed reasoning." Poor self-esteem distorts their ability to accurately assess their perceptions of their bodies, leading to self-destructive eating behaviors (Berry et al., 1995; Brewerton et al., 1992; Everill, et al., 1995 cited in Lester, 1997).

Within this framework, an anorectic's understanding of her illness may be dismissed as illogical and childlike. Behaviors of anorectics and bulimics are often described as manipulative, secretive, and deceitful—and clearly pathological. The feelings of rage expressed by anorectics against those who try to force them to eat are considered inappropriate. But from a feminist perspective, women with eating disorders do not improperly assess their bodies; they have learned perfectly well how the dominant culture expects them to perceive it. These women are not pathological (non-normal); they accurately internalize their culture's assessment of women. Their endless dieting, rigorous exercise, or bingeing and purging are rational (though counterproductive) coping strategies within a culture that constantly tells them that as women they take up too much space, eat too much, want too much. Many women in this culture experience themselves (and perceive that men experience them) as wanting too much affection, having too many needs, or being too loud or simply too much there (Bordo, 1993b).

Wooley warns that cognitive-behavioral therapy that seeks simply to control eating disorder symptoms and behaviors may teach women to suppress emotions, encouraging a restriction of affect that is central to the problem (Sesan, 1994). Feminist therapy recognizes that the low self-esteem, feelings of powerlessness, lack of entitlement, and lack of comfort in their bodies that women with eating disorders bring to therapy are the results of cultural oppression of women. Taking women's perceptions seriously means helping them to explore inherent contradictions in their prescribed social roles and encouraging them to work to change rather than to adapt to these roles (Bordo, 1993a; Peters & Fallon, 1994; Sesan, 1994). We will explore this transformative task further in the last step of the feminist ethics decision process.

✓ DESIGN WAYS TO RESTRUCTURE OR RESIST THE OPPRESSIVE PRACTICE

The perspective of feminist ethics suggests two areas of the dominant Western response to eating disorders that should be restructured: (1) developing primary prevention programs and (2) transforming treatment programs to reflect the significant effects of women's cultural oppression. Both require challenging major Western assumptions and values and encouraging competencies that women need in order to gain control of their lives.

Challenge the Beauty Myth

Effective prevention programs will challenge cultural norms about "ideal" female adulthood. Women are taught that their success in relationships and in work, their approval by others, and their self-esteem depend on their physical appearance. Prevention programs need to educate young women to decode the messages behind the media images of "attractive" thin women and to explore the effects of these images on women's physical and mental health (Kilbourne, 1994). Steiner-Adair (1994) argues that tapping into the passion of teens and children by addressing eating disorders as a social justice issue is a more effective strategy than scare tactics that emphasize the medical damages of dieting, bingeing, and purging. Looksism and weightism are forms of prejudice, and, like racism, anti-Semitism, and homophobia, they need to be considered within a political framework. Presenting them as such locates the primary disorder in the culture and identifies a problem that requires collective resistance. Furthermore, considering the issue in terms of social justice mitigates the individual shame and isolation that are a part of eating disorders. The injustice of weightism and looksism needs to be included in curriculum in very early years and continued through college years (Shisslak & Crago, 1994; Steiner-Adair, 1994).

Young people—male and female—can be taught to identify and critique looks-ist thinking. They can be encouraged to ask who benefits from cultural norms of ultrathinness for women. Young men and women alike should be taught to critically examine the conflicting role prescriptions for women. They need to recognize that the expectation that women will be good wives/mothers *and* successful in education and careers is unrealistic and unfairly holds women to a different standard than men (Shisslak & Crago, 1994; Steiner-Adair, 1994). Discussion groups using older peer role models can be useful for exploring the implications of these double standards.

Build Solidarity Among Women and Within Communities

Broader definitions of normal weight, body size, and eating need to be communicated. But women will likely be able to accept these definitions only if they also learn to value themselves and other women for reasons other than physical appearance. Many young women feel discomfort within women-only groups, especially groups of adult women. Adult women who have assumed traditional female roles may be associated with many aspects of femininity that are devalued in the culture. Steiner-Adair (1994) notes that we have no positive terms to describe and value women who are at home and raising children. On the other hand, young women may resent being told by women who have successful careers that women must make choices, that it is not possible to be the superwoman who "has it all" without risking physiologic and psychosocial health. Determined to believe that the days of such compromises are now over, young women sometimes perceive these messages as negative.

Some theorists believe that bulimia is a woman's attempt to negotiate the impossibly confused and unrealistic sex role expectations for women—to be a man (career oriented) by day and a woman (sex object and mother) by night. Others view anorexia as a life-threatening split between being female and being an adult (Steiner-Adair, 1994). Clearly, the passage from female child to female adult is a treacherous one. It is essential that young women not be cut off from critical older mentors and support from adult women. Building solidarity among women across age groups and life commitments is an important resource for empowering women. Support groups can help women value their diverse competencies and empower them to honor feminine values that are devalued in patriarchal cultures. Support groups can enable women to perceive one another as trusted allies working together to resist looksism. Collective political action teaches women that their primary power is reflected not by their ability to lose weight but to transform their society.

Two additional advantages of addressing eating disorders as a social justice issue should be noted. A broadly focused program that deals with eating disorders as a cultural disorder seems more likely to avoid a problem uncovered by several research studies. When educational programs focus on dieting and dietary restraint, they may unwittingly teach young women the very skills for reducing weight that these programs intend to prevent (Chally, 1998; White, 2000). Second, shifting focus from individual to cultural dysfunction offers parents the opportunity to become advocates for their daughters.

The feminist analysis of gender construction can be threatening for men and women. But when parents recognize eating disorders as the internalization of social prejudice, they can become fierce champions of the rights of their children. Focusing on social justice brings people together into collective action, affirming the value of interdependence. The national program, Eating Disorders Awareness and Prevention, Inc. (EDAP), headquartered in Seattle, Washington, is an excellent example of a program that promotes education and social action involving students, parents, health professionals, and community members. Their activities include a media advocacy project that encourages individuals and communities to pressure advertisers and other media organizations to present more realistic and diverse body images (EDAP, 2000).

Educate Early

Nurses are positioned to play a key role in this prevention and education. They can be teachers or resources for teachers in a wide variety of settings. These may include school programs, Girl Scouts and 4H clubs, church-sponsored youth programs, workshops sponsored by municipal athletic programs, and so on. Nurses could also develop content to help identify young people at risk for eating disorders and to be incorporated into health classes and discussions. Some of this material could be included in broader discussions on risky behaviors (White, 2000).

Nurses can also provide essential education for parents and other mentors for young women. Professional and volunteer women's organizations often want speakers on health topics. Similarly, opportunities to educate mothers and fathers through workplace wellness programs or parenting classes should not be overlooked. Day care workers, coaches, and fitness instructors are other groups that need to be reached. Nurses' holistic approach makes them credible advocates who can address both the sociocultural as well as the physiological/psychological components of eating disorders.

Nurses in the clinical setting also play an important role in shaping the attitudes of young women and men about body satisfaction. Some traditional practices may need to be reconsidered. For instance, consider that the first task when patients visit their physician or nurse practitioner is often to get weighed. Is checking weight always necessary, especially for patients who make frequent office visits? When it is not absolutely necessary, patients could be offered the option to be weighed or not. If collecting this data is important, nurses could explain to patients why they are being weighed. Furthermore, it may be appropriate to reconsider whether this must be the first interaction between patient and health care provider. In a thinness-obsessed culture, weighing patients as they enter the clinic may inadvertently reinforce the cultural message that appearance and body size are the most significant facts about people. Even if patients were weighed after the initial greeting, instead of as a component of the greeting, that would be progress. The process of weighing patients provides an opportunity for supportive dialogue. An attitude of acceptance is important, and disapproval, whether communicated overtly or subtly, can be damaging and thus is inappropriate. The dialogue that accompanies this ritual is an opportunity for the nurse to demonstrate acceptance and support, to encourage positive and discourage unhealthy patient response, and to uncover a potential eating disorder.

Reembodiment

Political action that challenges the toxicity of patriarchal culture is essential if women are to become whole and at home in their bodies and in society. But attention and energy must also be invested in helping all women to heal the disordered relationships between their bodies and themselves. Although many women are extremely body conscious, few are genuinely embodied. Hutchinson describes embodiment as experiencing the body as the center of existence. The body is a reference point for *being in* the world. To be embodied means to be in touch with emotions, needs, pleasures, pains, and perceptions as they are experienced in the body (Hutchinson, 1994).

Negative body images are the result of a lifetime of internalized messages. These may include internalized judgments by significant others, body shame that may have been modeled in our families, traumatic life experiences that we carry in our bodies, and the relentless media campaign to convince women that they need to buy something to measure up. We learn to protect ourselves from these assaults by numbing ourselves to somatic experiences. The body becomes an alien object to shape, criticize, and deprive. All women, especially those with eating disorders, need to reimagine their body image. Guided imagery, group work to relieve isolation, and neuromuscular reeducation that enables women to reconnect to their bodies through physical movement are tools that can help to heal the split between self and the body (Hutchinson, 1994). Participation in rituals and spirituality that reaffirm women's feminine embodied nature may also promote this healing process (Shisslak & Crago, 1994).

Restructuring Inpatient Treatment

Treatment for eating disorders should always be provided in the least restrictive environment required. The variety of outpatient settings available today makes hospitalization a last resort. The treatment approach in most inpatient settings emphasizes deprivation. Hospitalized women are often denied private access to bathrooms, placed on restrictive meal plans, or "force fed." Behavior that violates strict rules is often punished by restricting women to their rooms or denying privileges such as participating in social activities. Feminist therapists challenge approaches that substitute self-control with externally imposed control that prevents women from exploring their own needs. Feminists advocate a treatment model that encourages women to attend to their feelings and to experience emptiness and fullness (Kearney-Cooke, 1991; Sesan, 1994; Wooley & Wooley, 1985). Such programs promote opportunities to break through the isolation and shame associated with eating disorders, encouraging women to reach out to others prior to a binge or purge rather than endure these feelings in isolation.

Feminist therapists also strive to minimize the power relationships between therapists and clients and among those who staff inpatient programs. Despite the use by most treatment programs of a team approach, traditional male-dominated hierarchy is often reproduced. A male physician, psychiatrist, or psychologist is often the treatment leader, while other team members are typically female nurses, social workers, and counselors, all with lower status. In many cases, the team leader appears for a one-hour weekly therapy session or a medication check, while female staff members tend to day-to-day patient needs. Consequently, these treatment settings reproduce typical power imbalances between men and women (and between masculine work and feminine work), impeding efforts to educate patients about the role of gender devaluation in their illness.

Feminist therapists advocate more egalitarian relationships among staff and between staff and patients. Patients should be included in treatment team meetings, their expertise regarding their illness should be valued, and their collaboration in their treatment plans encouraged. These measures help to build trust and openness between staff and patients and encourage patients to learn to set their own goals/boundaries and value their own insights (Sesan, 1994).

Discussion and feminist analysis needs to be stimulated among those involved in treating eating disorders. Feminist therapists have power to effect change in treatment programs, while nurses and nurse practitioners can educate themselves and their patients about options available in their communities. Through ongoing education, prevention, and more effective treatment, our communities can empower women and men to value themselves and others for their personal strengths and individuality rather than for their physical appearance.

Step 5. Implement the Plan and Evaluate the Results

Each of the proposals for developing primary prevention programs and transforming treatment programs needs to be monitored and evaluated at regular intervals. Assessment by women in and outside treatment programs will be an essential component of this evaluation. Results of new research must be incorporated into the ongoing modification of prevention and treatment programs.

Further Connections

A feminist ethics approach will illuminate new aspects of traditional health care issues. For instance, the effects of gender on the dynamics surrounding physician-assisted death and euthanasia should be considered. The fact that women experience less aggressive management of their pain, a higher incidence of depression, a higher rate of poverty, and greater difficulty accessing good medical care indicates the need to include a gender analysis (Wolf, 1996). A feminist ethics approach will also uncover new ethical issues in health care related to gender oppression and associated oppression based on race, ethnicity, sexual orientation, and class. Ethical issues in three areas involving familiar and new topics will be considered briefly here.

Sexual Violence

Sexual violence, a patterned manifestation of the power structure in most societies, includes rape, intimate partner violence, sexual abuse, and sexual harassment. Sexual violence both reflects and helps to perpetuate the dominance of men (Dworkin, 1981; Herman, 1984; Sheffield, 1992). Intimate partner violence is the number one cause of injury to women in the United States. Although men are sometimes the victims of domestic violence, women's use of violence is more likely to be defensive and less severe than men's. The typical medical approach treats battering as a physical crisis, reduces male violence to individual, situational factors (e.g., stress in family, husband unemployed), and focuses prevention on the individual level. It fails to recognize that battering is a social process rooted in gender inequality. Feminists recommend an extension of treatment and intervention from the emergency room to primary care clinics including obstetrical services, community health facilities, and mental health centers. In all settings, nurses play a critical role as advocates for victims of intimate partner violence and educators of parents and community members. And they empower women when they strive to boost awareness of sexist attitudes in their practice settings.

Sexual harassment is a problem faced by women, including nurses, in the workplace. It includes a wide range of unwelcome sexually oriented and gender-offensive behaviors that contribute to a hostile work environment. Nurses are harassed by physicians, co-workers, and patients. Sexual harassment is about the abuse of power and status, and it must be viewed within the context of institutionalized male power. In a patriarchal society, nurses are vulnerable to abuse not only as women but also as members of a mostly female profession struggling for respect within the male-dominated health care industry. Sexual harassment can adversely affect physiological and psychological health as well as work performance. The issue must be addressed at organizational as well as individual levels to reduce this major occupational stressor.

Nurses should also recognize that sexual harassment is a potential health-related problem for all women. The majority of women will experience workplace sexual harassment at some point in their working lives. (Ninety percent of sexual harassment claims are filed by women but men can be subjects of sexual harassment as well.) Although women of all ages and in all types of jobs are affected, many often do not initially recognize sexual harassment for what it is. At first, women may be aware only of stress symptoms such as headaches, anxiety, and feeling reluctant to go to work. Those in health care should recognize these symptoms as potential indicators of sexual harassment.

Although significant attention has been given to harassment of adult women in the workplace, little research has been done on the health effects of same-age sexual harassment among adolescent females. Recent studies (e.g., American Association of University Women [AAUW], 1993) demonstrate that this is an everyday reality for many adolescent girls (and some boys). Nurses who provide care for this population should be aware of this increasing problem.

Disability as Socially Constructed

Disability, like gender, is socially constructed from biological reality. Some of the same cultural attitudes about the body that contribute to women's oppression also contribute to the oppression of disabled people. Disabled persons are constructed as "the other," representing failure of control, dependence, the threat of pain, and death (Wendell, 1992). Furthermore, Western culture tends to assume that the "real self" is the rational mind and that gender is a nonessential aspect of the person. Similarly, it is often assumed that disabilities are incidental to a person's identity and that there is a fuller, better "real self" inside that person (Wilkerson, 1998).

Disability activists have noted that concepts of health and disability are to a large degree created by the expectations of particular societies and by environmental, social, and economic elements of these societies. As genetic research and technology continue to evolve, issues surrounding the social construction of disability and disease will become increasingly germane to a broader population. Communities will struggle with questions about personal responsibilities to eradicate and prevent disease and "disability" and communal responsibility to care for the ill and disabled. The search for the "normal" human genome could challenge our capacity to appreciate and incorporate diversity into our communal life.

Western medicine's perception of its main purpose as control of the body ("making it better") contributes to the perception of those who cannot be "repaired" as symbols of medical failure. Persons with disabilities are often depersonalized and desexualized in health care (Wendell, 1992; Wilkerson, 1998). Most people, including many in health care, know little about how to live with chronic conditions or how to live with limitations and pain.

Nurses, physiotherapists, and other less "prestigious" health care professionals do much of the work of rehabilitation and management of long-term illnesses or disabilities. Physically disabled persons have experiences and knowledge about embodiment, dependence/independence, and the relativity of control. The commitment of nurses to patient advocacy, holistic care, and empowering patients to strive for optimal well-being makes them important apprentices to—as well as advocates for—their expert patients. Disabled persons may be better positioned to transcend cultural ideology about the body; their full integration into society may help liberate all persons from the restrictions of this cultural mythology.

Democratizing and Demedicalizing Health Care

The relationship- and context-oriented outlook of feminist ethics will lead feminists to reject a concept of health that is limited to physiologic health. Relationships among physical, mental, and social well-being are complex. On the other hand, feminists are cautious about the increasing tendency to medicalize human behavior. Women's lives often have been controlled through medical determinations of "illness," "pathology," and "normal health." As a result, feminists will encourage individuals and communities to carefully assess the impact of social and political arrangements on physiologic and mental health without medicalizing these social conditions. Thus, the impact of such areas as housing, poverty, automobile safety, lack of appropriate recreation for teens, and violence in the media should be addressed as communal problems that require public discussion and intervention.

When social conditions create or intensify health problems, health care institutions and those who work within them should develop partnerships with a wide variety of community stakeholders such as neighborhood centers; religious and other charitable organizations; schools; and social work, teaching, and parenting associations. Through these partnerships, health care organizations assume responsibility for working with community members to assess, prioritize, and address their health-related needs. Democritizing and demedicalizing "social health" is consistent with feminism's commitment to empowering marginalized groups to assume responsibility for social transformation and with nursing's commitment to empowering individuals, families, and communities to provide self-care.

Conclusion

This chapter demonstrates that feminist ethical analysis can illuminate aspects of ethical issues that are unnoticed or obscured by other perspectives. Oppression permeates relationships, organizations, and social institutions. Thus, although issues of oppression are not the only important ethical issues, they are issues that significantly impact and shape all of our lives. Feminist ethics is committed to revealing the harms done to women and others by oppressive power imbalances. Furthermore, as this chapter has illustrated, feminist ethical analysis should also lead us to design alternative practices and processes that will free us all to live richer and more authentic lives.

KEY POINTS

- Feminists recognize the complexity of eating disorders but assert that we cannot adequately understand their nature and incidence without a feminist analysis.
- Western culture's relentless focus on women's appearance and the promotion of an unrealistic ideal of thinness are new forms of social control of women in response to women's changing roles in society.
- Eating disorders are an extreme expression of discomfort with the female body, a feeling shared by most women in Western cultures. This discomfort is the result of a cultural ideology that associates the body with femininity, characterized by attributes such as incompetence, lack of control, and lust.
- Effective prevention and treatment programs for eating disorders will challenge the cultural norms of "ideal" female beauty and identify lookism as a form of social and political prejudice requiring collective resistance.
- Women can heal the disordered relationships between themselves and their bodies by learning to honor the feminine values that are devalued in patriarchal cultures and by learning how to be genuinely embodied.

REFLECT AND DISCUSS

1. Most women in Western cultures are not at home in their bodies. How is this discomfort with their bodies reflected?
2. The dominant treatment mode for eating disorders in the United States is a cognitive-behavioral approach. What causes eating disorders, according to this approach, and what is the primary goal of treatment for cognitive therapists?

3. Why do feminists believe that both the psychodynamic and the cognitive-behaviorist accounts of eating disorders are inadequate?
4. What do feminists believe are the causes of eating disorders in Western cultures? Why do feminists believe that factors that promote eating disorders in some women harm *all* women? What implications does this account have for prevention and treatment programs? Is the feminist viewpoint persuasive? Why or why not?
5. What messages do health care professionals communicate to women (and to men) about their bodies and appearance? How might the feminist analysis of eating disorders and looksism influence your interactions with your patients, especially women?

REFERENCES

American Anorexia Bulimia Association (2000). Bulimia nervosa. Available: http://www.aabainc.org [2000, September 9].

American Association of University Women (1991). Shortchanging girls, shortchanging America. Washington, DC: American Association of University Women Educational Foundation Press.

American Association of University Women (1993). Hostile hallways: The AAUW survey on sexual harassment in American schools. Washington, DC: American Association of University Women Educational Foundation Press.

Anderson, A. E. (1992). Males with eating disorders. In J. Yager, H. E. Gwirtsman, & C. K. Edelstein (Eds.), *Special problems in managing eating disorders* (pp. 87–118). Washington, DC: American Psychiatric Press.

Anderson, A. E., & DiDomenico, L. (1992). Diet vs. shape content of popular male and female magazines: A dose-response relationship to the incidence of eating disorders. *International Journal of Eating Disorders, 11,* 238–287.

Anorexia nervosa is a disease, not a protest (1984, February 12). *Newsday*, p. 2.

Berry, F. M., Fried, S., & Edelstein, E. L. (1995). Abnormal oral sensory perception in patients with a history of anorexia nervosa. *Psychotherapy and Psychomatics, 63*(1), 32–37.

Bordo, S. (1993a). Whose body is this? Feminism, medicine, and the conceptualization of eating disorders. In S. Bordo (Ed.), *Unbearable weight: Feminism, Western culture, and the body* (pp. 45–69). Berkeley, CA: University of California Press.

Bordo, S. (1993b). Anorexia nervosa: Psychopathology as the crystallization of culture. In S. Bordo (Ed.), *Unbearable weight: Feminism, Western culture, and the body* (pp. 139–163). Berkeley, CA: University of California Press.

Brewerton, T. D., et al. (1992). CSF beta-endorphins and dynorphin in bulimia nervosa. *American Journal of Psychiatry, 149*(8), 1886–1890.

Brownell, K. D., & Foreyt, J. P. (1986). *Handbook of eating disorders.* New York: Basic Books.

Bruch, H. (1973). *Eating disorders.* New York: Basic Books.

Bruch, H. (1979). *The golden cage.* NewYork: Vintage Books.

Bruch, H. (1985). Four decades of eating disorders. In D. Garner & P. Garfinkel (Eds.), *Handbook of psychotherapy for anorexia nervosa and bulimia* (pp. 7–18). New York: Guilford Press.

Brumberg, J. J. (1988). *Fasting girls: The emergence of anorexia nervosa as a modern disease.* Cambridge: Harvard University Press.

Carlat, D. J., Camargo, C. A., & Herzog, D. B. (1971). Eating disorders in males: A report on 135 patients. *American Journal of Psychiatry, 154,* 1127–1132.

Chally, P. S. (1998). An eating disorders prevention program. *Journal of Child and Adolescent Psychiatric Nursing, 11*(2), 51–60.

Chodorow, N. (1978). *The reproduction of mothering.* Berkeley, CA: University of California Press.

Crago, M., Shisslak, C. M., & Estes, L. S. (1996). Eating disturbances among American minority groups: A review. *International Journal of Eating Disorders, 19*(3), 239–248.

Department of Health and Human Services: Office on Women's Health (2000). Eating disorders. Available: http://www.4woman.gov [2000, September 9].

Dworkin, A. (1981). *Pornography: Men possessing women.* New York: G. P. Putnam's Sons.

Eating Disorders Awareness and Prevention, Inc. (2000). EDAP homepage. Available: http://edap inc/goals.html [2000, September 21].

Emmons, L. (1996). The relationship of dieting to weight in adolescents. *Adolescence, 31,* 167–168.

Everill, J., Water, G., & Macdonald, W. (1995). Dissociation in bulimic and non-eating-disordered women. *International Journal of Eating Disorders, 17*(2), 127–134.

Fairburn, C. G. (1992, October 25–27). Sexual abuse and eating disorders. Paper presented at the Eleventh National Conference on Eating Disorders, Columbus, OH.

Faludi, S. (1991). *Backlash: The undeclared war against American women.* New York: Crown.

Ferguson, A. (1991). *Sexual democracy: Women, oppression, and revolution.* Boulder, CO: Westview Press.

Frederick, C. M., & Grow, V. M. (1996). A mediational model of autonomy, self-esteem, and eating disordered attitudes and behaviors. *Psychology of Women Quarterly, 20,* 217–228.

Gilligan, C. (1982). *In a different voice.* Cambridge, MA: Harvard University Press.

Grothaus, K. L. (1998). Eating disorders and adolescents: An overview of a maladaptive behavior. *Journal of Child and Adolescent Psychiatric Nursing, 11*(4), 146–156.

Herman, D. (1984). The rape culture. In J. Freeman (Ed.), *Women: A feminist perspective* (pp. 20–38). Mountain View, CA: Mayfield Publishing.

Hesse-Biber, S. (1989). Eating patterns and disorders in a college population: Are college women's eating problems a new phenomenon? *Sex Roles, 20,* 71–89.

Hesse-Biber, S., Marino, M., & Watts-Roy, D. (1999). A longitudinal study of eating disorders among college women: Factors that influence recovery. *Gender & Society, 13*(3), 385–408.

Hollander, A. (1978). *Seeing through clothes.* New York: Viking Press.

Hooks, B. (1995). *Killing rage/ending racism.* New York: Henry Hold & Co.

Hsu, L. K. G. (1990). *Eating Disorders.* New York: Guilford.

Hutchinson, M. G. (1994). Imagining ourselves whole: A feminist approach to treating body image disorders. In P. Fallon, M. A. Katzman, & S. C. Wooley (Eds.), *Feminist perspectives on eating disorders* (pp. 152–170). New York: Guilford Press.

Jane, D. M., Hunter, G. C., & Lozzi, B. M. (1999). Do Cuban American women suffer from eating disorders? Effects of media exposure and acculturation. *Hispanic Journal of Behavioral Sciences, 21*(2), 212–218.

Kearney-Cooke, A. (1988). Group treatment of sexual abuse among women with eating disorders. *Women and Therapy, 7*(1), 5–21.

Kilbourne, J. (1994). Still killing us softly: Advertising and the obsession with thinness. In P. Fallon, M. A. Katzman, & S. C. Wooley (Eds.), *Feminist perspectives on eating disorders* (pp. 395–418). New York: Guilford Press.

Koff, E., & Rierdan, J. (1991). Perceptions of weight and attitudes toward eating in early adolescent girls. *Journal of Adolescent Health, 22,* 307–312.

Lennon, S. Lillethun, A., & Buckland, S. (1999). Attitudes toward social comparison as a function of self-esteem: Idealized appearance and body image. *Family and Consumer Sciences Research Journal, 27*(4), 379–405.

Lester, R. (1997). The (dis)embodied self in anorexia nervosa. *Social Science & Medicine, 44*(4), 479–489.

Levy, P. A. & Hadley, B. J. (1998). Family-of-origin relationships and self-differentiation among university students with bulimic-type behaviors. *Family Journal, 6*(1), 19–23.

Lugones, M. C., & Spelman, E. V. (1986). Have we got a theory for you! In M. Pearsall (Ed.), *Women and values* (pp. 19–31). Belmont, CA: Wadsworth.

Miller, K. J., Gleaves, D. H., Hirsch, T. G., Green, B. A., Snow, A. C., & Corbett, C. C. (2000). Comparisons of body image dimensions by race/ethnicity and gender in a university population. *International Journal of Eating Disorders, 27*(3), 310–316.

National Institute of Mental Health (1993). Eating disorders. Available: http://www.nimh.gov [2000, September 9].

Orbach, S. (1986). *Hunger strike: The anorectic's struggle as a metaphor for our age.* New York: W.W. Norton.

Peters, L., & Fallon, P. (1994). The journey of recovery: Dimensions of change. In P. Fallon, M. A. Katzman, & S. C. Wooley (Eds.), *Feminist perspectives on eating disorders* (pp. 339–354). New York: Guilford Press.

Pipher, M. (1994). *Reviving Ophelia: Saving the selves of adolescent girls.* New York: Ballantine Books.

Pope, H. G., & Hudson, J. I. (1992). Is childhood sexual abuse a risk factor for bulimia nervosa? *American Journal of Psychiatry, 149*(4), 455–463.

Raymond, N. C., Mitchell, J. E., P. Fallon, & M. A. Katzman (1994). A collaborative approach to the use of medication. In P. Fallon, M. A. Katzman, & S. C. Wooley (Eds.), *Feminist perspectives on eating disorders* (pp. 231–250). New York: Guilford Press.

Root, M. P. P., & Fallon, P. (1988). The incidence of victimization experiences in a bulimic sample. *Journal of Interpersonal Violence, 3*(2), 161–173.

Rothblum, E. (1994). "I'll die for the revolution but don't ask me not to diet": Feminism and the continuing stigmatization of obesity. In P. Fallon, M. A. Katzman, & S. C. Wooley (Eds.), *Feminist perspectives on eating disorders* (pp. 53–76). New York: Guilford Press.

Seid, R. P. (1994). Too "close to the bone": The historical context for women's obsession with slenderness. In P. Fallon, M. A. Katzman, & S. C. Wooley (Eds.), *Feminist perspectives on eating disorders* (pp. 3–16). New York: Guilford Press.

Sesan, R. (1994). Feminist inpatient treatment for eating disorders: An oxymoron? In P. Fallon, M. A. Katzman, & S. C. Wooley (Eds.), *Feminist perspectives on eating disorders* (pp. 251–271). New York: Guilford Press.

Sheffield, C. (1992). Sexual terrorism. In J. Kourany, J. Sterba, & R. Tong (Eds.), *Feminist philosophies.* Upper Saddle River, NJ: Prentice Hall.

Shisslak, C., & Crago, M. (1994). Toward a new model for the prevention of eating disorders. In P. Fallon, M. A. Katzman, & S. C. Wooley (Eds.), *Feminist perspectives on eating disorders* (pp. 419–437). New York: Guilford Press.

Shisslak, C., Crago, M., & Estes, L. (1995). The spectrum of eating disorders. *International Journal of Eating Disorders, 18,* 209–219.

Solomon, M. R. (1992). *Consumer behavior: Buying, having, and being.* Boston: Allyn and Bacon.

Steiner-Adair, C. (1986). The body politic: Normal female adolescent development and the development of eating disorders. *Journal of American Psychoanalysis, 14,* 95–114.

Steiner-Adair, C. (1994). The politics of prevention. In P. Fallon, M. A. Katzman, & S. C. Wooley (Eds.), *Feminist perspectives on eating disorders* (pp. 381–393). New York: Guilford Press.

Stephens, D. L., Hill, R. P., & Hanson, C. (1994). The beauty myth and female consumers: The controversial role of advertising. *Journal of Consumer Affairs, 28*(1), 137–152.

Storber, M. (1986). Anorexia nervosa: History and psychological concepts. In K. Brownell & J. Foreyt (Eds.), *Handbook of eating disorders* (pp. 231–246). New York: Basic Books.

Strong, S. M., Williamson, D. A., Netemeyer, R. G., & Geer, J. H. (2000). Eating disorder symptoms and concerns about body differ as a function of gender and sexual orientation. *Journal of Social and Clinical Psychology, 19*(2), 240–255.

Tiggemann, M., & Stevens, C. (1999). Weight concern across the life-span: Relationship to self-esteem and feminist identity. *International Journal of Eating Disorders, 26*(1), 103–106.

Thompson, B. (1994). Food, bodies, and growing up female: Childhood lessons about culture, race, and class. In P. Fallon, M. A. Katzman, & S. C. Wooley (Eds.), *Feminist perspectives on eating disorders*. New York: Guilford Press.

Vanderlinden, J., Norre, J., & Vandereychen, W. (1992). *A practical guide to the treatment of bulimia nervosa*. New York: Bronner/Mazel.

Waller, G. (1992). Sexual abuse and bulimic symptoms in eating disorders: Do family interaction and self-esteem explain the links? *International Journal of Eating Disorders, 12*(3), 235–248.

Wendell, S. (1992). Toward a feminist theory of disability. In H. B. Holmes, & L. M. Purdy (Eds.), *Feminist perspectives in medical ethics* (pp. 63–81). Bloomington, IN: Indiana University Press.

White, J. H. (2000). The prevention of eating disorders: A review of the research on risk factors with implications for practice. *Journal of Child and Adolescent Psychiatric Nursing, 13*(2), 76–88.

Wilkerson, A. L. (1998). *Diagnosis difference: The moral authority of medicine*. Ithaca, NY: Cornell University Press.

Wolf, N. (1994). Hunger. In P. Fallon, M. A. Katzman, & S. C. Wooley (Eds.), *Feminist perspectives on eating disorders* (pp. 94–114). New York: Guilford Press.

Wolf, S. M. (1996). Introduction: Gender and feminism in bioethics. In S. M. Wolf (Ed.), *Feminism & bioethics: Beyond reproduction* (pp. 3–46). New York: Oxford University Press.

Wooley, S. C. (1994). Sexual abuse and eating disorders: The concealed debate. In P. Fallon, M. A. Katzman, & S. C. Wooley (Eds.), *Feminist perspectives on eating disorders* (pp. 171–211). New York: Guilford Press.

Wooley, S. C., & Wooley, O. W. (1985). Intensive outpatient and residential treatment for bulimia. In D. M. Garner, & P. E. Garfinkel (Eds.), *Handbook of psychotherapy for anorexia nervosa and bulimia* (pp. 391–430). New York: Guilford Press.

8

Care for the Frail Elderly: A Comparative Analysis

*E*ach theoretical perspective that we have explored—rule ethics, virtue ethics, and feminist ethics—provides critical insights into the nature of ethical judgments. These three perspectives are not mutually exclusive; the ethical questions they raise and the guidance they provide may at times overlap and/or complement one another. They may also challenge us by framing ethical issues in strikingly different ways. This chapter provides an opportunity to compare these theoretical perspectives through the examination of ethical issues related to the increasing dependence of the frail elderly on formal and informal care in the community.

As demographic changes and advances in medicine have combined to create an increasing percentage of elderly who live longer on average, the needs of the dependent elderly raise far-reaching ethical issues. These issues are related to fundamental beliefs and attitudes about the personal and social value of caregiving, dependency and autonomy, intergenerational responsibilities, just distribution of family and community resources, and the relative responsibilities of families and society. After identifying and analyzing key ethical issues in a selected case scenario, the chapter will consider how the perception of ethical issues changes as we shift ethical theories. Although space does not permit an exhaustive analysis, key questions and issues will be drawn from each theoretical perspective.

The Frail Elderly: Context

The elderly population in the United States, people over 65, has increased tenfold since 1900. Thirty-five million people, or nearly 13 percent of the population today, are over 65. By 2050, this figure will grow to 20 percent. The fastest growing segment of the population is the group aged 85 and older, the "oldest old." This population has tripled since 1960, to more than 4.2 million Americans or 1.6 percent of the U.S. population, and will more than quadruple again by 2050 (Administration on Aging, 1997a; Federal Interagency Forum on Aging-Related Statistics, 2000). The rapid growth of this age group is particularly significant in terms of health care and assistance needs, since these individuals are likely to have multiple health problems that result in physical and mental frailty and subsequent dependency on formal and informal sources of care.

Family caregivers play a vital role as more of them increasingly assume nursing tasks. Eighty percent of all care received by the elderly comes from family or other informal systems (Blaser, 1998). Wives, daughters, and daughters-in-law most commonly provide this care. The other 20 percent of care is provided by formal health care services, particularly by nurses. Although family caregiving has always existed, its nature has changed significantly as a result of recent trends. First, pressures to control health care costs have resulted in an increasing effort to locate services outside expensive institutions. Second, chronic disease has become the dominant pattern of illness, resulting in a significant increase in disability among the frail elderly. Finally, an increasing number of medical treatments previously performed only in the hospital are now provided in the home as a result of technological developments (Ward-Griffin & McKeever, 2000).

The term *frail elderly* will be used here to refer to adults aged 65 and older with significant physical or mental frailty. Of the 34 million elderly who live at home or with family members, approximately 20 percent have at least one limitation in their ability to perform activities of daily living (ADL). Approximately 4 percent , or 1.4 million, are severely disabled and thus unable to perform major activities without assistance from others. These populations will double by 2040 (Administration on Aging, 1997b). Those who are aged 85 and older are four to five times more likely to be disabled and to require assistance with their personal care than those aged 65 to 74. Consequently, nearly 57 percent of the oldest old experience limitations in daily activities (Administration on Aging, 1999).

The need for long-term care varies by gender, race, and income. Life expectancy varies by gender and race. Men tend to die earlier than women as a result of major chronic illnesses such as heart disease, stroke, and cancer. As a result, the ratio of men to women in the 65 to 74 group is 82.2:100 and decreases to 40.5:100 among those who are 85 and older. The gap is expected to decrease, however, with projected ratios of 92.6:100 and 62.9:100 in 2050 (Administration on Aging, 1997a). At present, women are over 40 percent more likely to report limitations in daily activities than men (Administration on Aging, 1999).

Elderly people of color experience greater degrees of functional impairment than whites and rely more heavily on informal care providers (Hooyman & Gonyea, 1995). Black, non-Hispanic elderly are over two thirds more likely to experience two or more ADL limitations than white, non-Hispanic elderly persons (Administration on Aging, 1999). The greater degree of disability among elderly persons of color is linked to the fact that among the elderly, income level is also highly correlated with disability. Elderly persons below the poverty level are more than twice as likely to report two or more ADL limitations than those with incomes at or above the poverty threshold (Administration on Aging, 1999). Because poverty rate increases by age, gender, and race, so does the degree of disability. Fourteen percent of those over 85 are poor, compared with 9 percent of those aged 65 to 74. More older women than older men are below the poverty line—13 percent versus 7 percent . The combined effects of age, gender, and race are evident from the fact that in 1998 divorced black women aged 65 to 74 had a poverty rate of 47 percent, which is among the highest of any subset of older people (Federal Interagency Forum on Aging-Related Statistics, 2000).

Medicare and Medicaid provide some financial support for elder care. Medicare is the largest single payer of home care services. In the 1990s, Medicare home health spending rose an average of 30 percent per year (National Center for Policy Analysis, 1999). This increase is reflected not only in total dollars spent but also in the portion of Medicare dollars spent on home health, which grew from 2.5 percent in 1989 to 9.0 percent in 1997 (Allen, 1999; National Association for Home Care [NAHC], 2000b). Yet Medicare home health benefits are primarily intended for post–acute care rather than long-term care for chronic disabilities (Hooyman & Gonyea, 1995).

Medicaid is a federal and state means-tested welfare program for medical assistance for the categorically needy. Only about 10 percent of Medicaid expenditures are allocated to home care services (including home health, personal care, and community-based waiver services) (NAHC, 2000a); the bulk of Medicaid funds are spent on the elderly to pay for nursing home costs despite the fact that only 4 to 5 percent of those over 65 live in nursing homes.

The following case scenario illustrates a number of issues related to care for the frail elderly.

EXPERIENTIAL ACCOUNT: Caring for Mom

Louise Meyer, 78 years old, was married to George for 55 years. Together, they managed a wheat farm and raised three children, Joe, Elaine, and Peter. After George died 18 months ago, Louise lived alone. Elaine checked on her daily by telephone and visited every weekend. A recent fall and hospitalization, however, helped Elaine to persuade her mother to come and live with her and her two sons, 16 and 17 years old, 20 miles from the family farm.

For the past 19 years, Louise has been treated for Type 2 diabetes, and for the last eight years, she has been insulin dependent. She explains that she has no primary care physician because "a doctor can't do anything for me." Every two to three years, Louise has driven several hours to visit a large diabetes clinic in a major city for management of her condition. Because her driver's license was revoked four months ago, she now depends on Elaine to drive.

Over the years, Louise has developed a series of complications related to her diabetes. Because she is a poor surgical risk, she has inoperable cataracts. She suffers from lower extremity diabetic neuropathy. Symptoms of this include sharp pain in her legs, increasing muscle weakness, and some insensitivity to temperature. As a result, it is difficult for Louise to move. Increasingly her balance and coordination have also been affected.

In the past year, she has experienced a number of falls, the most recent resulting from an episode of dizziness that caused her to lose her balance when she was on a ladder. She was taken to the emergency room, where it was discovered that her blood pressure was 200/160. She also experienced right side numbness and weakness and slightly slurred speech. She was admitted for observation because of increasing pain in her lower right calf, an area injured in the fall. Ultrasound confirmed the presence of a small embolism, and she was started on heparin therapy. Two days later, she was discharged from the hospital with a percutaneous intravenous catheter line and a pump to administer intravenous antibiotics. Outpatient instructions included self-administering two subcutaneous injections of Lovenox, twice daily. Two medications to control her blood pressure were also prescribed, with instructions to take her blood pressure twice daily for the next six weeks. Her once-per-day dose of insulin was increased to a 50–50 mixture of insulin as well as her preloaded maintenance dose.

A nurse showed Elaine how to monitor and record Louise's blood pressure, how to draw up the two different insulins into the same syringe, where to inject the insulin, and how to administer the Lovenox into her mother's abdomen. Arrangements were made for a visiting nurse to come to the house once a week or as needed to change the dressing on the PIC line as well as deliver the IV antibiotics bags. On her first visit, Rachel Ward, RN, demonstrated how to change the IV bags that contained the antibiotics as well as flush the line. She explained that she would be out to visit Louise once a week until the order was discontinued three to four weeks later.

Elaine Bauer is 47 years old, divorced, and works as an office manager for a small-town insurance agency. She has assumed significant responsibility for her mother's personal care. She helps her to get in and out of the bathtub and family car and to navigate stairs. She manages her nutritional intake and medications, because Louise often forgets to eat or follow her medication regimen. Louise also resists some of her dietary restrictions and Elaine plays a critical role as coach and monitor. She records Louise's blood sugar reading twice a day, because she is unable to read the results on the monitor.

Bringing her mother to live with her has not been easy for Elaine. Her sons are busy with sports, friends, and part-time jobs. Her older son is researching college possibilities; Elaine has high hopes for him, but worries that unless he receives significant scholarship support he will be unable to attend the schools he is considering. While both of her sons are good kids, she worries that she does not spend enough time with them. The increased responsibilities of caring for her mother have added another layer of anxiety to her busy life. Although they cannot really afford it, she has cut back on her hours at work.

Initially, Elaine was petrified by the prospect of giving her mother injections. She is less fearful about this now but is generally anxious about her new responsibilities in managing Louise's diabetes. During one of the nurse's recent visits, Elaine expressed feelings of frustration, fear, and being overwhelmed by the responsibility of administering medications and maintaining the IV pump and stated, "Why can't you do these things?"

Elaine wonders whether Louise should move into a skilled nursing facility. She worries about her safety during the day when she is at work. She has raised the possibility of a nursing home with her brothers, Joe and Peter. They express concerns about the quality of care that their mother would receive as a Medicaid-dependent resident. Although Louise continues to mourn the loss of her husband and the farm community where she lived for decades, she enjoys the independence and companionship afforded her by living in her daughter's home.

Through the Rule Ethics Lens

Rule ethics seeks to determine what actions are right or wrong through the logical application of moral rules to particular cases. The Meyer case challenges us to apply rules of autonomy, beneficence, and justice to elder care. Among many ethical issues that arise in the Meyer case, three are primary from a rule ethics perspective: (1) balancing the value of independence versus safety, (2) family and society's responsibilities for long-term care for the frail elderly, and (3) responsibilities in the nurse–family caregiver relationship.

Conflicting Values: Independence Versus Safety

Clearly, Louise has substantial health care needs at this point. The first consideration from a rule ethics perspective is the responsibility of Louise's caregivers to protect her from harm, which is one of the rules of beneficence. Louise's dizziness, lack of balance and coordination, and difficulty in walking all raise safety concerns. Nurse Ward, the visiting nurse, must be concerned about Louise's falls and the many hours that she is alone. Like many elderly in the United States, however, Louise values the independence of noninstitutional living. Such independence is clearly an expression of her autonomy. Moving from her own home and the farm was a major dislocation for Louise. Further disconnection from her family and community would be extremely difficult. Living with two teenagers is no doubt chaotic and noisy at times, but preferable for Louise to the more regimented lifestyle of a nursing home.

Nurse Ward, Louise, and Elaine must consider whether the present arrangement imposes unreasonable risks of harm for Louise. Although nurses have a duty of beneficence to make reasonable efforts to protect patients from harm, this duty must be balanced against the value of independence as well as financial considerations (another aspect of patient well-being). Staying with her family and maintaining relative independence is important to Louise Meyer. Nurse Ward should help Louise and Elaine to recognize and evaluate the risks that are involved in remaining in the home, ensuring that they genuinely understand them in order to generate possible solutions. Louise and Elaine are competent decision makers, but they need to be informed decision makers.

Elaine seems generally capable of providing necessary care for her mother, but she feels anxious and a bit overwhelmed by the increased responsibilities for her care. Many laypeople would be anxious about giving injections. Administering the preloaded insulin dose is fairly straightforward, but she also faces the more challenging task of accurately drawing up the correct amounts of insulin and Lovenox. She will need support and positive affirmation from Nurse Ward for her efforts. In light of Louise's recent fall and embolism, Elaine may also be worried about further complications or deterioration of Louise's condition. She needs assistance in learning as much as possible about diabetes and its complications. Louise needs to see a primary care provider who could regularly monitor her diabetes and general health status. Perhaps Nurse Ward can persuade her to establish a relationship with a local provider. She may also be able to help Louise and Elaine locate sources of education and support for patients with diabetes and their caregivers.

Family and Societal Responsibilities

Caring for Louise in her home adds significant physical, emotional, and financial burdens to Elaine's life. Caregivers of the elderly, when compared with matched noncaregivers, report more chronic illness, poorer overall health, and greater use of prescription drugs (Hooyman & Gonyea, 1995). There are several justice issues raised in our case scenario. The first concerns the distribution of caretaking responsibilities among the three Meyer siblings. We do not know what decision process led to Elaine inviting her mother into her home, but the result is a common one. Seventy-two percent of unpaid family caregivers are women, the majority of them midlife daughters or daughters-in-law (Holstein & Mitzen, 1998; Robinson, 1997). There may have been perfectly good reasons why Elaine, rather than Joe or Peter, assumed the responsibility. Nonetheless, Joe and Peter owe their mother and their sister their support. They can provide financial assistance as well as help with house maintenance, transportation, and respite time for Elaine.

A broader issue from a rule ethics perspective is how we should understand the relation between the duties (of beneficence) of families to care for their elderly relatives and society's responsibilities to provide care. In some ethnic cultures, the responsibility of children to care for their parents is taken for granted and welcomed. In mainstream U.S. Caucasian culture, in which independence and mobility are highly valued, the degree of children's responsibility for their elderly parents is ambiguous. The reality is that this issue has generated insufficient consideration.

Many operate out of rather vague expectations that the elderly will take care of themselves with just a little help from family and neighbors until they are dying or very ill. They tend to envision this as a relatively short period in which the ill elderly will assuredly receive professional and likely institutional care. In short, American society has not come to terms with the fact that the elderly live longer and with more chronic conditions than a generation ago.

Meanwhile, professionals and policymakers have concluded that the elderly should be cared for in the least restrictive environment possible. Despite the significant increase in the over-65 population, the percentage of elderly Americans living in nursing homes declined from 4.6 percent in 1985 to 4.2 percent in 1995 (Reuters Health, 2000). While community-based care and in-home care are frequently better for the bodies and spirits of older people, the question of who is responsible for their care has not been addressed. Are children obliged to care for their parents in old age to the same degree that parents are obliged to care for their children? Is it realistic to assign children this responsibility in light of the time and money required for adequate care?

Clearly, our society does recognize some responsibility to care for ill and disabled elderly through programs such as Medicare and Medicaid. As the number of elderly has grown, federal dollars spent on these programs have soared, yet they are not designed to address the needs of homebound elderly. Both programs focus on acute and institutional health care. As the trend toward providing health care services in the home has accelerated in the past decade, the funds to support community-based and in-home care for the elderly have not followed (Levin-Epstein, 2000; NAHC, 2000b; Robinson, 1997; Weinberg, 1998; Wuest, 2000).

Increasing pressure to move care out of the hospital or the skilled nursing facility into the home is at least in part motivated by efforts to control the escalating costs of elder care. Concerns about the increasing costs of home health care led Congress to enact changes in the Medicare law through the Balanced Budget Act of 1997. The effects have been dramatic. Home health spending from fiscal year 1997 (FY97) to FY99 was reduced 48 percent, and Medicare dollars spent on home health decreased from 9 percent in FY97 to 4 percent in FY2000 (NAHC, 2000b). A prospective payment system for home care was implemented in October 2000, and a further 15 percent cut in expenditures is scheduled for October 2001. Fewer clients have utilized Medicare home health benefits due to these budget cuts, while home visits per client and reimbursements per client have declined since the 1997 changes (American Association of Retired Persons [AARP], 1998; NAHC, 2000b).

Despite the escalating expenditures for long-term care, federal and state funding is not meeting needs of the frail elderly to an extent that would enable them to stay in their own homes or with family members. Although Elaine Bauer would like more nursing care for her mother, she and her mother require social care as much as nursing care. Elaine seems able, at least for now, to provide much of her mother's personal care, but assistance in other areas would benefit both Elaine and Louise. Transportation would enable Louise to participate in senior center activities, providing companionship and mental stimulation. As her health deteriorates, Louise may require a more supervised environment such as an adult day care setting. Alternatively, daily visits by an aide to check on her safety and provide some companionship would benefit Louise and relieve some of Elaine's anxiety about leaving her mother alone during the day. Other homebound elderly may need aides to provide personal care, home repair, and housekeeping.

Elaine would benefit from more information about her mother's illness and available resources in her community; help with managing her own adaptation to her new responsibilities, social contacts with people with similar experiences, and substitute and respite care to provide her with time for her own self-care (Hooyman & Gonyea, 1995).

Presently, although we have several mechanisms to pay for some long-term care services, there is no coordinated and cohesive system for this care, and major gaps in services and funding exist. Elaine Bauer cannot afford to pay for the kinds of services described here. These simple support services could significantly improve Louise's health and safety as well as extend Elaine's ability to care for her. Thus, despite a growing consensus that care for the frail elderly should take place in the least restrictive setting, recent cutbacks in funding for home health care may actually increase institutionalization of the elderly. As financial assistance for home care is reduced, placing a family member in a nursing home through Medicaid funding may be the only viable financial option for increasing numbers of families.

The crisis in elder care is one part of the larger crisis in the American health care system. Despite cost-control policies, health care costs continue to increase at four or five times the rate of inflation (Munson, 2000). Furthermore, many Americans continue to lack access to even a basic level of health care. A fundamental requirement of justice in rule ethics is that communities should develop processes to ensure fair access to and allocation of health care to all members of the community. While few disagree with this principle in the abstract, agreement at the level of concrete policy has been elusive. This principle simply states that those health care resources (including tax dollars) that belong to the collective community should be distributed fairly to all community members. Numerous ethical questions must still be resolved, including how much of a community's resources should be invested in health care (versus areas such as education, police protection, or the environment); what constitutes a "basic" level of health care; how health care should be delivered; and what responsibility government, employers, charitable organizations, families, and individuals should have for paying the costs of health care.

The growing pressure to provide home health care highlights another issue regarding health care priorities. Until recently, our current health care system has been driven largely by an acute care model of health care. It is obvious that the crisis in health care cannot be resolved without major rethinking of this model. We simply cannot expand publicly funded and employer-funded insurance to include the millions of uninsured and underinsured and at the same time expand federal and state funding for home health care for the increasing numbers of frail elderly. We must make some difficult choices about our priorities in health care. What kinds of health services do we most value? If we want more public funding for home health services, what other services are we willing to trade for this? Furthermore, the disproportionate focus in health care insurance on physical rather than mental disability and illness appears to be discriminatory and therefore unjust. But if we want more support for treatment of mental health problems, including care for the increasing numbers of elderly with dementia, what are we willing to trade for this?

These issues of distributing responsibilities and community health care benefits are questions of justice that need to be addressed through community dialogue. Rule ethics will emphasize the need for broad participation by all persons in the community. Health care professionals need to contribute their expert insights regarding health needs and the effects of current health care policies. The elderly and family caregivers can also provide input from their experiences. Yet, the issue of elder care affects all members of the community, and all groups need to be heard.

Nurses and Family Caregivers

The relationship that develops between nurses and family caregivers is multifaceted and dynamic. Nurses are expected to develop partnerships with family caregivers in all health care settings. The increasing shift of responsibilities from paid caregivers to unpaid family members reshapes potential nurse–family partnerships. In the majority of cases, nurses teach family caregivers a variety of technical skills and gradually transfer much of the actual care of elderly patients to family members. The nurse often assumes the role of care manager rather than hands-on care provider.

Rule ethics requires that nurses treat family caregivers with the same respect as they do their patients. A number of ethical issues emerge in the nurse–family relationship. The first concerns role expectations. Family caregivers may be confused and/or frustrated by the gradual reduction in the nurse's involvement in caregiving. Nurses need to discuss and clearly communicate expectations for their role and that of the family caregivers.

There are a number of ways in which nurses can support family caregivers. The first is to monitor the health of family caregivers, especially those who are themselves elderly with considerable health concerns. Seeking respite services and accessing community services to decrease the workload of family caregivers are also important responsibilities. In addition, nurses can support caregivers' efforts to maintain their own mental and physical well-being. Given the time and energy demands of her job, her sons, and her mother, Elaine Bauer may easily become socially isolated, one of the common sources of stress for family caregivers. She may need encouragement to maintain personal connections to support her own mental health.

Finally, both family caregivers and nurses may experience frustration with the limitations of public policies and the lack of resources to provide adequate care. Nurses may become the object of the frustrations of caregivers who become overwhelmed. Recommending a support group, for instance, may appear rather insignificant to a chronically exhausted caregiver who perceives her primary need as simply more physical help. Nurses need to acknowledge the stress experienced by families and help them to recognize that inadequate resources are a matter of mutual concern. Nurses must also advocate for individual patients at the policy level, but they can also build coalitions with families to strengthen further lobbying efforts.

Through the Virtue Ethics Lens

Although elements overlap in the rule ethics and virtue ethics perspectives, a shift of emphasis occurs. Virtue ethics transfers the focus from the application of rules to the development and support of good character. Virtue ethics challenges us to consider whether our current policies regarding elder care promote the kind of individual and community character that we want to exhibit. Three primary ethical issues from the virtue ethics perspective are (1) impediments to the expression of caregiver virtues, (2) a shift from a conception of elder care as a private family responsibility to a shared communal responsibility, and (3) redefinition of the nurse case manager role.

Virtues of Caring

While Nurse Ward will call on nearly all of the nursing virtues in her interaction with Louise Meyer and her daughter, Elaine, fidelity to trust and mediation are particularly important. Louise seems either to underestimate the potential complications of her diabetes or to be unnecessarily resigned to an inevitable decline in her health. If Nurse Ward can win her trust, she may be able to persuade her to take a more active role in promoting and preserving her health. Developing trust with Elaine is important but challenging as well. Elaine no doubt welcomed Nurse Ward into her home, grateful for her professional expertise. But Elaine perceives that Nurse Ward expects her to do more and more of the nursing tasks. Elaine may not feel that accepting responsibility for her mother's care is extraordinary but simply what daughters do. Nonetheless, she may feel abandoned by brothers who have contributed little, her government that has restricted home health care funding when many family members need more help, and now by this nurse who teaches and leaves. As a result, any tension in Nurse Ward's relationship with Elaine will need to be acknowledged and negotiated.

As noted earlier, Nurse Ward can help Elaine access resources and develop plans to reduce her workload. She also may be able to facilitate communication and cooperation between Elaine and her brothers, Joe and Peter. Perhaps she can initiate a family conference to discuss Louise's health and educate the brothers about her needs and Elaine's needs for assistance. This mediation role is critically important in home care.

Health care organizations increasingly employ nurses as case managers (NCMs) to coordinate services as well as to advocate for patients who encounter a perplexing array of agencies and programs. Community NCM programs are employed by organizations, including Medicare-funded managed care programs, to reduce expenses by preventing hospitalization or rapid rehospitalization. NCM programs have been widely acclaimed in nursing literature for their ability to improve quality of care while reducing costs, thus promoting the interests of both patients and payers. NCMs may be used to manage health care for the frail elderly living in the community, particularly those with complex health problems (Guttman, 1999; Padgett, 1998).

NCMs are expected to balance patient needs against the cost-saving interests of their employing agency or organization. There are, however, genuine conflicts of interests that cannot be resolved at the level of individual case management (Padgett, 1998). The imbalance of power between the patients and the employing organizations makes the task of balancing patient needs and employer interests often impossible. Structural constraints on caring that arise in NCM roles clearly undermine the ability of nurses to embody fidelity to trust, compassion, and mediation, potentially creating the feelings of abandonment experienced by Elaine Bauer.

Family Values and Community Values

Virtue ethics encourages us to consider what impediments or obstacles undermine people's efforts to embody their ideal virtues. The ability of both Elaine Bauer and Nurse Ward to embody the virtue of compassion in order to provide quality care for Louise Meyer is limited by the lack of a coherent social policy regarding elder care (Weinberg, 1998). Virtue ethics echoes the concerns about social policy noted in the rule ethics discussion. The debate is reframed, however, as we look through the virtue ethics lens.

Virtues reflect commitments to be a certain kind of person or to create a certain kind of community. Virtue ethics encourages us to reflect on what kind of community the United States wants to be with regard to care for the frail elderly. It is clear that many Americans value independence, self-determination, and privacy. These values are embodied in expectations that individuals will support themselves and avoid being a burden on others. A correlative belief is that a "good" family is one that takes care of its members. The value of individualism is further reflected in the belief that family life is private and that spouses, parents, and children caring for frail elders should be free as much as possible from government interference with how they fulfill their responsibilities and functions (McKeever, 1996; Hooyman & Gonyea, 1995). Within this conception of community, social institutions and policies should nurture individual autonomy and self-reliance.

Within this model of community, loss of dependence will be feared and the goal of assistance to individuals lacking independence will be oriented toward maintaining or restoring independence. Dependency will be perceived as a matter of misfortune, decline, or even personal failure within a model of community that so clearly defines the ideal and mature citizen as a self-reliant individual. Care for children, the physically and mentally disabled, or the frail elderly is perceived in this model as the responsibility of individual families. Families also are expected to be self-reliant and independent. Care outside of the family in institutions, whether day care for children, nursing homes, or institutional care for the mentally impaired, is perceived as an undesirable last resort (Hooyman & Gonyea, 1995; Wuest, 2000).

Virtue ethics should encourage communities to critically examine these assumptions. First, the presumptive definition of mature, normative human living as independent and self-reliant should be examined. Our fullest expressions of humanity are not limited to areas of individual achievement and self-improvement; they are also found in relationships characterized by reciprocity, mutuality, and interdependence. Furthermore, dependence and frailty are not limited to separate, special groups of people. They are an integral part of every person's life. Individuals experience periods of dependence and frailty throughout their lives due to illness, pregnancy, accidents, loss of employment, mental stress, depression, or grief. We are all dependent on others for friendship, companionship, and collective action in work, play, and politics. These are not extras or incidentals of a good human life—they are essential aspects of a mature, full life.

Second, the presumption that care for the frail and dependent is an individual family responsibility must be examined. Why is this a family responsibility rather than a community responsibility? Why do we assume that care provided in the family home is better than care provided in the community? A major motivation behind public policies that have shifted burdens for elder care from institutional settings to the home has been the effort to control costs. Uncompensated care to the frail elderly includes an average of 28 to 40 hours per week of custodial care. The estimated annual value of this kin care in 1990 was $18 billion (Robinson, 1997). We will return to this factor in the feminist discussion below. However, cost savings is not the only factor in the presumption that family care is the ideal.

Many believe that the family should take the primary responsibility for care because care provided at home by family members will be best for the persons receiving care. Family members will provide more personalized care both because of their personal knowledge of the elderly person and because family members share natural ties of gratitude and affection. The presumption, of course, is that care provided by nonrelatives in institutions or by agencies will be impersonal, performed as a job rather than out of personal attachment, and less individualized. Even if we accept the claim that the best care will be provided in the home by relatives, it need not be understood as only a private obligation.

Children owe their parents some support in their old age based on a sense of reciprocity and gratitude for earlier care received and sacrifices made. But children are not the only ones who owe a debt of gratitude to the elderly. All children benefit from the efforts of adults to create and preserve a community that provides for safety, education, a system of law, a stable economy, and a cultural inheritance of art and ideas. Certainly, adults are paid to perform some of this work, but sacrifices and effort go beyond paid work. In many cultures, the care of children and the frail is considered a shared responsibility of all adults in the community. All adults nurture, teach accountability, and share communal values/traditions with the young because these young people are the future of the entire community. Similarly, all adults (and children to some degree) honor, care for, and keep company with the elderly because every adult has inherited the community preserved and nurtured by these elders. Virtue ethics challenges the U.S. community to reconsider what kind of a community we want to be, whether one that elevates individuality and independence above all else, one that more fully values reciprocity and interdependence, or some other ideal.

The presumption that the best care will be provided in the home by family members warrants critical evaluation as well. Families are not always places of harmony and love. The level of child abuse, intimate partner violence, and elder abuse are testimony to this fact. On the other hand, paid caregivers outside of the home may provide compassionate and personalized care as a reflection of professional virtues and/or personal affection for those for whom they provide care. Whether care is provided by family members or paid caregivers, the quality of the care will suffer if there are insufficient resources allotted. Even the efforts of the most dedicated family members, such as Elaine Bauer, will be affected by the stress of multiple responsibilities, financial burdens, physical exhaustion, and social isolation. Home care is often contrasted with the specter of elderly persons abandoned, lonely, and sedated in nursing facilities. But the reality of home care for many like Louise Meyer may be long hours spent alone while family members are at work or school. Without transportation, Louise may have few opportunities to interact socially with her peers. Elaine may spend numerous hours uncovering available services that are then provided in multiple settings requiring time for transportation and coordination of services. Thus, while she and her sons may be best able to meet Louise's psychosocial needs, they may have little time or energy to devote to these aspects of care.

Alternatives to Individual Family Responsibility

Care for the elderly might be reconceptualized as a community responsibility much like the community responsibility for education of the young. Public education is a necessity in a community that values the dignity of every individual and supports the participation of each individual in the process of collective self-government. Democracies believe that every person should have the right to take part in the processes that determine how society will be structured and the norms for social interaction. A basic level of education is essential to this participation. Public education is also supported by the realization that our future well-being depends in part on the ability of these children in later years to be economically productive and to manage our social institutions. Public education is thus a collective responsibility of all community members.

A guarantee of a minimum level of care for the frail elderly might similarly be conceptualized as a collective responsibility. Bonds of reciprocity link younger community members to elders who have passed on responsibilities for communal governance and maintenance of our economic and social institutions. Just as public education enables all to participate in community life, care for the frail elderly is a reciprocal act that acknowledges the contributions already made. Furthermore, care for the chronically disabled who may never have been able to work or to serve the community is a communal responsibility based on our recognition of our common vulnerability to illness, accidents, or disabilities.

What are the implications of this model of communal responsibility? First, the role of families would be revisioned. Although family members have special bonds of reciprocity and affection, responsibility for elder care would not be a private responsibility of individual families. Care for the frail elderly would be a community responsibility, and family caregivers would be valued partners working with many others to fulfill the community's commitments. Caregiving provided by family members would be recognized and valued as a significant contribution to the community.

Second, the goal of public elder care policies would be expanded beyond avoiding hospitalization or nursing homes and enabling individuals to stay in their homes as long as possible. The goal would be to provide support necessary to meet at least the basic physiological and psychosocial needs of the frail elderly. Rather than a "drain on the economy," support for the elderly would be understood as one essential element of sustaining a humane community. Communities would develop a variety of culturally appropriate resources to provide adequate care for diverse groups of seniors. Seniors, families, professionals, and volunteers would work together to assess needs and to develop options. Families and individuals might choose from a variety of services that would combine informal and formal care. Artificial distinctions between medical and nonmedical needs would be eliminated and integrated services built around the functional needs of both the frail elderly and their caregivers developed (Hooyman & Gonyea, 1995; Neysmith, 1993).

Multiple options exist to provide and finance these services. As a communal dimension, elder care becomes the responsibility of the collective community and not simply the duty of government. Individuals, families, public and private organizations, and various levels of government might share the communal responsibility, but only the federal government could ultimately guarantee that the burdens are fairly distributed across the whole community.

Care Manager Role

The role of case manager would be restructured under a model of community responsibility for elder care. Although case managers who are employed by medical service providers often strive to advocate for their patients, their collaboration with families and frail elderly would be less constrained in a model of care management in which the managers work for the community. A primary role would be to educate the elderly and their families about the options for care available (Guttman, 1999). Such education should be provided proactively within a variety of settings such as through employee assistance programs, neighborhood centers, and church programs before crises occur and options become more limited. Together, families and care managers could tailor services to the needs and goals of patients and families. Follow-up education and further technical training as needs arise should be provided. Public education about the role of caregivers and their needs for support can help to promote the communal value of caregiving (Hooyman & Gonyea, 1995).

Effective care management would be systemic and include coordination and monitoring of care and titration of levels of support according to needs. Since care managers would coordinate a variety of social and health care services, nurses in these roles would need to embody virtues of collaboration and flexibility. Care managers would serve the community as well as dependent elderly and their families by advocating at the system level to adjust and develop appropriate services to meet the evolving needs of the frail elderly (Hooyman & Gonyea, 1995).

Through the Feminist Ethics Lens

Although feminist concerns will overlap with those of rule and virtue ethics, there are distinctly feminist ethical issues to consider. Thus, feminist ethics shifts our focus again by considering how current policies in elder care may perpetuate women's oppression and how relevant relationships, policies, and institutions could be restructured to empower both women and men. Feminists will (1) evaluate the gender inequities in caregiving, (2) note how the presumed separation of public and private spheres supports current elder care social policies and perpetuates gender imbalance of power, and (3) advocate for reinventing the workplace to facilitate adequate elder care.

Gender Inequities in Caregiving

Why is Elaine Bauer's role as the primary caregiver for her elderly mother, given that Louise Meyer also has two sons, so readily accepted in our society? What may seem unfair, however, is commonplace. As noted earlier, 72 percent of unpaid family caregivers are women. There is a hierarchy of social support in which gender supersedes kinship in all situations except care provided by married spouses. Thus, among the frail elderly, spouses provide the most care for married persons, daughters and daughters-in-law for the widowed, and sisters for the unmarried and childless. When men assume the caregiver role for their parents, it is generally by default. Eighty-eight percent of the time, it is because they are the only living child, in a family with all brothers, or the only geographically available adult. Although sons are as likely as daughters to have a parent living with them, they are much less likely to provide hands-on care (Robinson, 1997). Daughters and daughters-in-law are, in fact, three times as likely as sons and sons-in-law to provide personal care assistance to aging parents (Hooyman & Gonyea, 1995). Feminist ethics challenges us to consider the disproportionate responsibilities for elder care assumed by daughters like Elaine Bauer. It also challenges us to ask whether there are social or institutional policies that restrict the ability of men to assume these roles.

While the significant shift of caregiving responsibilities from paid professional caregivers to families is widely recognized, the gender inequities in caregiving are frequently unacknowledged. In light of the fact that the frail elderly require 28 to 40 hours of custodial care per week, the effects of this gender inequity are significant (Robinson, 1997). Elder care policies in the United States continue to presume a middle-class model of the nuclear family in which men are the wage earners and women are at home with free time for caregiving. However, most women are not at home—more than 71 percent of all women aged 16 and over were employed outside the home in 1998. They averaged 38 hours per week, and 51 percent worked full time. Marriage clearly has little effect on paid work status since 69 percent of married women worked outside the home also, averaging 36 hours per week, with 47 percent working full time. The only significant difference was found among women with children under six years of age, where the rate of employment dropped to 58 percent and the percentage working full time dropped to 35 percent (Cohen & Bianchi, 1999).

This is not a new state of affairs: Women's labor force participation rates have changed little over the last 20 years, except in terms of race. Until the late 1980s, black women aged 30 to 44 had the highest labor force participation rates, but by the 1990s the participation rates of white, non-Hispanic women and black women were similar. Rates for Hispanic women are only slightly lower. Significant changes in women's employment have occurred, however, since 1950. Women's participation in the paid labor force has increased 26 percent since 1950. Furthermore, the difference between men's and women's aggregate participation rates have changed dramatically from a 50 percentage point difference in 1950 to only 15 percentage points in 1998. The closing of this gap is due to women's increasing employment and also due to the 12 percent drop in men's employment rates since 1950 (Fullerton, 1999).

Women are disproportionately the caregivers for dependent children and adults with developmental disabilities, in addition to being the primary caregivers for the frail elderly. Some women like Elaine Bauer carry the double responsibilities of caring for children and a frail parent without the physical, emotional, or financial support of a male partner. An estimated 25 percent of U.S. households with children under age 18 are single parent, and 80 percent of these are female headed in 2000 (U.S. Census Bureau, 1998).

Although a significant proportion of women report positive benefits of caring for frail spouses and parents, there are also significant burdens associated with the caregiving role. These burdens include effects on physical health, increased stress, disruptions and strains on family relations, restrictions in social and leisure activities, employment restrictions, and financial effects (Braithwaite, 1992; McKeever, 1996; Hooyman & Gonyea, 1995).

Clearly, women are carrying more than their share of the burdens of caregiving in our society. Most are not at home with "free time." Women are already responsible for a disproportionate amount of the work of child care and housework. Most women have few extra resources to take on additional responsibilities for the frail elderly. Feminists both note the inequality of the caregiving responsibilities and encourage us to ask why our society continues to promote public policies that perpetuate this gender inequality.

The Presumption of Separate Spheres

Since the Industrial Revolution, Western cultures have divided social life into public and private spheres. The private sphere of the home and family has traditionally been identified as women's responsibility, while the public realm of the marketplace and government has presumptively been claimed as men's sphere of responsibility. Feminists suggest that the misfit between social policies regarding elder care that heavily depend on family caregivers, in spite of the fact that most women are employed, is a reflection of ideological beliefs about women's roles in the family. Caregiving is presumed to be primarily women's responsibility (McKeever, 1996; Robinson, 1997; Hooyman & Gonyea, 1995). Women should ideally be in the home as caregivers for children, husbands, and dependent adult relatives. Women are perceived as natural carers because of their expressive, nurturing characters, whereas men are responsible for supporting the family due to their goal-oriented dispositions. Most feminists reject the claim that women are more natural caregivers than men, arguing that the gender division of labor is the result of patriarchal imbalances of power that encourage distinct socialization processes for males and females. Women are more likely to develop better caregiving skills than men because they are expected to do this work and are socialized to do so.

Feminists reject the false division between the public and private spheres, noting numerous ways in which the two spheres are interdependent. There are significant interdependencies between the workplace and the home, for instance. The structure of the corporate world assumes that workers have "wives" who take care of domestic chores and child care so that workers can devote themselves to their careers or jobs. It is assumed that someone other than the worker is picking up children after school, nursing them when they are home sick, attending teacher–student conferences, preparing meals, doing housework, caring for elderly parents, arranging for home repairs, and so on. But increasingly there is no "wife" at home doing all of these things. As women have entered the paid workforce in increasing numbers, however, their responsibilities for child care and housework have not significantly decreased. Employed wives spend nearly twice the number of hours per week on these domestic tasks than employed husbands do (Rodgers, 1992).

The effects of this "double burden" of work and family on women include chronic fatigue and marital stress as well as economic disadvantages. Women are disadvantaged in the workplace by the more limited time available to them to devote to their jobs/careers as well as by the need to leave their jobs periodically for pregnancies or to care for ill or frail dependents (Okin, 1989). Nearly 12 percent of the earnings gap between men and women is explained by women's time spent out of the labor market on domestic work. Salary disparities over time contribute to the situation in the United States in which female-headed families represent 53 percent of all poor families (Hooyman & Gonyea, 1995).

Public policies on care for the frail elderly similarly affect the private sphere of the home. Research demonstrates that 9 percent of family caregivers leave the labor force to provide care, 29 percent adjust their work schedules, and 18 percent take time off without pay (Robinson, 1997). Workers with elder care responsibilities reduce their work hours an average of five hours per week (Mutschler, 1994). Because women are disproportionately these caregivers, their economic status is further undermined by these policies. Once again, the workplace makes no provisions for the realities of aging parents who require care. Nor do most public policies such as the system of unemployment compensation that provides no benefits for a woman who quits her job due to the lack of elder care or inappropriate hours relative to her family responsibilities.

The tensions between paid work and caregiving have long-term economic effects on women. Because of the interruptions in their employment history due to caregiving responsibilities, older women are less likely to have an adequate Social Security benefit or a private pension. Social Security benefits for retired women are 75 percent of that for retired men; only 18 percent of women receive private pensions compared to 34 percent of men over 65, and women's pensions on average are 57 percent of men's (Johnson, 1999).

The heavy burdens of elder care impact individual women, but the gender inequities in caregiving also perpetuate the gender power imbalance of patriarchy. Women carry disproportionate responsibilities for unpaid caregiving in the home, in part because they have less power to insist that the burdens be more evenly distributed. But the effects of caregiving responsibilities increase women's economic disadvantage and limit their participation in other social institutions as well. Some state programs in the United States pay family caregivers. Box 8–1 considers whether this is an appropriate means to alleviate women's economic disadvantage.

Reinventing the Workplace

Current public and workplace policies regarding long-term care clearly place a disproportionate burden on women who already carry more than their share of caregiving responsibilities. The exacerbation of gender inequities alone is a sufficient reason

Box 8–1   Communities in Dialogue:

Financial Assistance for Family Caregivers

As the number of people requiring extensive home care accelerates, strategies to reduce the long-term economic effect on caregivers, most of whom are women, must be considered. The financial impact of caring for dependent relatives is significant. Yet American society is deeply ambivalent about providing government payments to people to fulfill their family responsibilities. If we agree that family members have an obligation to provide care for dependent relatives, it does not follow that they should be expected to sacrifice financial security to provide care. For the roughly 30 percent of family caregivers who are at or near the poverty level, financial support can make the difference in their ability to sustain care. Nonetheless, financial compensation for family caregivers is controversial in the United States.

Thirty-five states in the U.S. provide some form of financial payment to relatives, including cash allowances, vouchers for specific services, or grants for certain out-of-pocket expenses, though eligibility is restricted. Some 15 states explicitly exclude payments to relatives for caregiving.

In contrast to limited U.S. assistance, at least 59 other industrialized countries provide significantly superior financial support for caregivers. Direct cash payments to individuals who require care, the most common model, permits consumers to use their own discretion to purchase services that best meet their needs, including payment to family caregivers. In Scandinavian countries, family caregivers receive actual wages for their services.

Many people prefer family caregivers because they believe them to be more knowledgeable about a relative's preferences and needs, more reliable, and more caring than unrelated workers. A dependent relative may feel more secure having a family member rather than a stranger in the home. Concerns about reliability and competence are justifiable in light of the clearly inadequate wages paid to home care workers and consequent staff turnover.

Some argue that family caregivers should be paid because they perform an important social function and forfeit other opportunities to ensure their own financial security. This is particularly important for women who are already economically disadvantaged by their disproportionate caregiving responsibilities. Some oppose compensation on ideological grounds that providing care for dependent relatives is a moral obligation that should be motivated by love and gratitude. The presumption, apparently, is that caregiving cannot be simultaneously loving and paid or that payment will inevitably transform personal caring relationships into impersonal business transactions. Although these assumptions

Box 8–1   Communities in Dialogue:

Financial Assistance for Family Caregivers

should be questioned, there are legitimate concerns about the potential for financial fraud and abuse when family caregivers are compensated. The most common form of financial fraud occurs when family members employed by home care agencies collude with the client to report services that were not delivered. In other cases, the family caregiver defrauds agencies without client involvement or the dependent relative is coerced into signing the service receipt. Neglect is the most common type of abuse; family members may provide early morning or late evening care, leaving the impaired elder alone while working a full-time job. Concerns about abuse and neglect cannot be easily dismissed in light of the well-documented history of similar mistreatment in foster care and Aid to Dependent Children systems. At the least, these concerns point to the need for vigilant monitoring.

Feminists who support financial compensation for family caregivers as a matter of gender justice must also consider that this policy may indirectly perpetuate the exploitation of all in-home workers, most of whom are women. Home care workers are underpaid, receive few benefits, and have little or no opportunity for career advancement. The policy of paying family members to provide care for minimum wage may reduce pressures to increase wages and benefits for all in-home workers. Job seekers may choose jobs with higher compensation levels, leaving impaired elders and their families with little choice but a family caregiver.

Compensation for family caregivers must be considered as one part of a larger set of policies and programs to ensure adequate support and care for impaired elders and their families. Community dialogue regarding paid family caregivers must consider and balance the demands of communal responsibility, filial obligations, and gender justice.

Questions

1. Can the concerns about fraud and abuse of dependent relatives be adequately addressed in a cost-effective manner?

2. Are there alternative methods for supporting family caregivers that would provide economic, emotional, and practical support for these caregivers?

3. How might women who are caregivers for family members and other paid in-home care providers support each other in advocating for fair compensation and improved working conditions?

to change public policies. But these policies also harm the dependent elderly, create domestic tension, and impair worker productivity. Feminists support the view that care for the elderly should be recognized as a social responsibility and not merely a private one. Economic and social supports for caregivers and community-based alternatives are needed for the well-being of both caregivers and their dependents. In addition, feminists argue that gender equity and quality of life for all community members depends on reinventing the workplace (Hochschild, 1997; Hooyman & Gonyea, 1995; Okin, 1989; Parker & Hall, 1993).

Although some progressive employers have developed family-responsive benefits such as family and medical leave, flexible work arrangements and employer-provided elder care services, these solutions treat the problems of family responsibilities as simply an individual worker's problem rather than a social problem. Furthermore, since these benefits continue to be used disproportionately by women, they reinforce the cultural assumption that family issues are women's responsibilities. Women (and men) who use these benefits may be perceived as less committed to their careers and consequently shunted into a "mommy track."

Feminists propose that corporate America needs to recognize the multiple changes in family structure and develop benefits and policies that support employees with diverse lifestyles and family structures (including informal domestic partnerships). Corporate policies should emphasize employee choice and empowerment and should seek to develop employer–community partnerships to address the social responsibilities of caregiving. More fundamentally, feminists promote the restructuring of the work–family relationship to recognize that family life is not peripheral but an essential component of their employees' lives. Corporate policies should embrace the full reality of human lives and acknowledge that workers have a variety of family responsibilities that change over time. Workers should be offered options for structuring their work week and their long-term career (Bailyn, 1992). People will be more engaged in their work when they are permitted to express, rather than suppress, their full identities in the workplace. A more flexible workplace enables employees to bring their full selves to work and to be psychologically engaged in the tasks and relationships that make up their jobs, knowing that their family responsibilities are supported and valued (Parker & Hall, 1993). The need for work–family balance must be extended to lower- income wage earners, including the large group of underpaid and undervalued nursing aides who provide most of the hands-on institutional care for the elderly. The needs of contingent workers—part-timers, temporary employees, and those who provide services that are contracted for outside of corporations—who now represent 30 percent of the workforce also must be addressed.

Corporations will need government support for these changes. A combination of incentives and mandates will likely be necessary. Corporations may not perceive these changes as serving their economic interests. In the short run, this is clearly true. But the need to value the work of caregiving and those who provide this care is in the long-term interests of business and society. Restructuring the workplace is an investment in human capital that will promote greater productivity and quality of community life.

Nursing and Long-Term Care

As noted earlier, health care organizations increasingly employ nurses as NCMs to improve quality care in complex cases while also reducing costs. Although NCMs play important roles as coordinators and brokers of services as well as patient advocates, feminists caution that managed care organizations may also exploit gender-linked abilities to achieve their economic interests. NCMs are encouraged to use their skills of communication, mediation, and coordination to humanize the not infrequently harsh realities of managed care. But the conflicts between the economic interests of the NCMs' employers and their patients are more than mere communication problems; there are genuine conflicts of interests that severely limit the ability of NCMs to promote their patients' best interests (Padgett, 1998). Furthermore, as nurses become the facilitators, mediators, and coordinators that attempt to guide patients through a flawed system, they may also inadvertently become enablers of an unjust system that promotes cost effectiveness over patient quality. Thus, nurses who take on the NCM role in order to improve quality care for patients may find their gender-linked expressive/caring abilities exploited in ways that undermine their own professional values and quality patient care.

Feminists, consequently, support the redefinition of the case management role described earlier in which a care manager is employed by the community rather than by specific medical service providers. As nurses recognize that conflicts of interests between patients and medical service providers are built into the structure of these health care systems, they may also play an important role in developing support groups for consumers of elder care services. The purpose of these support groups would be to promote social change by enabling family caregivers to understand how their caring role is devalued and undermined by social attitudes and policies. One example of such a group is the California-based support group "Women Who Care," composed of caregivers of the elderly. The group educates and encourages caregivers to seek common solutions for the problems they face and to move from being individual victims of circumstances to being advocates for social change (Hooyman & Gonyea, 1995).

Nurses also have an important role to play in developing relationships of solidarity with those—mostly women, and disproportionately women of color—who provide care for the elderly in nursing homes and in private homes. They are underpaid, often limited to part-time status that offers no benefits, and often lack adequate supervision and training. Their caregiving work, like that of family caregivers, is essential to the economy, but is largely invisible and devalued in the marketplace and society. Nurses need to recognize their common interests with nursing aides and develop groups devoted to collective action to improve the treatment of all caregivers.

Conclusion

The issues regarding elder care are complex; much more could be said about how rule ethics, virtue ethics, and feminist ethics could be applied. Nonetheless, as we examine the issues of elder care through each of these lenses, we see that different aspects of the issue come into focus and some aspects are reframed. Box 8–2 provides a comparative summary of the ethical analysis of these three theories.

Box 8–2 Looking at Elder Care Through Three Ethical Lenses

Fundamental questions	Rule Ethics	Virtue Ethics	Feminist Ethics
	How do the rules of autonomy, beneficence, and justice apply to elder care?	What does elder care reflect about our character as individuals and communities?	How do current beliefs and policies perpetuate women's oppression?
Primary ethical issues	1. Balancing the value of independence vs. safety 2. Family and society's responsibilities for care of the frail elderly 3. Responsibilities in the nurse–family caregiver relationship	1. Impediments to expression of caregiving virtues 2. Shift from elder care as a private family responsibility to a shared communal one 3. Redefinition of the nurse case manager role	1. Evaluating gender inequities in caregiving 2. Separation of public and private spheres supports elder care social policies and perpetuates gender imbalances of power 3. Need to reinvent the workplace to facilitate adequate elder care
Key challenges	Reordering health care priorities in order to provide more public funds for home health services	Creating social institutions and policies needed to promote a community of reciprocity that supports dependent elderly and formal and informal caregivers	Restructuring familial relationships, paid workplace, and public policies to eliminate gender inequities and empower men and women to integrate work and family

Each theory challenges our community to ask essential questions: How do the rules of autonomy, beneficence, and justice apply to elder care? What kind of social institutions and policies are needed to promote a community of reciprocity that supports the dependent elderly and their formal and informal caregivers? How can familial relationships, the paid workplace, and public policies be restructured to eliminate gender inequities and empower women and men to integrate work and family responsibilities? Answering these questions will require sustained dialogue within families, health care organizations, all levels of government and civic communities, and workplaces. Nurses will play a vital role as educators, mediators, and facilitators within families, health care organizations, and communities. This dialogue is one part of the ongoing communal dialogue of ethics in which we consider what values and principles are needed to make our lives and society as civil and fruitful as possible.

KEY POINTS

- With the need for elder care rapidly increasing, family caregivers, especially women, are assuming a greater responsibility for home care of the frail elderly.
- While the trend toward providing health care services in the home has accelerated in the past decade, the funds to support community-based and in-home care for the elderly have not followed.
- Rule ethics, virtue ethics, and feminist ethics produce overlapping and complementary assessments of the ethical issues of elder care, but in some areas their analyses are strikingly different as well.
- Each ethical theory challenges our communities to engage in conversations regarding fundamental values and assumptions affecting elder care. These include a reassessment of:
  - How we have prioritized health care needs
  - Our assumption that elder care is primarily a private, family responsibility
  - How family and workplace structures perpetuate gender oppression as well as undermine the ability of women and men to integrate family and work
- The ability of nurses to advocate for their frail elderly patients may be compromised by organizations providing home health care services and public policies. Nurses must recognize the potential conflicts, advocate for restructuring of their roles as care managers, and play active roles in promoting communal dialogues in order to adequately meet the growing need for elder care.

REFLECT AND DISCUSS

1. What do you regard as the most critical ethical issues in elder care and why? Are there ethical issues that were not raised in this chapter that you regard as critical?
2. Nurses interact with people across the life span who experience and adapt to dependence and frailty. How do you regard the value that is placed on independence within American culture and within nursing philosophy?
3. The analysis of ethical issues in elder care using three ethical theories points to the

need for communal dialogue about responsibilities for elder care and the priorities of our health care system. What role do you think that nurses can and should play in generating this dialogue? In what contexts do you think that nurses can best contribute to these dialogues?

4. It is generally assumed that expanding funding for elder care will require reductions in other areas of health care or increasing taxes. Between 1979 and 1996, average U.S. family income declined by 10.5 percent for the poorest 20 percent, increased a mere 2.4 percent for the middle 20 percent, and increased 28.3 percent for the wealthiest 20 percent. Public funding for elder care (including services for mental disability) could be expanded without cutting other areas if the wealthiest 20 percent paid a significantly greater percentage of taxes. Do you think that fairness requires wealthier Americans to bear a greater burden in public funding of health care?

5. The three ethical theories illuminate different aspects of elder care. Are the analyses provided by these different perspectives entirely complementary, or are there points at which they conflict? If conflicts exist, how does the position of cultural pluralism help us to think about them?

REFERENCES

Administration on Aging (1997a). Table 1—Projections of the population, by age and sex: 1995 to 2050. Available: http://www.aoa.dhhs.gov/aoa/stats/aginb21/table1.html [2000, October 27].

Administration on Aging (1997b). Table 19—Projections of the noninstitutional population 65 years and over with ADL limitations: 1990 to 2040. Available: http://www.aoa.dhhs.gov/aoa/stats/aging21/table19.html [2000, October 27].

Administration on Aging (1999). Number and percent of persons reporting problems with two or more activities of daily living. http://www.aoa.dhhs.gov/aoa/stats/Disabilities/2plusadls.html [2000, October 27].

Allen, T. (1999). Preserving home health care: There's no place like home. Available: http://www.house.gov/apps/list/hearing/me01_allen/homehealth92599.html [2000, November 4].

AARP (1998). FYI: Who uses Medicare's home health benefit? Available: http://research.aarp.org/health/fyi_hhealth.html [2000, November 5].

Bailyn, L. (1992). Issues of work and family in different national contexts: How the United States, Britain, and Sweden respond. *Human Resource Management, 31,* 201–208.

Blaser, C. J. (1998). The case against paid family caregivers: Ethical and practical issues. *Generations, 22*(3), 65–89.

Braithwaite, V. (1992). Caregiver burden: Making the concept scientifically useful and policy relevant. *Research on Aging, 14,* 3–27.

Cohen, P., & Bianchi, S. (1999). Marriage, children, and women's employment : What do we know? *Monthly Labor Review, 122*(12), 22–31.

Federal Interagency Forum on Aging-Related Statistics (2000). Older Americans 2000: Key Indicators of Well-Being. Available: http://www.agingstats.gov/chartbook2000/pr081000.html [2000, October 27].

Fullerton, H., Jr. (1999). 75 years of change, 1950–1998 and 1998–2025. *Monthly Labor Review, 122*(12), 3–10.

Guttman, R. (1999). Case management of the frail elderly in the community. *Clinical Nurse Specialist, 13*(4), 174–178.

Hochschild, A. R. (1997). *The time bind: When work becomes home and home becomes work*. New York: Henry Holt and Company.

Holstein, M., & Mitzen, P. (1998). Care of elders in the community: Moral lives, moral quandaries. *Generations, 22*(3), 64–65.

Hooyman, N. R., & Gonyea, J. (1995). *Feminist perspectives on family care: Policies for gender justice*. Thousand Oaks, CA: Sage Publications.

Johnson, R. W. (1999). The gender gap in pension wealth: Is women's progress in the labor market equalizing retirement benefits? The Urban Institute. Available: http://www.urban.org/retire ment/briefs/1/brief_1.html [2000, November 12].

Levin-Epstein, M. (2000). As Congress deals with home health, all of managed care holds its breath. Available: http://www.managedcaremag.com/archive MC/0006/0006.homehealth.html.

McKeever, P. (1996). The family: Long term care research and policy formulation. *Nursing Inquiry, 3*, 200–206.

Munson, R. (2000). Social context: The crisis isn't over. In R. Munson (Ed.), *Intervention and reflection: Basic issues in medical ethics* (6th ed.) (pp. 805–813). Belmont, CA: Wadsworth.

Mutschler, P. H. (1994). From executive suite to production line: How employees in different occupations manage elder care responsibilities. *Research on Aging, 16*, 7–26.

National Association for Home Care (2000a). Basic statistics about home care. Available: http://www.nahc.org/Consumer/hcstats.html [2000, November 5].

National Association for Home Care (2000b). Crisis in home care: Dismantling of the Medicare home health benefit. Available: http://www.nahc.org/NAHC/LegReg/Crisis/crisishh.html [2000, November 4].

National Center for Policy Analysis (1999). Home-care costs out of control. Available: http://www.ncpa.org/health/pdh43.html [2000, November 4].

Neysmith, S. (1993). Developing a home care system to meet the needs of aging Canadians and their families. In J. Hendricks & C. Rosenthal (Eds.), *The remainder of their days: Domestic policy and older families in the U.S. and Canada* (pp. 145–168). New York: Garland.

Okin, S. M. (1989). *Justice, gender, and the family*. New York: Basic Books.

Padgett, S. M. (1998). Dilemmas of caring in a corporate context: A critique of nursing case management. *Advanced Nursing Science, 20*(4), 1–12.

Parker, V., & Hall, D. (1993). Workplace flexibility: Faddish or fundamental? In P. H. Mirvis (Ed.), *Building the competitive workplace: Investing in human capital for corporate success* (pp. 122–155). New York: John Wiley.

Reuters Health (2000). Numbers of elderly living in nursing homes on decline. Available: http://www.nurseweek.com/news/00–01/013100i.html [2000, November 5].

Robinson, K. M. (1997). Family caregiving: Who provides the care, and at what cost? *Nursing Economics, 15*(5), 243–247.

Rodgers, C. S. (1992). The flexible workplace: What have we learned? *Human Resource Management, 31*, 183–199.

U.S. Census Bureau (1998). Population projections. Available: http://www.census.gov/population/ projections/nation/hh-fam/table5n.text [2000, November 12].

Ward-Griffin, C., & McKeever, P. (2000). Relationships between nurses and family caregivers: Partners in care? *Advances in Nursing Science, 22*(3), 89–103.

Weinberg, J. K. (1998). Balancing autonomy and resources in healthcare for elders. *Generations, 22*(3), 92–95.

Wuest, J. (2000). Repatterning care: Women's proactive management of family caregiving demands. *Health Care for Women International, 21*, 393–411.

APPENDIX A

The ICN Code of Ethics for Nurses

INTERNATIONAL COUNCIL OF NURSES (2000)

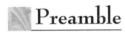 Preamble

Nurses have four fundamental responsibilities: to promote health, to prevent illness, to restore health and to alleviate suffering. The need for nursing is universal.

Inherent in nursing is respect for human rights, including the right to life, to dignity and to be treated with respect. Nursing care is unrestricted by considerations of age, colour, creed, culture, disability or illness, gender, nationality, politics, race, or social status.

Nurses render health services to the individual, the family, and the community and coordinate their services with those of related groups.

The Code

The *ICN Code of Ethics for Nurses* has four principal elements that outline the standards of ethical conduct.

Elements of the Code

1. NURSES AND PEOPLE

The nurse's primary professional responsibility is to people requiring nursing care.

In providing care, the nurse promotes an environment in which the human rights, values, customs, and spiritual beliefs of the individual, family, and community are respected.

The nurse ensures that the individual receives sufficient information on which to base consent for care and related treatment.

The nurse holds in confidence personal information and uses judgement in sharing this information.

The nurse shares with society the responsibility for initiating and supporting action to meet the health and social needs of the public, in particular those of vulnerable populations.

The nurse also shares responsibility to sustain and protect the natural environment from depletion, pollution, degradation, and destruction.

2. Nurses and practice

The nurse carries personal responsibility and accountability for nursing practice, and for maintaining competence by continual learning.

The nurse maintains a standard of personal health such that the ability to provide care is not compromised.

The nurse uses judgement regarding individual competence when accepting and delegating responsibility.

The nurse at all times maintains standards of personal conduct which reflect well on the profession and enhance public confidence.

The nurse, in providing care, ensures that use of technology and scientific advances are compatible with the safety, dignity, and rights of people.

3. Nurses and the profession

The nurse assumes the major role in determining and implementing acceptable standards of clinical nursing practice, management research, and education.

The nurse is active in developing a core of research-based professional knowledge.

The nurse, acting through the professional organisation, participates in creating and maintaining equitable social and economic working conditions in nursing.

4. Nurses and co-workers

The nurse sustains a cooperative relationship with co-workers in nursing and other fields.

The nurse takes appropriate action to safeguard individuals when their care is endangered by a co-worker or any other person.

Reprinted with permission of the International Council of Nurses.

APPENDIX B

Code for Nurses with Interpretive Statements

AMERICAN NURSES ASSOCIATION (1985)

Introduction

A code of ethics indicates a profession's acceptance of the responsibility and trust with which it has been invested by society. Under the terms of the implicit contract between society and the nursing profession, society grants the profession considerable autonomy and authority to function in the conduct of its affairs. The development of a code of ethics is an essential activity of a profession and provides one means for the exercise of professional self-regulation.

Upon entering the profession, each nurse inherits a measure of both the responsibility and trust that have accrued to nursing over the years, as well as the corresponding obligation to adhere to the profession's code of conduct and relationships for ethical practice. The *Code for Nurses with Interpretive Statements* is thus more a collective expression of nursing conscience and philosophy than a set of external rules imposed upon an individual practitioner of nursing. Personal and professional integrity can be assured only if an individual is committed to the profession's code of conduct.

A code of ethical conduct offers general principles to guide and evaluate nursing actions. It does not assure the virtues required for professional practice within the character of each nurse. In particular situations, the justification of behavior as ethical must satisfy not only the individual nurse acting as a moral agent but also the standards for professional peer review.

The *Code for Nurses* was adopted by the American Nurses Association in 1950 and has been revised periodically. It serves to inform both the nurse and society of the profession's expectations and requirements in ethical matters. The code and interpretive statements together provide a framework within which nurses can make ethical decisions and discharge their responsibilities to the public, to other members of the health team, and to the profession.

Although a particular situation by its nature may determine the use of specific moral principles, the basic philosophical values, directives, and suggestions provided here are widely applicable to situations encountered in clinical practice. The *Code for Nurses* is not open to negotiation in employment settings, nor is it permissible for individuals or groups of nurses to adapt or change the language of this code.

The requirements of the code may often exceed those of the law. Violations of the law may subject the nurse to civil or criminal liability. The state nurses' associations in fulfilling the profession's duty to society, may discipline their members for violations of the code. Loss of the respect and confidence of society and of one's colleagues is a serious sanction resulting from violation of the code. In addition, every nurse has a personal obligation to uphold and adhere to the code and to ensure that nursing colleagues do likewise.

Guidance and assistance in applying the code to local situations may be obtained from the American Nurses Association and the constituent state nurses' associations.

Code for Nurses

1. The nurse provides services with respect for human dignity and the uniqueness of the client, unrestricted by considerations of social or economic status, personal attributes, or the nature of health problems.
2. The nurse safeguards the client's right to privacy by judiciously protecting information of a confidential nature.
3. The nurse acts to safeguard the client and the public when health care and safety are affected by the incompetent, unethical, or illegal practice of any person.
4. The nurse assumes responsibility and accountability for individual nursing judgments and actions.
5. The nurse maintains competence in nursing.
6. The nurse exercises informed judgment and uses individual competence and qualifications as criteria in seeking consultation, accepting responsibilities, and delegating nursing activities to others.
7. The nurse participates in activities that contribute to the ongoing development of the profession's body of knowledge.
8. The nurse participates in the profession's efforts to implement and improve standards of nursing.
9. The nurse participates in the profession's efforts to establish and maintain conditions of employment conducive to high quality nursing care.
10. The nurse participates in the profession's effort to protect the public from misinformation and misrepresentation and to maintain the integrity of nursing.
11. The nurse collaborates with members of the health professions and other citizens in promoting community and national efforts to meet the health needs of the public.

Code for Nurses with Interpretive Statements

1. The nurse provides services with respect for human dignity and the uniqueness of the client, unrestricted by considerations of social or economic status, personal attributes, or the nature of health problems.

1.1 Respect for Human Dignity

The fundamental principle of nursing practice is respect for the inherent dignity and worth of every client. Nurses are morally obligated to respect human existence and the individuality of all persons who are the recipients of nursing actions. Nurses therefore must take all reasonable means to protect and preserve human life when there is hope of recovery or reasonable hope of benefit from life-prolonging treatment.

Truth telling and the process of reaching informed choice underlie the exercise of self-determination, which is basic to respect for persons. Clients should be as fully involved as possible in the planning and implementation of their own health care. Clients have the moral right to determine what will be done with their own person; to be given accurate information, and all the information necessary for making informed judgments; to be assisted with weighing the benefits and burdens of options in their treatment; to accept, refuse, or terminate treatment without coercion; and to be given necessary emotional support. Each nurse has an obligation to be knowledgeable about the moral and legal rights of all clients and to protect and support those rights. In situations in which the client lacks the capacity to make a decision, a surrogate decision maker should be designated.

Individuals are interdependent members of the community. Taking into account both individual rights and the interdependence of persons in decision making, the nurse recognizes those situations in which individual rights to autonomy in health care may temporarily be overridden to preserve the life of the human community; for example, when a disaster demands triage or when an individual presents a direct danger to others. The many variables involved make it imperative that each case be considered with full awareness of the need to preserve the rights and responsibilities of clients and the demands of justice. The suspension of individual rights must always be considered a deviation to be tolerated as briefly as possible.

1.2 Status and Attributes of Clients

The need for health care is universal, transcending all national, ethnic, racial, religious, cultural, political, educational, economic, developmental, personality, role, and sexual differences. Nursing care is delivered without prejudicial behavior. Individual value systems and life-styles should be considered in the planning of health care with and for each client. Attributes of clients influence nursing practice to the extent that they represent factors the nurse must understand, consider, and respect in tailoring care to personal needs and in maintaining the individual's self-respect and dignity.

1.3 The Nature of Health Problems

The nurse's respect for the worth and dignity of the individual human being applies, irrespective of the nature of the health problem. It is reflected in care given the person who is disabled as well as one without disability, the person with long-term illness as well as one with acute illness, the recovering patient as well as one in the last phase of life. This respect extends to all who require the services of the nurse for the promotion of health, the prevention of illness, the restoration of health, the alleviation of suffering, and the provision of supportive care of the dying. The nurse does not act deliberately to terminate the life of any person.

The nurse's concern for human dignity and for the provision of high quality nursing care is not limited by personal attitudes or beliefs. If ethically opposed to interventions in a particular case because of the procedures to be used, the nurse is justified in refusing to participate. Such refusal should be made known in advance and in time for other appropriate arrangements to be made for the client's nursing care. If the nurse becomes involved in such a case and the client's life is in jeopardy, the nurse is obliged to provide for the client's safety, to avoid abandonment, and to withdraw only when assured that alternative sources of nursing care are available to the client.

The measures nurses take to care for the dying client and the client's family emphasize human contact. They enable the client to live with as much physical, emotional, and spiritual comfort as possible, and they maximize the values the client has treasured in life. Nursing care is directed toward the prevention and relief of the suffering commonly associated with the dying process. The nurse may provide interventions to relieve symptoms in the dying client even when the interventions entail substantial risks of hastening death.

1.4 The Setting for Health Care

The nurse adheres to the principle of nondiscriminatory, nonprejudicial care in every situation and endeavors to promote its acceptance by others. The setting shall not determine the nurse's readiness to respect clients and to render or obtain needed services.

2. The nurse safeguards the client's right to privacy by judiciously protecting information of a confidential nature.

2.1 The Client's Right to Privacy

The right to privacy is an inalienable human right. The client trusts the nurse to hold all information in confidence. This trust could be destroyed and the client's welfare jeopardized by injudicious disclosure of information provided in confidence. The duty of confidentiality, however, is not absolute when innocent parties are in direct jeopardy.

2.2 Protection of Information

The rights, well-being, and safety of the individual client should be the determining factors in arriving at any professional judgment concerning the disposition of confidential information received from the client relevant to his or her treatment. The standards of nursing practice and the nursing responsibility to provide high quality health services require that relevant data be shared with members of the health team. Only information pertinent to a client's treatment and welfare is disclosed, and it is disclosed only to those directly concerned with the client's care.

Information documenting the appropriateness, necessity, and quality of care required for the purposes of peer review, third-party payment, and other quality assurance mechanisms must be disclosed only under defined policies, mandates, or protocols. These written guidelines must assure that the rights, well-being, and safety of the client are maintained.

2.3 Access to Records

If in the course of providing care there is a need for the nurse to have access to the records of persons not under the nurse's care, the persons affected should be notified and, whenever possible, permission should be obtained first. Although records belong to the agency where the data are collected, the individual maintains the right of control over the information in the record. Similarly, professionals may exercise the right of control over information they have generated in the course of health care.

If the nurse wishes to use a client's treatment record for research or nonclinical purposes in which anonymity cannot be guaranteed, the client's consent must be obtained first. Ethically, this ensures the client's right to privacy; legally, it protects the client against unlawful invasion of privacy.

3. The nurse acts to safeguard the client and the public when health care and safety are affected by incompetent, unethical, or illegal practice by any person.

3.1 Safeguarding the Health and Safety of the Client

The nurse's primary commitment is to the health, welfare, and safety of the client. As an advocate for the client, the nurse must be alert to and take appropriate action regarding any instances of incompetent, unethical, or illegal practice by any member of the health care team or the health care system, or any action on the part of others that places the rights or best interests of the client in jeopardy. To function effectively in this role, nurses must be aware of the employing institution's policies and procedures, nursing standards of practice, the *Code for Nurses,* and laws governing nursing and health care practice with regard to incompetent, unethical, or illegal practice.

3.2 Acting on Questionable Practice

When the nurse is aware of inappropriate or questionable practice in the provision of health care, concern should be expressed to the person carrying out the questionable practice and attention called to the possible detrimental effect upon the client's welfare. When factors in the health care delivery system threaten the welfare of the client, similar action should be directed to the responsible administrative person. If indicated, the practice should then be reported to the appropriate authority within the institution, agency, or larger system.

There should be an established process for the reporting and handling of incompetent, unethical, or illegal practice within the employment setting so that such reporting can go through official channels without causing fear of reprisal. The nurse should be knowledgeable about the process and be prepared to use it if necessary. When questions are raised about the practices of individual practitioners or of health care systems, written documentation of the observed practices or behaviors must be available to the appropriate authorities. State nurses associations should be prepared to provide assistance and support in the development and evaluation of such processes and in reporting procedures.

When incompetent, unethical, or illegal practice on the part of anyone concerned with the client's care is not corrected within the employment setting and continues to jeopardize the client's welfare and safety, the problem should be reported to other appropriate authorities such as practice committees of the pertinent professional organizations or the legally constituted bodies concerned with licensing of specific categories of health workers or professional practitioners. Some situations may warrant the concern and involvement of all such groups. Accurate reporting and documentation undergird all actions.

3.3 Review Mechanisms

The nurse should participate in the planning, establishment, implementation, and evaluation of review mechanisms that serve to safeguard clients, such as duly constituted peer review processes or committees and ethics committees. Such ongoing review mechanisms are based on established criteria, have stated purposes, include a process for making recommendations, and facilitate improved delivery of nursing and other health services to clients wherever nursing services are provided.

4. The nurse assumes responsibility and accountability for individual nursing judgments and actions.

4.1 Acceptance of Responsibility and Accountability

The recipients of professional nursing services are entitled to high quality nursing care. Individual professional licensure is the protective mechanism legislated by the public to ensure the basic and minimum competencies of the professional nurse. Beyond that, society has accorded to the nursing profession the right to regulate its own practice. The regulation and control of nursing practice by nurses demand that individual practitioners of professional nursing must bear primary responsibility for the nursing care clients receive and must be individually accountable for their own practice.

4.2 Responsibility for Nursing Judgment and Action

Responsibility refers to the carrying out of duties associated with a particular role assumed by the nurse. Nursing obligations are reflected in the ANA publications *Nursing: A Social Policy Statement* and *Standards of Clinical Nursing Practice*. In recognizing the rights of clients, the standards describe a collaborative relationship between the nurse and the client through use of the nursing process. Nursing responsibilities include data collection and assessment of the health status of the client; formation of nursing diagnoses derived from client assessment; development of a nursing care plan that is directed toward designated goals, assists the client in maximizing his or her health capabilities, and provides for the client's participation in promoting, maintaining, and restoring his or her health; evaluation of the effectiveness of nursing care in achieving goals as determined by the client and the nurse; and subsequent reassessment and revision of the nursing care plan as warranted. In the process of assuming these responsibilities, the nurse is held accountable for them.

4.3 Accountability for Nursing Judgment and Action

Accountability refers to being answerable to someone for something one has done. It means providing an explanation or rationale to oneself, to clients, to peers, to the nursing profession, and to society. In order to be accountable, nurses act under a code of ethical conduct that is grounded in the moral principles of fidelity and respect for the dignity, worth, and self-determination of clients.

The nursing profession continues to develop ways to clarify nursing's accountability to society. The contract between the profession and society is made explicit through such mechanisms as (a) the *Code for Nurses,* (b) the standards of nursing practice, (c) the development of nursing theory derived from nursing research in order to guide nursing actions, (d) educational requirements for practice, (e) certification, and (f) mechanisms for evaluating the effectiveness of the nurse's performance of nursing responsibilities.

Nurses are accountable for judgments made and actions taken in the course of nursing practice. Neither physicians' orders nor the employing agency's policies relieve the nurse of accountability for actions taken and judgments made.

5. The nurse maintains competence in nursing.

5.1 Personal Responsibility for Competence

The profession of nursing is obligated to provide adequate and competent nursing care. Therefore it is the personal responsibility of each nurse to maintain competency in practice. For the client's optimum well-being and for the nurse's own professional development, the care of the client reflects and incorporates new techniques and knowledge in health care as these develop, especially as they relate to the nurse's particular field of practice. The nurse must be aware of the need for continued professional learning and must assume personal responsibility for currency of knowledge and skills.

5.2 Measurement of Competence in Nursing Practice

Evaluation of one's performance by peers is a hallmark of professionalism and a method by which the profession is held accountable to society. Nurses must be willing to have their practice reviewed and evaluated by their peers. Guidelines for evaluating the scope of practice and the appropriateness, effectiveness, and efficiency of nursing practice are found in nursing practice acts, ANA standards of practice, and other quality assurance mechanisms. Each nurse is responsible for participating in the development of objective criteria for evaluation. In addition, the nurse engages in ongoing self-evaluation of clinical competency, decision-making abilities, and professional judgments.

5.3 Intraprofessional Responsibility for Competence in Nursing Care

Nurses share responsibility for high quality nursing care. Nurses are required to have knowledge relevant to the current scope of nursing practice, changing issues and concerns, and ethical concepts and principles. Since individual competencies vary, nurses refer clients to and consult with other nurses with expertise and recognized competencies in various fields of practice.

6. *The nurse exercises informed judgment and uses individual competency and qualifications as criteria in seeking consultation, accepting responsibilities, and delegating nursing activities.*

6.1 Changing Functions

Nurses are faced with decisions in the context of the increased complexity of health care, changing patterns in the delivery of health services, and the development of evolving nursing practice in response to the health needs of clients. As the scope of nursing practice changes, the nurse must exercise judgment in accepting responsibilities, seeking consultation, and assigning responsibilities to others who carry out nursing care.

6.2 Accepting Responsibilities

The nurse must not engage in practices prohibited by law or delegate to others activities prohibited by practice acts of other health care personnel or by other laws. Nurses determine the scope of their practice in light of their education, knowledge, competency, and extent of experience. If the nurse concludes that he or she lacks competence or is inadequately prepared to carry out a specific function, the nurse has the responsibility to refuse that work and to seek alternative sources of care based on concern for the client's welfare. In that refusal, both the client and the nurse·are protected. Inasmuch as the nurse is responsible for the continuous care of patients in health care settings, the nurse is frequently called upon to carry out components of care delegated by other health professionals as part of the client's treatment regimen. The nurse should not accept these interdependent functions if they are so extensive as to prevent the nurse from fulfilling the responsibility to provide appropriate nursing care to clients.

6.3 Consultation and Collaboration

The provision of health and illness care to clients is a complex process that requires a wide range of knowledge, skills, and collaborative efforts. Nurses must be aware of their own individual competencies. When the needs of the client are beyond the qualifications and competencies of the nurse, consultation and collaboration must be sought from qualified nurses, other health professionals, or other appropriate sources. Participation on intradisciplinary teams is often an effective approach to the provision of high quality total health services.

6.4 Delegation of Nursing Activities

Inasmuch as the nurse is accountable for the quality of nursing care rendered to clients, nurses are accountable for the delegation of nursing care activities to other health workers. Therefore, the nurse must assess individual competency in assigning selected components of nursing care to other nursing service personnel. The nurse should not delegate to any member of the nursing team a function for which that person is not prepared or qualified. Employer policies or directives do not relieve the nurse of accountability for making judgments about the delegation of nursing care activities.

7. The nurse participates in activities that contribute to the ongoing development of the profession's body of knowledge.

7.1 The Nurse and Development of Knowledge

Every profession must engage in scholarly inquiry to identify, verify, and continually enlarge the body of knowledge that forms the foundation for its practice. A unique body of verified knowledge provides both framework and direction for the profession in all of its activities and for the practitioner in the provision of nursing care. The accrual of scientific and humanistic knowledge promotes the advancement of practice and the well-being of the profession's clients. Ongoing scholarly activity such as research and the development of theory is indispensable to the full discharge of a profession's obligations to society. Each nurse has a role in this area of professional activity, whether as an investigator in furthering knowledge, as a participant in research, or as a user of theoretical and empirical knowledge.

7.2 Protection of Rights of Human Participants in Research

Individual rights valued by society and by the nursing profession that have particular application in research include the right of adequately informed consent, the right to freedom from risk of injury, and the right of privacy and preservation of dignity. Inherent in these rights is respect for each individual's rights to exercise self-determination, to choose to participate or not, to have full information, and to terminate participation in research without penalty.

It is the duty of the nurse functioning in any research role to maintain vigilance in protecting the life, health, and privacy of human subjects from both anticipated and unanticipated risks and in assuring informed consent. Subjects' integrity, privacy, and rights must be especially safeguarded if the subjects are unable to protect themselves because of incapacity or because they are in a dependent relationship to the investigator. The investigation should be discontinued if its continuance might be harmful to the subject.

7.3 General Guidelines for Participating in Research

Before participating in research conducted by others, the nurse has an obligation to (a) obtain information about the intent and the nature of the research and (b) ascertain that the study proposal is approved by the appropriate bodies, such as institutional review boards.

Research should be conducted and directed by qualified persons. The nurse who participates in research in any capacity should be fully informed about both the nurse's and the client's rights and obligations.

8. *The nurse participates in the profession's efforts to implement and improve standards of nursing.*

8.1 Responsibility to the Public for Standards

Nursing is responsible and accountable for admitting to the profession only those individuals who have demonstrated the knowledge, skills, and commitment considered essential to professional practice. Nurse educators have a major responsibility for ensuring that these competencies and a demonstrated commitment to professional practice have been achieved before the entry of an individual into the practice of professional nursing.

Established standards and guidelines for nursing practice provide guidance for the delivery of professional nursing care and are a means for evaluating care received by the public. The nurse has a personal responsibility and commitment to clients for implementation and maintenance of optimal standards of nursing practice.

8.2 Responsibility to the Profession for Standards

Established standards reflect the practice of nursing grounded in ethical commitments and a body of knowledge. Professional standards or guidelines exist in nursing practice, nursing service, nursing education, and nursing research. The nurse has the responsibility to monitor these standards in daily practice and to participate actively in the profession's ongoing efforts to foster optimal standards of practice at the local, regional, state, and national levels of the health care system.

Nurse educators have the additional responsibility to maintain optimal standards of nursing practice and education in nursing education programs and in any other settings where planned learning activities for nursing students take place.

9. *The nurse participates in the profession's efforts to establish and maintain conditions of employment conducive to high quality nursing care.*

9.1 Responsibility for Conditions of Employment

The nurse must be concerned with conditions of employment that (a) enable the nurse to practice in accordance with the standards of nursing practice and (b) provide a care environment that meets the standards of nursing service. The provision of high quality nursing care is the responsibility of both the individual nurse and the nursing profession. Professional autonomy and self-regulation in the control of conditions of practice are necessary for implementing nursing standards.

9.2 Maintaining Conditions for High Quality Nursing Care

Articulation and control of nursing practice can be accomplished through individual agreement and collective action. A nurse may enter into an agreement with individuals or organizations to provide health care. Nurses may participate in collective action such as collective bargaining through their state nurses' association to determine the terms and conditions of employment conducive to high quality nursing care. Such agreements should be consistent with the profession's standards of practice, the state law regulating nursing practice, and the *Code for Nurses.*

10. *The nurse participates in the profession's effort to protect the public from misinformation and misrepresentation and to maintain the integrity of nursing.*

10.1 Protection from Misinformation and Misrepresentation

Nurses are responsible for advising clients against the use of products that endanger the clients' safety and welfare. The nurse shall not use any form of public or professional communication to make claims that are false, fraudulent, misleading, deceptive, or unfair.

The nurse does not give or imply endorsement to advertising, promotion, or sale of commercial products or services in a manner that may be interpreted as reflecting the opinion or judgment of the profession as a whole. The nurse may use knowledge of specific services or products in advising an individual client, since this may contribute to the client's health and well-being. In the course of providing information or education to clients or other practitioners about commercial products or services, however, a variety of similar products or services should be offered or described so the client or practitioner can make an informed choice.

10.2 Maintaining the Integrity of Nursing

The use of the title *registered nurse* is granted by state governments for the protection of the public. Use of that title carries with it the responsibility to act in the public interest. The nurse may use the title *R.N.* and symbols of academic degrees or other earned or honorary professional symbols of recognition in all ways that are legal and appropriate. The title and other symbols of the profession should not be used, however, for benefits unrelated to nursing practice or the profession, or used by those who may seek to exploit them for other purposes.

Nurses should refrain from casting a vote in any deliberations involving health care services or facilities where the nurse has business or other interests that could be construed as a conflict of interest.

11. The nurse collaborates with members of the health professions and other citizens in promoting community and national efforts to meet the health needs of the public.

11.1 Collaboration with Others to Meet Health Needs

The availability and accessibility of high quality health services to all people require collaborative planning at the local, state, national, and international levels that respects the interdependence of health professionals and clients in health care systems. Nursing care is an integral part of high quality health care, and nurses have an obligation to promote equitable access to nursing and health care for all people.

11.2 Responsibility to the Public

The nursing profession is committed to promoting the welfare and safety of all people. The goals and values of nursing are essential to effective delivery of health services. For the benefit of the individual client and the public at large, nursing's goals and commitments need adequate representation. Nurses should ensure this representation by active participation in decision making in institutional and political arenas to assure a just distribution of health care and nursing resources.

11.3 Relationships with Other Disciplines

The complexity of health care delivery systems requires a multidisciplinary approach to delivery of services that has the strong support and active participation of all the health professions. Nurses should actively promote the collaborative planning required to ensure the availability and accessibility of high quality health services to all persons whose health needs are unmet.

Reprinted with permission of the American Nurses Association.

Note: The ANA Code for Nurses is being revised. Drafts of the revised code are available at http://www.ana.org/ethics/code9.htm.

APPENDIX C

Code of Ethics for Registered Nurses

Canadian Nurses Association (1997)

Preamble

The *Code of Ethics for Registered Nurses* gives guidance for decision making concerning ethical matters, serves as a means for self-evaluation and reflection regarding ethical nursing practice, and provides a basis for peer review initiatives. The code not only educates nurses about their ethical responsibilities, but also informs other health care professionals and members of the public about the moral commitments expected of nurses.

The Canadian Nurses Association (CNA) periodically revises its code to address changing societal needs, values, and conditions that challenge the ability of nurses to practice ethically. Examples of such factors are: the consequences of economic constraints; increasing use of technology in health care; and, changing ways of delivering nursing services, such as the move to care outside the institutional setting. This revised *Code of Ethics for Registered Nurses* provides nurses with direction for ethical decision making and practice in everyday situations as they are influenced by current trends and conditions. It applies to nurses in all practice settings, whatever their position and area of responsibility.

Ethical problems and concerns, as well as ethical distress at the individual level, can be the result of decisions made at the institutional, regional, provincial, and federal levels. Differing responsibilities, capabilities, and ways of working toward change also exist at the client, institutional and societal levels. For all contexts the code offers guidance on providing care that conforms with ethical practice, and on actively influencing and participating in policy development, review, and revision.

The complex issues in nursing practice have both legal and ethical dimensions. The laws and ethics of health care overlap, as both are concerned that the conduct of health professionals show respect for the well-being, dignity, and liberty of clients. An ideal system of law would be compatible with ethics, in that adherence to the law ought never require the violation of ethics. Still, the domains of law and ethics remain distinct, and the code addresses ethical responsibilities only.

279

Elements of the Code

A value is something that is prized or held dear; something that is deeply cared about. This code is organized around seven primary values that are central to ethical nursing practice:

Health and well-being
Choice
Dignity
Confidentiality
Fairness
Accountability
Practice environments that are conducive to safe, competent, and ethical care.

Each value is articulated by responsibility statements that clarify its application and provide more direct guidance. Where it is clear that an action or inaction would involve an **ethical violation** (i.e., the neglect of a moral obligation), the level of guidance is prescriptive. The statement is intended to tell the nurse and others what is ethically acceptable and what is not. Where the situation involves an **ethical problem** or dilemma, guidance is advisory. No ready-made answers can be offered and thoughtful consideration is required to increase the quality of decision making. Where the situation provokes feelings of guilt, concern, or distaste, it is a situation of ethical distress. In instances of **ethical distress** the level of guidance is more limited but there remains a responsibility for the nurse to examine the situation in light of the provisions of the code. Decisions will be influenced by the particular circumstances of the situation. Ethical reflection and judgement are required to determine how a particular value or responsibility applies in a particular nursing context.

There is room within the profession for disagreement among nurses about the relative weight of different ethical values and principles. More than one proposed intervention may be ethical and reflective of good practice. Discussion is extremely helpful in the resolution of ethical issues. As appropriate, clients, colleagues in nursing and other disciplines, professional nurses' associations and other experts are included in discussions about ethical problems. In addition to this code, legislation, and the standards of practice, policies, and guidelines of professional nurses associations may also assist in problem solving.

The values articulated in this code are grounded in the professional nursing relationship with clients and indicate what nurses care about in that relationship. For example, to identify health and well-being as a value is to say that nurses care for and about the health and well-being of their clients. The nurse–client relationship presupposes a certain measure of trust on the part of the client. Care and trust complement one another in professional nursing relationships. Both hinge on the values identified in the code. By upholding these values in practice, nurses earn and maintain the trust of those in their care. For each of the values, the scope of responsibilities identified extends beyond individuals to include families, communities, and society.

Health and Well-Being

Nurses value health and well-being and assist persons to achieve their optimum level of health in situations of normal health, illness, injury, or in the process of dying.

1. Nurses provide care directed first and foremost toward the health and well-being of the client.
2. Nurses recognize that health is more than the absence of disease or infirmity and assist clients to achieve the maximum level of health and well-being possible.
3. Nurses recognize that health status is influenced by a variety of factors. In ways that are consistent with their professional role and responsibilities, nurses are accountable for addressing institutional, social, and political factors influencing health and health care.
4. Nurses support and advocate a full continuum of health services including health promotion and disease prevention initiatives, as well as diagnostic, restorative, rehabilitative and palliative care services.
5. Nurses respect and value the knowledge and skills other health care providers bring to the health care team and actively seek to support and collaborate with others so that maximum benefits to clients can be realized.
6. Nurses foster well-being when life can no longer be sustained, by alleviating suffering and supporting a dignified and peaceful death.
7. Nurses provide the best care circumstances permit even when the need arises in an emergency outside an employment situation.
8. Nurses participate, to the best of their abilities, in research and other activities that contribute to the ongoing development of nursing knowledge. Nurses participating in research observe the nursing profession's guidelines, as well as other guidelines, for ethical research.

Choice

Nurses respect and promote the autonomy of clients and help them to express their health needs and values, and to obtain appropriate information and services.

1. Nurses seek to involve clients in health planning and health care decision making.
2. Nurses provide the information and support required so that clients, to the best of their ability, are able to act on their own behalf in meeting their health and health care needs. Information given is complete, accurate, truthful, and understandable. When they are unable to provide the required information, nurses assist clients in obtaining it from other appropriate sources.
3. Nurses demonstrate sensitivity to the willingness/readiness of clients to receive information about their health condition and care options. Nurses respect the wishes of those who refuse, or are not ready, to receive information about their health condition.

4. Nurses practice within relevant legislation governing consent or choice. Nurses seek to ensure that nursing care is authorized by informed choice, and are guided by this ideal when participating in the consent process in cooperation with other members of the health team.

5. Nurses respect the informed decisions of competent persons to refuse treatment and to choose to live at risk. However, nurses are not obliged to comply with clients' wishes when doing so would require action contrary to the law. If the care requested is contrary to the nurse's moral beliefs, appropriate care is provided until alternative care arrangements are in place to meet the client's needs.

6. Nurses are sensitive to their position of relative power in professional relationships with clients and take care to foster self-determination on the part of their clients. Nurses are sufficiently clear about personal values to recognize and deal appropriately with potential value conflicts.

7. Nurses respect decisions and lawful directives, written or verbal, about present and future health care choices affirmed by a client prior to becoming incompetent.

8. Nurses seek to involve clients of diminished competence in decision-making to the extent that those clients are capable. Nurses continue to value autonomy when illness or other factors reduce the capacity for self-determination, such as by providing opportunities for clients to make choices about aspects of their lives for which they maintain the capacity to make decisions.

9. Nurses seek to obtain consent for nursing care from a substitute decision-maker when clients lack the capacity to make decisions about their care, did not make their wishes known prior to becoming incompetent, or for any reason it is unclear what the client would have wanted in a particular circumstance. When prior wishes of an incompetent client are not known or are unclear, care decisions must be in the best interest of the client and are based on what the client would want, as far as it is known.

Dignity

Nurses value and advocate the dignity and self-respect of human beings.

1. Nurses relate to all persons receiving care as persons worthy of respect and endeavor in all their actions to preserve and demonstrate respect for each individual.

2. Nurses exhibit sensitivity to the client's individual needs, values, and choices. Nursing care is designed to accommodate the biological, psychological, social, cultural, and spiritual needs of clients. Nurses do not exploit clients' vulnerabilities for their own interests or gain, whether this be sexual, emotional, social, political, or financial.

3. Nurses respect the privacy of clients when care is given.

4. Nurses treat human life as precious and worthy of respect. Respect includes seeking out and honoring clients' wishes regarding quality of life. Decision making about life-sustaining treatment carefully balances these considerations.

5. Nurses intervene if others fail to respect the dignity of clients.

6. Nurses advocate the dignity of clients in the use of technology in the health care setting.

7. Nurses advocate health and social conditions that allow persons to live with dignity throughout their lives and in the process of dying. They do so in ways that are consistent with their professional role and responsibilities.

Confidentiality

Nurses safeguard the trust of clients that information learned in the context of a professional relationship is shared outside the health care team only with the client's permission or as legally required.

1. Nurses observe practices that protect the confidentiality of each client's health and health care information.

2. Nurses intervene if other participants in the health care delivery system fail to respect client confidentiality.

3. Nurses disclose confidential information only as authorized by the client, unless there is substantial risk of serious harm to the client or other persons, or a legal obligation to disclose. Where disclosure is warranted, both the amount of information disclosed and the number of people informed is restricted to the minimum necessary.

4. Nurses, whenever possible, inform their clients about the boundaries of professional confidentiality at the onset of care, including the circumstances under which confidential information might be disclosed without consent. If feasible, when disclosure becomes necessary, nurses inform clients what information will be disclosed, to whom, and for what reasons.

5. Nurses advocate policies and safeguards to protect and preserve client confidentiality and intervene if the security of confidential information is jeopardized because of a weakness in the provisions of the system, e.g., inadequate safeguarding guidelines and procedures for the use of computer databases.

Fairness

Nurses apply and promote principles of equity and fairness to assist clients in receiving unbiased treatment and a share of health services and resources proportionate to their needs.

1. Nurses provide care in response to need regardless of such factors as race, ethnicity, culture, spiritual beliefs, social or marital status, gender, sexual orientation, age, health status, lifestyle, or the physical attributes of the client.

2. Nurses are justified in using reasonable means to protect against violence when they anticipate acts of violence toward themselves, others, or property with good reason.

3. Nurses strive to be fair in making decisions about the allocation of services and goods that they provide, when the distribution of these is within their control.
4. Nurses put forward, and advocate, the interests of all persons in their care. This includes helping individuals and groups gain access to appropriate health care that is of their choosing.
5. Nurses promote appropriate and ethical care at the institutional/agency and community levels by participating, to the extent possible, in the development, implementation, and ongoing review of policies and procedures designed to make the best use of available resources and of current knowledge and research.
6. Nurses advocate, in ways that are consistent with their role and responsibilities, health policies and decision-making procedures that are fair and comprehensive, and that promote fairness and inclusiveness in health resource allocation.

Accountability

Nurses act in a manner consistent with their professional responsibilities and standards of practice.

1. Nurses comply with the values and responsibilities in this *Code of Ethics for Registered Nurses* as well as with the professional standards and laws pertaining to their practice.
2. Nurses conduct themselves with honesty and integrity.
3. Nurses, whether they are engaged in clinical, administrative, research, or educational endeavors, have professional responsibilities and accountabilities toward safeguarding the quality of nursing care clients receive. These responsibilities vary but are all oriented to the expected outcome of safe, competent, and ethical nursing practice.
4. Nurses, individually or in partnership with others, take preventive as well as corrective action to protect clients from unsafe, incompetent, or unethical care.
5. Nurses base their practice on relevant knowledge, and acquire new skills and knowledge in their area of practice on a continuing basis, as necessary for the provision of safe, competent, and ethical nursing care.
6. Nurses, whether engaged in clinical practice, administration, research or education, provide timely and accurate feedback to other nurses about their practice, so as to support safe and competent care and contribute to ongoing learning. By so doing, they also acknowledge excellence in practice.
7. Nurses practice within their own level of competence. They seek additional information or knowledge; seek the help, and/or supervision and help, of a competent practitioner; and/or request a different work assignment, when aspects of the care required are beyond their level of competence. In the meantime, nurses provide care within the level of their skill and experience.
8. Nurses give primary considerations to the welfare of clients and any possibility of harm in future care situations when they suspect unethical conduct or incompetent or unsafe care. When nurses have reasonable grounds for concern about the behavior of colleagues in this regard, or about the safety of condi-

tions in the care setting, they carefully review the situation and take steps, individually or in partnership with others, to resolve the problem.

9. Nurses support other nurses who act in good faith to protect clients from incompetent, unethical, or unsafe care, and advocate work environments in which nurses are treated with respect when they intervene.

10. Nurses speaking on nursing and health-related matters in a public forum or a court provide accurate and relevant information.

Practice Environments Conducive to Safe, Competent, and Ethical Care

Nurses advocate practice environments that have the organizational and human support systems, and the resource allocations necessary for safe, competent, and ethical nursing care.

1. Nurses collaborate with nursing colleagues and other members of the health team to advocate health care environments that are conducive to ethical practice and to the health and well-being of clients and others in the setting. They do this in ways that are consistent with their professional role and responsibilities.

2. Nurses share their nursing knowledge with other members of the health team for the benefit of clients. To the best of their abilities, nurses provide mentorship and guidance for the professional development of students of nursing and other nurses.

3. Nurses seeking professional employment accurately state their area(s) of competence and seek reasonable assurance that employment conditions will permit care consistent with the values and responsibilities of the code, as well as with their personal ethical beliefs.

4. Nurses practice ethically by striving for the best care achievable in the circumstances. They also make the effort, individually or in partnership with others, to improve practice environments by advocating on behalf of their clients as possible.

5. Nurses planning to participate in job action, or who practice in environments where job action occurs, take steps to safeguard the health and safety of clients during the course of the action.

Reprinted with permission of the Canadian Nurses Association.

APPENDIX D

Health Care Ethics Resources
on the Internet

Literature Searches

MEDLINE

Created by the National Library of Medicine, this database provides bibliographic information and abstracts for nearly nine million articles from medical journals.
http://www.nlm.nih.gov

National Reference Center for Bioethics Literature

Maintained by the Joseph P. and Rose F. Kennedy Institute of Ethics, this site provides extensive searches in health care ethics.
www.bioethics.georgetown.edu

PubMed

Provides direct links to publisher Web sites for the full text of selected journals.
http://www.ncbi.nlm.gov/PubMed

Health Care Ethics Centers or Institutes

Centre for Applied Ethics, University of British Columbia

Provides links to dozens of health care ethics institutions and organizations, publications, and online forums for discussing bioethics.
http://www.ethics.ubc.ca/resources/biomed

MacLean Center for Clinical Medical Ethics at the University of Chicago

Presents diverse views on practical, ethical concerns confronting health care professionals and patients. It also provides hundreds of links to Internet sites devoted to a wide range of topics such as genetics, death and dying, home care, and alternative medicine.
http://ccme-mac4.bsd.uchicago.edu/CCME.html

Midwest Bioethics Center

Provides bioethics consultation and general information on ethics.
http://www.midbio.org ; http://www.midbio.com

National Catholic Bioethics Center

Provides information on ethics in health care.
http://www.ncbcenter.org

National Human Genome Research Institute

Discussion of the ethical issues involved in human genetics research, news about genetic discoveries, fact sheets, and links to other Internet sites that offer genetic and genomic resources. The institute is part of the National Institutes of Health.
http://www.nhgri.nih.gov

The Center for Bioethics at the University of Pennsylvania

Features discussions of health care ethics issues for professionals and non-professionals.
http://www.med.upenn.edu/~bioethic

The Center for Ethics & Human Rights

Operated by the American Nurses Association, this excellent site provides links to dozens of Internet ethics sites. Topics include caregiving, genetics, death and dying, hospice, patients rights, and spiritual issues.
http://www.ana.org/ethics/elinks.htm

University of Buffalo Center for Clinical Ethics and Humanities in Health Care

Provides links to many health care ethics journal articles and documents as well as an excellent collection of links to other Internet sites devoted to health care ethics issues. Topics include physician-assisted death, hospital and palliative care, advanced directives, medical record privacy, and genetics.
http://wings.buffalo.edu/faculty/research/bioethics

E-mail Listserve

BIOMED-L

Subscribers to this list discuss health care ethics issues. Subjects have included the right to die, fetal cell transplant, patient autonomy, and respirator withdrawal. Send an e-mail message to listserv@listserv.nodak.edu; subject line message: subscribe BIOMED-L *firstname lastname*

Index

Bentham, Jeremy, 31–33
Bias, 15, 161, 163–165
Binge eating, 206–209
    See also Eating disorders
Bioethics, 3
Birth control, 11
Body mass indexes (BMIs), 212, 214
Boston Women's Health Book Collective, 167, 187
Boundaries in home health nursing, setting professional
    context, analyze the, 146–147
    decision process
        character development, institutional support for, 152
        character development, remove impediments to, 151
        communities, identify relevant, 147
        moral considerations, identify relevant, 147–148
        practical reasoning to modify moral concepts, 151
        virtues, identify and apply relevant, 148–151
    implement plan and evaluate the results, 152
    options, explore, 147
    problem identification, 144–145
Buddhism, 96, 98
Budgetary management, 180
Bulimia nervosa, 206–209
    See also Eating disorders
Burnout, 150

Canada, 84, 85, 100
Canadian Nurses Association (CNA), 4
Cardiac disease and gender-biased treatment, 182
Caring, virtues of, 246–247
    See also care ethics *under* Feminist ethics
Categorical imperative, 47–50
Centers for Disease Control (CDC), 160, 183
Changing landscape of nursing, 6–7
Character, 3, 95, 141–144, 151–152
    See also character, developing and sustaining *under* Virtue ethics

Christian Scientists, 10
Circumcision, female, 11
City-states, Greek, 96–97
Class and quality of care, 184, 187–188
Code for Nurses: Ethical Concepts Applied to Nursing, 4, 25, 26, 101, 134, 137, 165
Code for Nurses with Interpretative Statements, 4
Code of Ethics for Registered Nurses, 4, 25
Codes of ethics, 3–5
Cognitive-behavioral approach and eating disorders, 224–225
Cohesion within nursing groups, lack of, 176
Collaborative profession, 3–4
Color, treatment of women of, 183–185
    See also Cultural issues; Race
Co-mentoring, 121–122
Commercialization of health care, 153
Communal dialogue. *See* Dialogue, ethics as communal
Community
    employer-community partnerships, 256
    feminist ethics, 226–227, 257
    frail elderly, 245, 247–250, 257
    leaders and culturally based beliefs about health/illness, 8
    neglect of relationships and, 61
    virtue ethics, 96–97, 99–102, 138–139, 147, 247–250
Compassion, 103, 107–113, 139, 149–150
Competence, 57
Confidentiality, 60, 83–84
Conflict, physician–nurse. *See* Pain medication in the NICU
Conflicts of interest, 151
Conflict within oppressed groups, 175–176
Confucianism, 96
Consent, informed, 19–20
Consequences and utilitarianism, 30, 39–41, 77–82
Contextual factors of the case and ethical analysis, 17, 67–69, 136–137, 146–147

Evaluation process and virtue ethics, 132
  See also Boundaries in home health
    nursing, setting professional; Pain
    medication in the NICU
Experience and contextual judgment, 117
Experiences as resources, diverse, 15,
    173–174
Expert practitioners in ethics, 120–121
Externalization and social construction of
    reality, 186
Extraordinary/ordinary distinction, 52–54

Fairness, 47, 74–75, 148
Families
  advance directives, 25
  eating disorders, 210–212, 227
  employer-community partnerships, 256
  financial assistance for family caregivers,
    254–255
  frail elderly, 238, 242–245, 247–249,
    254–255
  life support measures and family
    disagreements, 24–26
  utilitarian approach to medical decisions,
    80
  Western medicine, clashes between
    parents and representatives of, 8–10
Fashion and eating disorders, 213–214, 220
Fat as a moral issue, female, 220
Fatigue, emotional/physical, 150
Fatphobia, 213
Fecundity, 37–38
Female circumcision, 11
Feminine caregiver, residual effects from the
    nineteenth century idea of the, 107,
    146–147, 150, 151, 176
Feminist ethics
  care ethics
    distortions of feminine caring,
      174–176
    essentialism, gender, 172–173
    experiences in nurturing roles, focusing
      on women's, 173–174
    *In a Different Voice: Psychological Theory
      and Women's Development* (Gilligan),
      168–169, 171–172

institutional constraints, 177–178
masculine but not feminine values,
    tendency to emphasize, 178–179
masculine virtues, distortions of,
    176–177
overview, 168–170
power imbalance, effects of, 174
voice, ethics in a different, 170–171
common project to which a number of
    theorists are committed, 205
concepts of feminism and, 160–162
conclusions, 197–198, 232
contexts in philosophy and nursing
  bias in traditional ethics, gender,
    163–165
  critical analysis/debate regarding
    relevance of gender to ethics,
    162–163
  feminism and nursing, 166–167
  health, women's, 167
  transition, nursing in, 165–166
defining feminism, 160
experiential account, 159–160
key points in chapter, 198–199, 232
new ethical issues
  democratizing and demedicalizing
    health care, 231–232
  disability as socially constructed,
    230–231
  sexual violence, 229–230
patriarchy, understanding, 167–168
restructuring, models for, 194–197
review questions, 199–200, 232–233
shared themes
  epistemology, contributions of feminist,
    193–194
  hierarchies of power, perpetuating,
    179–185
  justice, relational account of,
    185–186
  social construction of reality, health care
    and the, 186–193
  See also Eating disorders; Frail elderly
Financial assistance for family caregivers,
    254–255
Flourishing, human, 97–98

Neonatal intensive care unit (NICU). *See* Pain medication in the NICU

Netherlands, 84

Neuromuscular reeducation and combating eating disorders, 228

NICU (neonatal intensive care unit). *See* Pain medication in the NICU

Nightingale, Florence, 100, 165

Nightingale Pledge, 101

Nonmaleficence, 24–25, 30–31, 50, 55

Notification issues and HIV (human immunodeficiency virus), 153

Nurse case managers (NCMs), 153, 246–247, 250, 257

Nursing's Agenda for Health Care Reform, 125

Nurturing roles, focusing on women's experiences in, 173–174

Oaths, professional, 101–102

Objectivation and social construction of reality, 186

Objectivism, ethical, 14–15

On Liberty (Mill), 45

Oppression, 176–177, 183, 197, 206
See also Eating disorders; Feminist ethics

Options/solutions and ethical analysis, 18, 69, 77, 137–138, 147, 218–219

Ordinary/extraordinary distinction, 52–54

Organ donations and utilitarianism, 79

Origin of the Family, Private Property and the State (Engels), 163

Our Bodies, Ourselves, 167

Pain medication in the NICU
case description, 134–136
contextual factors of the case, 136–137
decision process
character development, institutional support for, 142–144
character development, remove impediments to, 141–142
communities, identify relevant, 138–139
moral considerations, identify relevant, 139
peer groups, conflict resolution, 143–144

practical reasoning to modify moral concepts, 140–141
protocol, develop a pain management, 143
virtues, identify and apply relevant, 139–140
implementing programs, 144
options, explore, 137–138
problem identification, 136

Partner notification and HIV (human immunodeficiency virus), 153

Partner violence, 229–230

Part-timers, 256

Paternalism, 27

Patient-to-nurse ratio, 7

Patriarchy, 161, 167–168, 177, 220–223
See also Feminist ethics

Peer groups, conflict resolution, 143–144

Peer monitoring, 125

Perception, 108, 112–113

Perfect duties, 51–52, 73–74

Persistent vegetative states (PVS), 114–117

Peru, 84

Philosophical ethics, 6

Physician–nurse conflict. *See* Pain medication in the NICU

Placebo effect, 34–43

Plato, 96, 216

Pleasure and utilitarianism, 31–34

Pluralism, ethical, 12–16

Pluralism of values, 27

Pluralistic nature of Western societies
See also Cultural issues

Policy-making bodies, 4

Power, perpetuating hierarchies of, 179–186

Power imbalance, gender and, 174, 178, 194–195, 220–221, 228–229
See also Feminist ethics

Practical reasoning, 104, 132, 140–141, 151, 153
See also under Virtue ethics

Predicting consequences, 40–41

Principles, 2

Principles of Biomedical Ethics (Beauchamp & Childress), 24, 127

People don't care what you know until they know you care.

– Bill Hill, owner of Bill Hill's College of Cosmetology
in Davenport, Iowa (my beauty school)

This book is dedicated to my family support system.

**In memory of
Doug Chaplin**

THE DEAN'S LIST™
of DaddyDos

A COLORING + ACTIVITY BOOK   BY DEAN BANOWETZ

FOR MOMMIES TOO!

TABLE OF CONTENTS

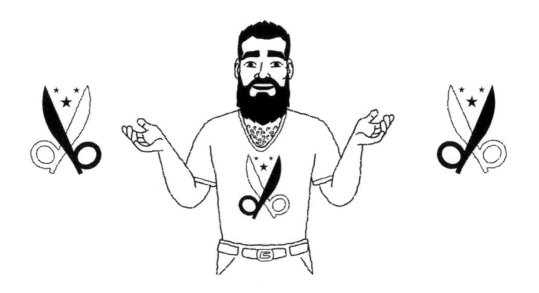

INTRODUCTION

My partner and I spent an hour and a half curling our daughter's hair and all we got was a bad attitude!

– Eric Metten, Dean's friend who was hair challenged. Until now.

There are times in a man's life when his true mettle is tested. It's not providing money for the family, mowing the lawn or checking that strange noise in the middle of the night. The true test of any Dad is when their precious young daughter comes up to him and says in that sweet, hopeful voice, "Daddy, can you do French braids?" When a befuddled Dad looks like you just asked him to do nuclear fusion, that little girl is likely to burst into projectile tears. That is a Daddy *Don't.*

Daddy Dos is the help that you've needed for years. Creating amazing hairstyles for your daughters and sons or the little girls in your life. It's for every single time the Chief Hairstylist of the House (a.k.a. probably the woman) has left the nest and someone under five feet tall is having a

9-1-1 hair emergency. Do you want an issue with tissues? Or do you want to get the job done?

There will be no more pleading, "Wait until Mommy gets home."

There will be no more wishing, "Why can't my own mother just materialize?"

There will be no more thinking, "I can rebuild a car, but I'm afraid of a bobby-pin."

It's time to be the man I know you can be. In other words, just 'do it! This book will show you how.

I wrote this for husbands, boyfriends, fathers and even some women who are *not so gifted* in the art of hair—ladies, I know you're out there, and there is no shame in being a CEO who can't make a bun. In fact, the other day, I had a lesbian and her partner approach me with tears in their eyes. They weren't the victims of prejudice and they didn't just have one of those annoying couple's spats over which paint color goes up in the living room. One of the partners was pregnant and both confided something that rocked them to the core about having a child. College fund? Nope. "I can't even do a ponytail without the kid's head looking lopsided, or like she has a weird growth coming out of one side," said one of the women with a look of horror. That was her biggest parenting fear! Dean to the rescue. It was time for these lovely ladies to rise to an important challenge: ensuring the child has the most amazing hairstyle on the block. We're talking about a final result that prompts someone to stop you and ask, "What salon did you take little Penelope to today?" You'll be able to look back at them with equal parts smug and joy and say, "That would be the salon down the hall from the kitchen called our bathroom."

Snap! But don't get too smug just yet. We got a lot of 'dos to cover.

In this book, I will teach you over 30 basic 'dos for little girls ranging from the time they actually grow hair to those testing years of dance classes, ballet recitals, school dances (yes, those excruciating social rituals still exist), graduations, the horrible visit from Aunt Bev, and many other social occasions when you're judged by how your child looks. Most importantly, she'll experience the joy that comes with looking her best. I will also break this down to the most common questions I'm actually asked as a Hollywood hairstylist, including: "What is a bobby pin?" or "What is that @$%# French roll?" (swearing—never beautiful)

These dos are quick and easy. They'll cover your butt on the day you've got five minutes to get out of the house, while your child is looking like one of those street urchins from *Les Miz* (if you don't know the reference, Google it). No, your neighbors cannot call Child Protective Services for bangs that look like the cat cut them, but you're setting your little wonder up for tons of teasing and bullying at school, which sucks. Why not take the necessary steps to avoid the pain altogether?

I know the mommies and step-mommies will find this book useful, but the men really need the help. That's why I explain hair in "guy" lingo. Every style can be phrased in man-speak. Hair will no longer be a foreign language. Consider me your one-stop Rosetta Stone for the universal language of hair. Ready for some translations? Your brush is your tool (hold back your giggles). Your arsenal of hair products goes in your tackle box. Braiding hair is like dealing with cable wires. Three wires: white, red and yellow. I'll explain how to cross them to form the perfect braid. Defusing a bomb with a ten-second countdown, you are now Kiefer Sutherland saving the free world from impending doom. No, the bathroom won't explode, but your six-year-old might.

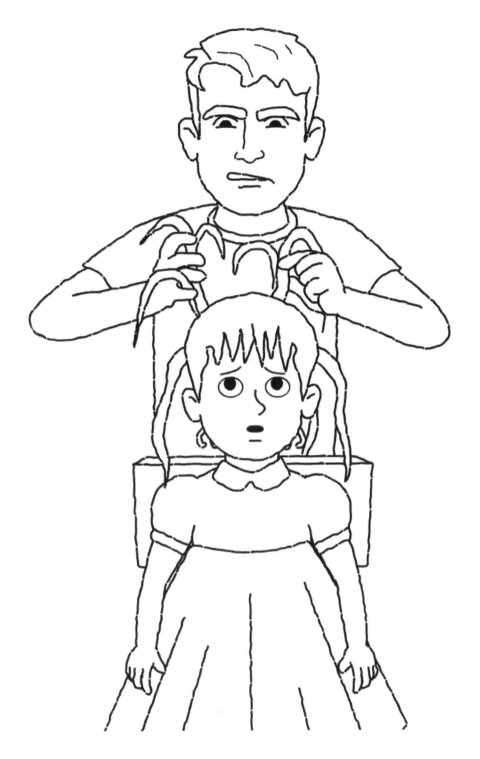

BREATHE AND FOCUS!

 @DBANO @DEANBANOWETZ

 #DADDYDOS

Activity Time!

Dads—you can't have all the fun. The illustration on the previous page (and throughout the book) is meant to be **colored**!

Rip it out, color away and throw it on the fridge when it's done. Better yet, snap a photo of you and little miss with your final masterpiece and share it!

Be sure to tag:

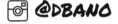 **@DBANO** 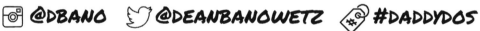 **@DEANBANOWETZ** 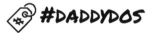 **#DADDYDOS**

I bet most men never knew that hair could be this action packed and exciting. Your buddy Dean here isn't just your teacher. I'm your hair commando. And just like that Tom Hanks movie, I want you to look at that paddle brush and coated rubber bands and say, "I am the captain now!"

Let's talk intentions for a moment. Why are you doing your daughter's hair in the first place? First of all, you don't want to look like a dork in front of your kid or your significant other. From stopping a speeding train, to that damn math homework, to trimming split ends, Daddy should be able to do anything. Second, when you're a parent and caregiver, you should be the "go to" because it establishes trust. You won't always have to say, "ask Mommy" or "ask your other Daddy" or "ask that nice lady down the street. She must know how to do hair." You wouldn't run next door if your child had a fever to ask "the nice lady" what to do. It's the same thing when your daughter wants a high pony or half-up, half-down. You don't need to call in the SWAT team – **s**pecial **w**omen **a**ll **t**attling on you. Get educated on these pages. You can do it yourself!

Not to make you feel guilty, but as a Dad, you're often considered the provider, safety net, emotional resource, dog walker, driver and the person your child can turn to on a Saturday morning when gymnastics is looming. Your baby will be able to say to you, "Today, let's make it a low braid with a pink bow. Thanks, Daddy! You're the best!"

By the way, there are perks to knowing how to style your child's hair. Your frazzled partner might take one look at you doing that curled pony and, despite that ripped, nacho stained college T-shirt you're wearing from 1992 and the fact you haven't been to the gym in two weeks (or years), actually say, "Baby, you are so damn helpful with hair that it's turning me on. Let's have a 'date' tonight." You can thank me later.

Before I show you the styles and restore happiness and harmony to many households, let me tell you a bit about myself. My name is Dean and I'm the 13th of 15 kids who grew up on a farm in De Witt, Iowa. My early life can be summed up in a few words: get up at the butt crack of dawn. Wait, there are more words: walk through wet fields of corn in the middle of summer where it was only 1,000 percent humidity. The only good thing about working the fields (oh yes, I did!) was the awesome farmer's tan.

My job in those days was detasseling the corn. In case you've never detassled anything in your life, this is not a stripper's term. No, it's all about corn, which grows in stalks and there is a tassel on top that once it's pollinated changes direction. You detassel to get more corn. Or basically, I had to rip the stuff off. Detasseling was a walk in the park vs. roughing a bean field. Oh, I know that you know that means walking through a soybean field and pulling out all the weeds in that row.

Right now, the jaws of my celebrity clients are dropping and quite a few must be making plans to have a benefit in my honor. Yes, your buddy Dean worked the land and worked it from dusk until dawn. People make about $35 to $45 a day for this backbreaking work, but I worked for free and my feed.

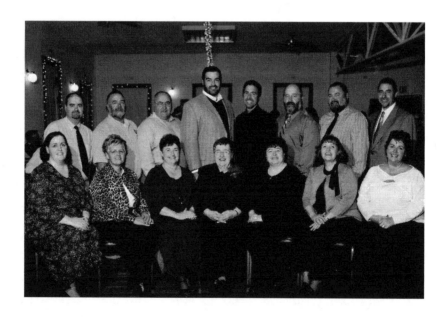

1st row: Annette (#11), Dee (#3), Judy (#1), Sally (mom), Alice (#2), Mary (#7) and Deb (#10) *2nd row:* Randy (#14), Alan (#6), Lloyd (#4), me (#13), Leon (#12), Steve (#5), Dick (#9) and Marvin (#8)

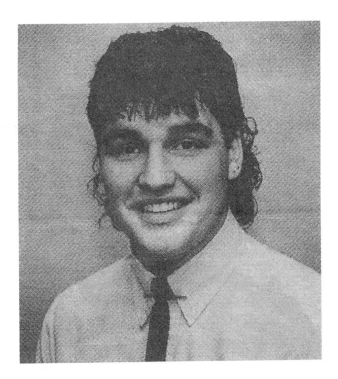

*Permed mullet. Eddie Murphy in Coming to
America influenced me.*

That's more farm talk. By the way, please feel free to call your parents and thank them for your childhood, which might have only involved mowing the backyard.

Now, back to style. In those days, my Dad was the family hairdresser and he would buzz us, so we didn't pass out on those hot summer workdays. Even worse was my high school look, which was your basic, curly, permed mullet. Take a moment to digest. Yes, I was close to six feet tall at age 16 and wore *a permed mullet.*

I took my mullet self during one of the summer months (Mom liked to get rid of us) to our family friends Alice and Charlie's farm. Some might call this a vacation, but I'm still not so sure. They had cows, and milking them was job number one. It was hideous work and the reason why I still don't drink milk. If there were a way to make some good ice cream without milk, I'd do that in a second. Until then I refuse to drink what came out of a cow's boob. Meanwhile, they had one horse and I'd ride him around the pasture—otherwise known in farm talk as "chillin' on a horse"—and this is where the magic began. Since there was absolutely no other way to possibly entertain myself, I would do a little French braid on the horse's mane. No one was happy about it, but I got in worse trouble when I braided the cow's tail. There are some very interesting styles you can do on a tail and I think the horse appreciated a way to break out of her generic equine look. It also redefines the idea of getting some tail on summer vacay.

Back on my own farm, I used to steal my sister's oh-so-chic Barbie dolls and do their hair. Again, these weren't paying customers, but everyone needs a little practice. My punishment for stealing these Barbie dolls was more time in the field working. I think my parents tried to work the gay away, but it didn't matter one bit. Left alone with those long corn tassels, I'd simply braid them. Then I'd grab bunches of long grass and create my own special plant ponytails. It was never ending. I'm not even kidding. *Really.*

My sister Annette is the one I call #11. Most of the time, my brothers and sisters and I call each other by our birth numbers. But I digress. #11 had me French braid her hair almost every single day before she went to school. I hated that she had to go to school so much earlier, but I still dragged myself out of bed to do her hair—my job and my joy.

When I lived with her after I got out of the U.S. Army, she would still bang on my bedroom door and beg me to do her hair. I'd do a French braid from the bottom up, and then my nieces started begging, "Uncle Dean, we want to make an appointment. We hear you work for free and hugs, which are free." Who was I to say no to all these amazing women in my family?

It got serious when I started doing several nieces' weddings. But it didn't have to be a special occasion to get me to backcomb. I was the one who started saying, "Do you know what a nice pony might do for that outfit?" I wasn't talking about anything that lived in the barn.

When I went to beauty school it was on! I learned my art at Bill Hill's College of Cosmetology in Davenport, Iowa, located in the back of a tasteful carpet and furniture retail store. Sure, it wasn't exactly a gorgeous place to train and you had to look past the hideous green shag carpeting and orange lawn chairs that were often on sale. Despite these obstacles, Bill Hill took our training seriously and made his students wear lab jackets over dress pants.

I'd go a step further and wear a button-down shirt with a tie during school hours. My goal was to always look like a cross between a famous author and a mad scientist with my long assed lab coat on. My unusual garb worked on several levels. People would come in and the receptionist would say, "So, who do you want to do your hair?"

"The tall guy in the lab coat," they would say. Maybe it was because I looked so professional. Or maybe they heard a good reference from a dairy cow on our farm or #11. Or perhaps in hair it's about how you carry yourself, and I've always had high confidence levels in this area.

DADDY DO TIP

Dads, if you look like you're scared to death, your girls won't trust you to touch a strand of their hair. Wipe that terrified expression off your face – stat.

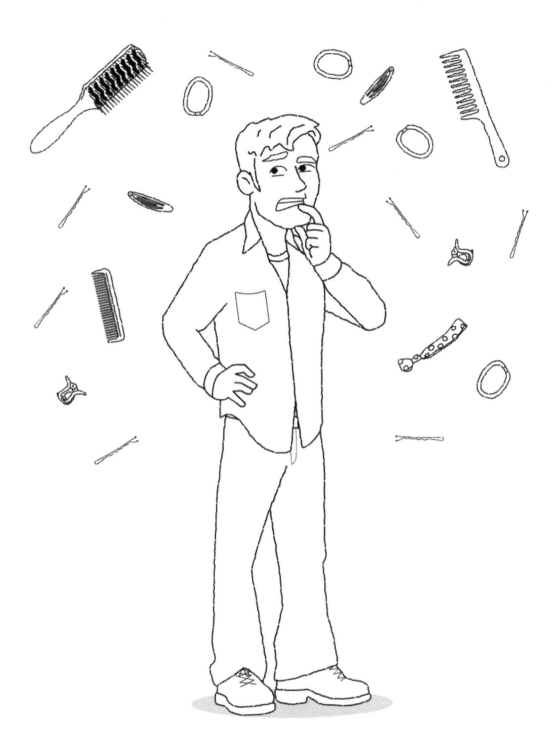

**CHOICES =
GOOD**

@DBANO @DEANBANOWETZ
#DADDYDOS

My professional training encouraged my family and soon even Judy (#1) had me cutting her bangs. My niece Cindy (#1.4 - the kids were the point whatever after their parents) made their appointments with Uncle Dean. Even Lloyd (#4) sent his wife Karry (#4.0) for a trim.

My sister Dee (#3) also went to beauty school to learn how to do hair, but only trusted me with her own personal haircuts. We'd joke about how doing hair with me was such a calm experience vs. our time spent with Dad the hair destroyer. When we were kids if Dad ever saw hair fall into our eyes (even for a second or in a tornado-like storm), he would get so pissed off that he'd line up the entire row of boys and take the clippers to us. Our hair was hostage to his moods and our ability to see to do chores while avoiding any high winds. You never wanted to see those clippers come out because for the rest of the summer, you would be a lopsided mess with origami hair patches.

Of course, his counterpart was my lovely Mom, a once-a-week shampoo and set lady, with a downtown hair appointment every Friday with Dee (#3). She looked at hair as a relaxing treat away from 14 of her kids, which was exactly the right attitude. Way to go, Mom! So what if she had her hair picked out and sprayed to death with that thick stuff that also clogs your lungs and doubles for glue during art projects. Mom had that hair cemented on her head and it never moved. It was almost like the hair was afraid. If it dared to break free, it would get another layer of shellac.

Hair was such serious business to her that I wasn't allowed to do my Mom's hair until after I graduated from beauty school. It might be good to mention here that my mom had dark brown hair that would be styled into a perfect bubble set with the curls taped to her skin around her hairline. I (#13) used that pink tape with the rickrack looking edges. She topped her hair creation off with a ton of spray and the sheer scarf tied under her chin to prevent the wind from even thinking about destroying it. Mom seemed to have made a deal with Mother Nature. Wind didn't bother her and Mom tried to only release her share of toxic spray chemicals into the ozone once a week. It was a win-win.

My Dad died when I was 15 years old, and Mom appreciated that I had direction in my life and later loved when I took over the entire family's follicles. The minute someone got engaged, I knew I'd be getting a call and I would always try to be available for the big day. It wasn't a wedding if I didn't 'do it, if you know what I mean.

I'd have my tackle box of tools with me, but more on that in a moment. At this point, I'm going to say enough about me. You can learn more later on.

In fact, just turn the page and let's get to it.

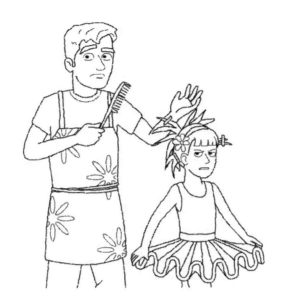

WHY THIS BOOK?

Here are the reasons why you need this book. YOU know who you are:

One: I'm sick of hearing hair horror stories from parents and children about how their day or event (dance competition, school dance, picture day) was wrecked by having sad/bad hair.

Two: I need to stop the insanity. The other day a Dad told me he cut the ponytail ties out of his daughter's hair because he was afraid of ripping out a strand. He ended up nicking her ear and wound up in the emergency room! You can't live in insane hair fear anymore when it comes to your child.

Three: I have a lot of gay friends who have adopted or have kids from a previous marriage. They are living the Number Two reason above and begged me to write this book. I feel their pain, and I'm here to serve.

Four: Straight people, and you know who you are, also don't know jack about doing their kids' hair. There are a lot of you out there, too!

Five: There is a lot of divorce. Divorce means kids with two homes and parents who quite often don't really communicate all that well anymore. If you ask your ex to do the hair in advance, it's just another thing she uses to say that you're a (insert swear word here). In each home, someone should be able to make the child look like she didn't spend the night hair-wise in a wind tunnel.

Six: It's time to realize that you can look manly and do hair. Skill is sexy! I'm somewhat butch and look like the bodyguard you want to have around you if you suddenly morphed into Beyonce overnight. And I do hair. I love doing hair. I'm great at doing hair. Enough said.

Seven: It's all about pride. I want your child to be able to say, "Yeah, my Dad did this style. He knows how to do hair. He takes care of me. Dad? I can always count on him."

Eight: I don't accept lame excuses. Don't hit me with the following: "Manly hands are too big to do hair or hold that brush." The last time I looked many brain surgeons held even smaller tools, and they're opening up a brain, not securing a bun. I have XXL-sized hands. If I can do hair with these bear paws, you *certainly* can too.

Nine: You will feel crazy accomplished. Happy! Overjoyed! There is nothing like putting a smile on the face of the one you love – and good hair equals smiles. In fact, studies show that when you feel beautiful then you have a better day. Don't you want your child to have the best day possible? Okay, I know that's a little Dean guilt and I'm sorry. (But it's true, so stop wrecking your child's day with bad hair and get on it!)

Ten: YOU CAN DO THIS. YES, YOU CAN. TURN THE PAGE! SORRY FOR YELLING AT YOU IN PRINT. If your wife/daughter doesn't trust you to do their hair, you have to practice. Grab a doll head and let's go.

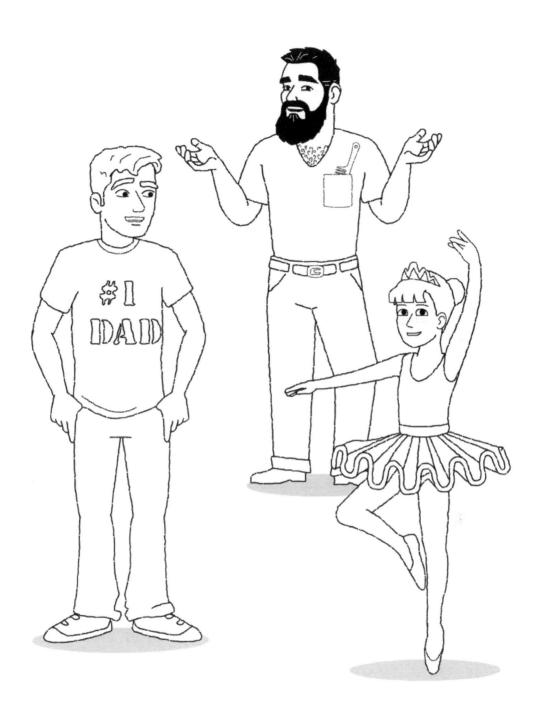

SEE! I TOLD YOU
TO TRUST ME.

@DBANO @DEANBANOWETZ
#DADDYDOS

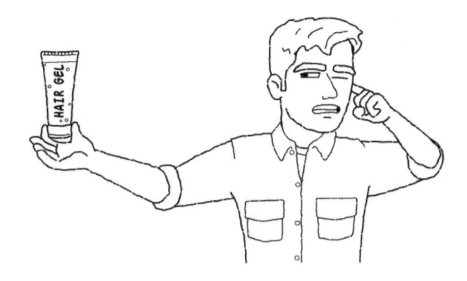

CHAPTER ONE:
GETTING OVER YOUR
HAIR FEARS

There are many men who would rather hold a grenade than a tube of hair gel. They're not afraid of cutting down a forest with blades the size of airplane propellers, but the idea of cutting bangs makes them break out in hives. How can a 250-pound man be fearful around a French braid? This book is all about challenging yourself and learning to get over your hair fears.

Remember that overcoming fear is called growth. Or you can quote my motto, "If you can fight a middle of the night intruder and swing a bat or kill really big bugs or deal with your mother then you can do a bun."

It's a guy thing to be responsible for another human being. This is why you will take your daughter's hair fate into your own hands. By the way, if you don't do her hair right your daughter can and possibly will look like a trashy 'ho and no one wants that description under their yearbook photo.

HOW TO GET STARTED

The good news is you don't have to find some swanky salon to prepare yourself for what you need to do the Daddy Dos. You can buy this stuff wherever you get your groceries. Trust me that the products are there even if you've never seen them. I also guarantee you that they're not in the beer and chips aisle, which is why you might have not spotted them in the past. Perhaps you've noticed things in the grocery store that read GOODY. They don't have that label because some sports team won the big game and everyone is shouting out that word. This brand means they're good at hair, although there are so many brands out there that equally fit the bill. In the Appendix section of this book, I'll provide you with my Dean's List of favorite products and links where to find them if you want to order them online. (Online ordering means you don't have a checkout person seeing you with bows, although many single Dads could play the caring, concerned, competent parent card there and even get a hot date for the weekend. Nothing says good Dad like new headbands for spring).

Please don't be shy about stocking up. Again, there is no shame in buying bobby pins even when you have a tat of a giant eagle on your shoulder and a Harley sits in your driveway. There is no shame in purchasing hairspray either because it indicates that you believe in personal hygiene and looking good, which are two traits that should be celebrated by all. Again, I'm a 300-pound guy (okay 230 is my goal weight) and some of the most famous hairdressers in the world are bald, manly-men who could take down a building and then style the little old ladies they've just rescued. We're manly, but we still know how to stock up on a great hair mousse when it's on sale.

NOW LET'S GET THIS PARTY GOING

I believe that most men know what it means when that first bell in a boxing match is rung or the coin flip in football decides what team will send out their defensive squad. Think of this moment in the same way:

Ding, ding, ding, it's time to start on your quest of being the best Daddy on the planet – and one who handles your little girl's hair.

Perhaps you're saying, "Dean, I don't know a damn thing about hair. In fact, I shaved mine off years ago because I couldn't even be bothered to own a comb." No matter if you're bald or you have a Fabio-like mane, we will begin at the starting line. There will also be time to learn your new craft. Think of doing your daughter's hair for the first time like that magical day when you popped open the hood of your first car and started to learn what was what. It's all about practicing until perfecting.

Of course, the first time you changed the oil in your car you spilled a little oil on the floor. I expect you to make mistakes. I want you to make mistakes. It won't take long before you're making very few mistakes, and your little girl is bouncing out of the house with a high pony swinging in the breeze.

DADDY DO TIP
Doing your daughter's hair is all about responsibility. You cook and clean. Those are necessities of life. So is doing your baby's hair.

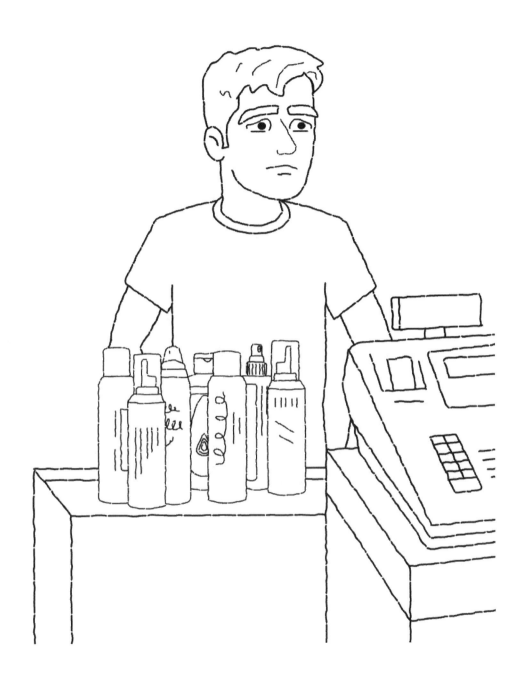

IT'S GOING TO
COST YOU SOME $

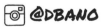 @DBANO 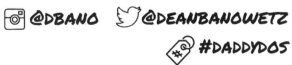 @DEANBANOWETZ

#DADDYDOS

The point here is you need to buck up. News flash: Women agree that one of the sexiest things a man can do is to take care of his children. I hate to bring this up so soon, but if you braid your kid's hair, your wife might be so thrilled that you'll have a very rocking evening when the kids are sleeping. In other words, you master the bun and you will master the buns later on.

I'm sorry, but I must drag sex into it. Hair is an easy thing to do in order to delight your partner and push them in the direction of having wild sex with you later as a thank you gift. I'm not even kidding here.

SIDEBAR: THE IMPORTANCE OF HAIR TO WOMEN

Time out, men! I know many of you are thinking, "Who cares about hair? Why is it such a big friggin' deal to the ladies?" As guys, we often like long, swinging, shiny locks on our ladies. With kids, isn't it enough to just have them put it in a messy pony and get on with it? No, no, no!

People ask, "Dean, why is hair so important?"

When your hair is done and you look good, you do feel better about the entire day. Even if something crappy happens (a teacher yells at you, you get a D in science), your child will still feel better about herself when she sees an amazing reflection staring back at her in the mirror. So what if she can't climb the damn rope in gym class? Who cares if that little turd Brandon told her she was stupid and has cooties. When little Amber looks in the mirror and sees a gorgeous braid, she still feels good about herself and realizes that Brandon is the sort of abusive little putz that Dr. Phil warns about on that great daytime talk show. She looks good, which makes her feel good, which equals she can take on the world.

Why is hair so important to our ladies, big and small? When you look good and feel better, you have more self-confidence and that equals success in life. There isn't a father I know who doesn't want his little girl to be a success in life and feel good about herself. We know about how life cuts you down and both females and males will be gunning for her self-confidence. Why not give her all the ammo possible to feel great on the inside, so those detractors just fall away like rain flowing down a gutter.

WHY DO YOU NEED DADDY-DAUGHTER HAIR TIME

It's all about the b-word: bonding. Many fathers and daughters don't get to spend quality time together and doing hair is a great, quiet time without anyone else around to have some private moments. Many dads aren't into doing little tea parties and sitting on the floor playing with dolls. Doing hair together is an actual activity that both of you can enjoy with amazing results.

If you're not convinced, I promise you will see joy on your little girl's face when you help her with her hair. The beautiful thing is this is a time to really chat and find out what's going on in your child's life. You might hear about how she thinks the dog is from outer space and that guy Matthew has a big crush on her. (What! The little bastard!) Hair is a way to accomplish a lot of things at one time, including actual grooming combined with touching base in our busy lives.

Many Dads wake up early and work all kinds of crazy hours. They're just not home. When you are home, it's great to have an important task to do with your daughter that guarantees some special time. Plus, there will still be some unenlightened Dads who don't read this book and who can't figure out how to get rid of one clump of frizz. You do hair now, and suddenly you're the coolest Dad on the entire block. Meanwhile, your partner doesn't resent you because he or she does most (if not all) of the child rearing duties. You've taken a task away, and have provided a much-needed break. This is a total win-win.

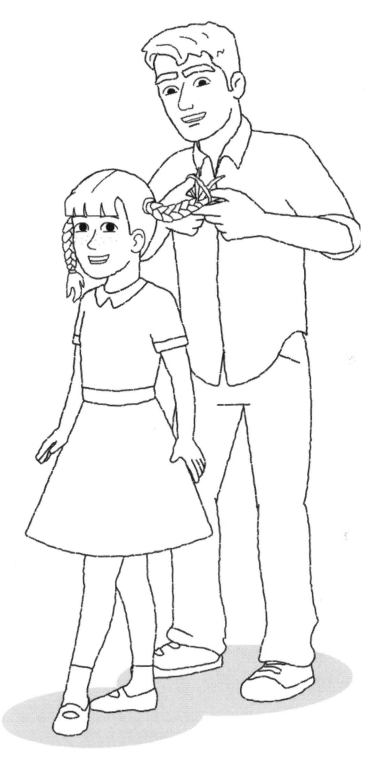

HAPPY KID =
HAPPY LIFE

📷 @DBANO 🐦 @DEANBANOWETZ

🏷️ #DADDYDOS

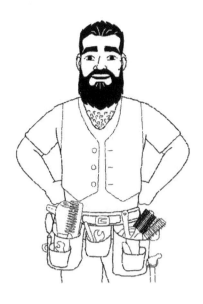

CHAPTER TWO:
YOUR HAIR TACKLE BOX

Just like when you fix a car, you don't just stand there empty-handed without any of your best tools. Hair is the same way.

It's all about having your arsenal of tools at the ready. I'd like you to buy a real tackle or a toolbox to keep your hair supplies in. You can find them for a few bucks at Target or Walmart in the camping section. You can also think of collecting your supplies as an interactive activity you can do with your daughter. Just say, "I've got a special mission we're going on today – together."

Imagine the shocked look on her precious little dimpled face when you say, "Saddle up, Sally! We're going to Target to get supplies so Daddy can do your hair." After you lift her gorgeous, future supermodel/scientist chin off the ground, proceed to the driveway. This is your territory and you know what to do: get in the car, fire up the ignition, put on a manly Van Halen tune and get ready to buy the following things that I'll list below.

By the way, I'm combat trained from my years in the Army. I always believe that it's best to be prepared and keep your supplies very handy, so you can always find them before you go into battle. To that end, here is your preparedness kit:

YOUR BASIC DADDY DO TOOL KIT:

1. Vent brush. Great to use on wet hair.

2. Paddle brush. Perfect for brushing dry hair.

3. Round brush. This is for advanced dads who are blowing out hair with a hair dryer. Not an air compressor.

4. Wide toothed comb. Great for detangling wet hair.

5. Coated rubber bands. Goody has some great options.

6. Bobby pins in the same color as your daughter's hair. I always have about 15 bobby pins stashed in the glove box or on my tie if I am going out. Cyndi Bands work great too.

7. Snap barrettes to pull back the little pieces. Plus, they're so cute. You can put them in a pony to lock it all in. Think of them like changing a tie. You can't have enough in different colors.

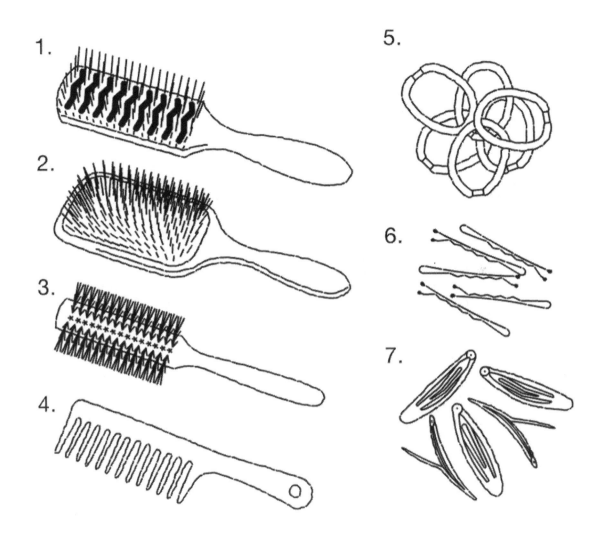

1.
2.
3.
4.
5.
6.
7.

THESE WILL SAVE YOU...

@DBANO   @DEANBANOWETZ
#DADDYDOS

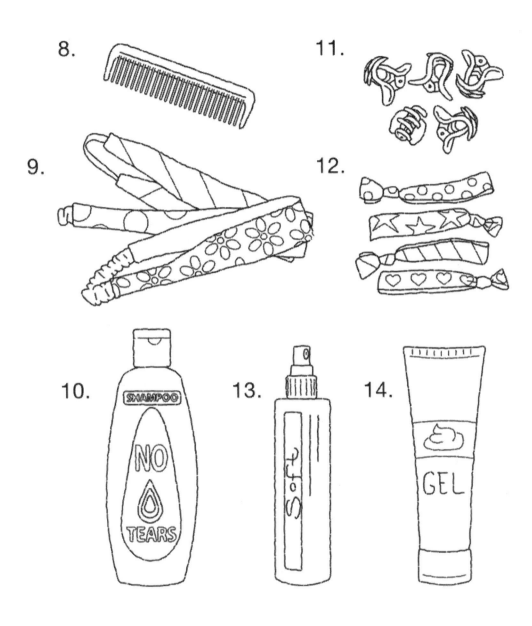

8.

11.

9.

12.

10.

13.

14.

... BUY THEM!

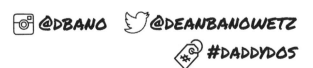

8. Standard comb. You kept this in your back pocket, remember?

9. Fabric headbands. They're quick and easy.

10. Baby shampoo and a gentle conditioner. Enough said.

11. Tiny jaw clamps. I use them on *American Idol, The X Factor* and *Dancing with the Stars* all the time. If your child is a dancer, you want to be able to lock her hair down while you style. It makes it easier.

12. Ties and colored bands. You can never have enough ponytail ties. (You'll end up finding them everywhere in the house and even on the gearshift of your car).

13. Spray leave-in conditioner. It can be a lifesaver. It tames the hair down and can help you get rid of tangles.

14. A medium-hold gel. Don't get anything too strong; it's too sticky. Gel is great to hold the little, runaway bits down.

DADDY DO TIP
People always ask me to divulge my go-to brands. Here they are in a nutshell: I love Johnson & Johnson's, Joico/Aquage products and Paul Mitchell's line. More about what I love product-wise in the Appendix of the book.

'DO DILEMMA: SHOULD YOU USE HAIR SPRAY ON KIDS?

Yes, you can use hair spray on kids, but it's not an everyday thing. This will depend upon the level of activity. If your daughter is a flower girl at a wedding use it to keep a style for a long time and for the photos. Or perhaps you'll use it for a graduation or a big dinner event.

DADDY DO TIP

When using hair spray on a child, I like to get a Kleenex and have your child hold it against their forehead. Drape the tissue down their face like a mask. You can have fun by saying they're hiding from you. Then use the spray. Remove the tissue when done. This is a great way to avoid getting the spray in the child's eyes or mouth—and it's much better than just asking them to shut their eyes. Kids love to peek!

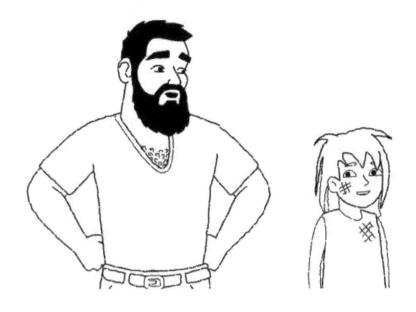

CHAPTER THREE:
KIDS R DIRTY – CLEAN 'EM

Let's talk about kiddie hygiene for a moment or what I like to call Basic Whipper Snapper Beauty School 101. No, you can't skip this chapter and get to the styles because understanding your daughter's hair and how to get it to behave under your care is crucial. Plus, I provide advice on how to get rid of tangles and the tears that go with them.

If you want to stop the waterworks keep reading. The last thing you need is a report to the home front female/male honcho saying, "Mommy, Daddy ripped out my hair trying to get my tangles out! He made me cry". Imagine your partner giving you the death ray stare here as she/he imagines you literally ripping every strand of hair out of her precious baby's head. That is just too much hassle, so please read this entire chapter.

LITTLE PRECIOUS AND HER HAIR TYPE

Your daughter either has straight or curly hair. It will be one of the two. If it's not straight then it's curly although there can be some variations on the two themes here. You can have straight/wavy, which is your basic surfer girl hair even if you live in the middle of Iowa. You also have to consider your daughter's hair texture, which should fall into the fine or course variety.

As a rule, curly hair is usually course and a lot of times straight hair is fine, but these aren't absolutes.

Ask yourself: Does your daughter's hair naturally curl? Is it stick straight? When dry is it thinner strands that lay straight and glossy or more coarse looking and a bit less shiny? Again, you can have straight, fine hair or curly fine hair or wavy coarse hair.

You'll also want to figure out if your daughter has oily or dry hair. Does it look a little greasy if you don't wash it every single day or like it could use a little conditioner? These are pretty easy concepts, and you can figure it out if you pretend like you're 24's Jack Bauer giving a report on a suspect to CTU (Counter Terrorism Unit). What are the particulars? Do a little detective work here, and if you just can't figure it out, you can ask a woman in your life like the woman who comes to clean once a week. Try to avoid asking your partner who will think you've lost your mind when you casually say, "What are we having for dinner and is little Ashley fine-curly or course-straight in the hair department?"

PRODUCTS FOR SHAMPOOING AND CONDITIONING

Fine, straight or curly, you just need a general shampoo and conditioner for your child. (Again, in the appendix of this book, I'll list a few personal favorites). Most likely your partner has purchased the goods, but you can do it with a little help from the Appendix section.

BEFORE YOU SHAMPOO

Before a drop of water hits little Ashley's head brush her hair out thoroughly. Don't just brush the outside layer. Get in there good and really brush all of her hair – outer and under hair. You'll want to do this with a good, vented paddle brush. After the hair is loosened, you can finish with a wide toothed comb. The rule: The curlier the hair, the wider the teeth in the comb. It follows that the thinner the hair, the smaller the teeth on the comb. Curly course hair equals a wide toothed comb. My fave is the Tangle Teezer or the Wet Brush.

NOW SHAMPOO

Getting your child's head clean is an easy task. Just wet your daughter's head in the sink or in the shower/tub and shampoo. Caution: Make sure you buy a product that doesn't burn the eyes and be careful not to use too much shampoo so it runs into the eyes. Just a glop the size of a pea will do to start. Use a little more if your child has long-long hair (past her shoulder blades).

Just rub the shampoo into your hands, rub your hands together and then start with your fingertips on the scalp of the hair and work it through. After the shampoo builds up a frothy lather, rinse it off completely. There is nothing worse than leftover caked on shampoo or conditioner. Give it an extra 30 seconds in the water if you're not sure and look down to make sure the water is running clean and not soapy. If you still see soapy then make sure to keep rinsing.

Prior to rinsing, make sure to get in there and shampoo the scalp, which should feel good and gets rid of sweat, dirt and even chlorine from the pool. It will also get rid of old products that are still there such as hair spray for special events.

Judge if your child needs one or two shampoo treatments. How? If your child hasn't had their hair washed in three days, two shampoo treatments would be necessary. Finish by using a quarter-sized amount of conditioner, which you will rub into your hands to emulsify. Start at the ends and work your way up with the conditioner. Never just glop it out of the bottle onto your child's head, which doesn't feel good. Work it upward and then allow it to sit for a minute or two – or until your child becomes a bit unglued. Then rinse completely. Quick tip: Get the shampoo halo or the baby pour cup. It will make your life so much easier.

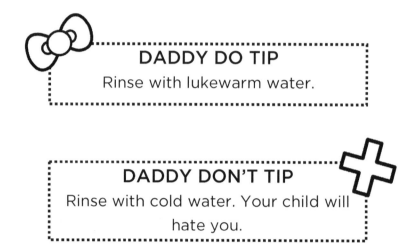

DADDY DO TIP
Rinse with lukewarm water.

DADDY DON'T TIP
Rinse with cold water. Your child will hate you.

By the way, you need conditioner. When you skip it, most kids get crazy tangles, which you then have to rip out with a brush. Conditioner gets rid of that painful activity and all the dirty looks that go with the fact that tangles, like homework and rain, are your fault as a parent.

A NOTE ABOUT SPECIALTY SHAMPOOS

There are times when you need a more specialized shampoo. I have friends with multi-racial kids, and they're constantly asking me for advice. I love a site called mixedchicks.net where they sell a product line specially developed for mixed race children. What makes their hair different is that it's a natural texture. If you use the wrong shampoo on natural textured hair, it will dry it out and make it even more difficult to manage. It also helps to use a leave-in conditioner (you don't wash it out, but this only works for brands that say leave in; you can't just leave *anything* in).

TIME TO DRY YOUR LITTLE PRINCESS' HAIR

Here's a good golden rule: Use a bath towel to dry the body; use a hand towel to dry the hair. You don't want to get oils from the body on her hair and vice versa. In older kids, including pre-teens, using the hair towel with the corresponding hair oils on their faces can even cause acne. I like to give the hair towel to the child. Let them learn how to dry their own hair with a towel, which is a worthwhile learning activity. You dry your own hair; they work on their own hair. They feel like they're participating, which makes them enjoy the activity. Your goal is to get 80 percent of the water out.

DADDY DO TIP

If you have a child with really long hair, towel dry first then go section by section starting at the nape of the neck and then comb from the roots to the end. Then take another section and go roots to the end. You keep doing each section until all of the hair is smooth and tangle free. You can also take all the hair and wrap it in a Bounty paper towel to really suck the water out. If you don't have a Bounty, I use a Kleenex. Use anything that's absorbent and quick.

To make it extra fun, I have my nieces scrunch their hair up when they get out of the shower just to see how much water is coming out. Got a shop cloth? Use it on your daughter's hair providing you didn't use it on your greasy car. A shop cloth really gets the moisture out.

VERY BIG DADDY DON'T TIP

IF YOU BLOW DRY SUPER WET HAIR, YOU ARE
BOILING IT. Plus, it will take a LOT longer to dry.
Take the time to dry it with a towel before you
blow-dry it. When you blow it just make sure you
use low heat and high air speed to help rough dry
the hair. Check out my new InBlu Turbo Ionic Hair
Dryer www.instyler.com

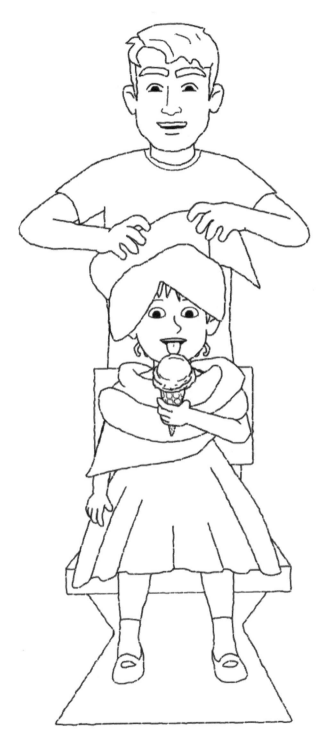

**ICE CREAM &
HAIR DON'T MIX!**

@DBANO   @DEANBANOWETZ
#DADDYDOS

DADDY DO TIP

If you want to try a great wavy style you will do a braid (see next chapter) and let your child sleep in the braid. In the morning, your daughter will have the most amazing wavy hair once you take the braids out. It's minimal effort and it looks like you did something major! The key to this is making sure the hair is 99% dry before you braid. Another tip is you can leave about 1 ½ of the section out of the braid. The straight ends will help make it look more trendy. #itlooksgreatwithaheadbandalso

TROUBLESHOOT THE TANGLES

Most kids have to deal with a terror called tangles. What I always do is find the tangle and "push it up." This means I grab the ends and slide the tangle toward the scalp, which helps to loosen it up. Then I push it through again, which you may have to do two or three times. It unlocks whatever is happening that's causing your daughter's hair to look like some sort of cemented together spaghetti dish. What do you do about a tangle that's stubborn and just not coming out? Despite your daughter's tears, because tangles are a very serious issue when you're eight or nine, you have to give the tangle special attention.

Here are my tips for getting rid of the most stubborn tangle. I call this tangle troubleshooting:

□ **Make short, calming strokes through the tangle to break it up.** Do this with a gentle brush or a wide toothed comb. I love using the tangle teaser brush or the wet brush (see page 20).

- **Still no relief? Actually put your fingers into the tangle and slide them around.** Make a motion inside that tangle with your fingers like you're opening an umbrella. Now that you've tried your fingers, go back to using the brush to try to break it up or comb it through to get rid of it.

- **You can use a leave-in conditioner (a few small sprays) to soften it up and thus break it up.** I like the BioMega Volumizing Moisture Spray.

- **I do love Paul Mitchell conditioner as a product to avoid tangles.** If your daughter has tangle-prone hair, you might want to make this one of your staples. Yes, man up and go buy it, keep it in the shower or on the tub and tell your child to use it. Your partner won't question you and think that he or she bought it in the first place.

Once you break up the tangled mess and the hair is smooth again, call your sister, wife or the gay down the street and reveal the big news. You're not just a Daddy and an accountant/CPA/ cop, but also a de-tangler. Well done!

OH, THE DRAMA OF IT ALL

One quick word when it comes to the emotional drama caused by hair tangles. As I said before—but it bears repeating—most little girls will go into either gales of tears or true hysteria when you even talk about getting the tangles out: Why? Probably they know it can hurt or someone has made it hurt in the past. Don't take this lightly because this is a serious emotional drama for your child. Even if your girl is upset, don't raise your voice because it just elevates the drama. And please don't burst into tears with her. Dr. Dean the hair doctor is here to help you get past the emotional soap opera of the tangle.

Use this script:

> *Your Little Girl (snot running, short hiccup-y breaths):*
> "Daddy, I have a tangle and you're not taking it out! I want Mommy!"

You (in a calm voice like you would use with your boss):
"Honey, let me help you. No, really, I'm pretty good at getting rid of tangles. You see how I untangle all the cords by the TV, right? And the TV isn't broken."

YLG (tears flowing):
"I still want Mommy!"

You (in your best never-say-die mode):
"Baby, we have to do this together. Maybe you could help me. Could you work on one section and I'll work on the other one."

YLG (somewhat intrigued):
"Help you?"

You (avoiding a desire to ditch this and clean the garage):
"Yes, Daddy needs tons of help here. Let's do this together. You can even be in charge."

By the way, do not resort to bribes. It doesn't help if you promise 31 Flavors for allowing you to get rid of tangles. This sets up sugary carbs as a treat for basic grooming. When in doubt, educate your daughter. If they still aren't sure you're a master de-tangler, simply say, "Honey, we have no choice. We have to get this tangle out. We want your hair to be super beautiful. If this tangle is there, it will bug us all day. So, let's get this tangle out, so we have a really amazing day." You're doing so much talking that most kids will throw in the towel at this point and allow you to just get to work.

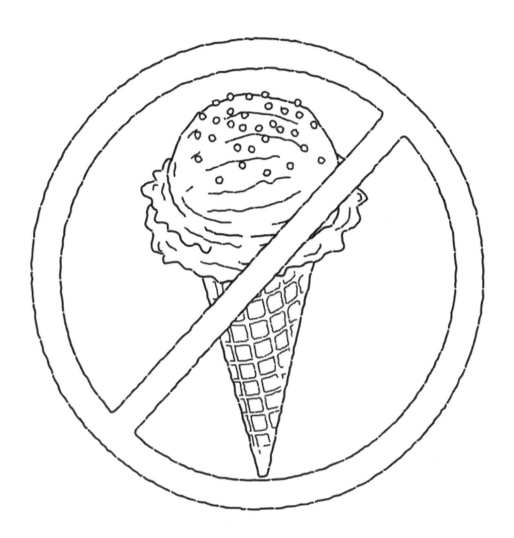

#FAIL

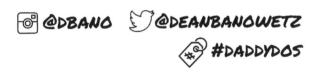

NOW LET'S PART THE HAIR

It's easy to make a great part in your child's hair. How do you do it? I take a comb and slide it down the scalp using my free hand to separate the hair. You can do these parts:

– Part down the middle
– Part on either side
– A diagonal or zigzag part

I have used a capped or upside down pen to create a part, sliding it through like you're writing a note. This is especially helpful when creating a zigzag look. Create the zigzag and use your other hand to separate it. You can even use a chopstick or a straw. Just make sure you're not using something sharp. This means no screwdriver or power tools.

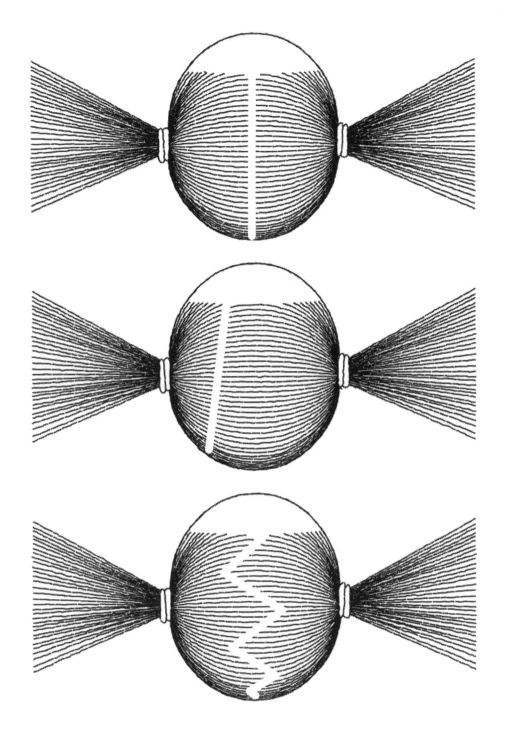

IT'S A
PART-Y!

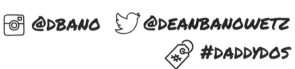

@DBANO @DEANBANOWETZ #DADDYDOS

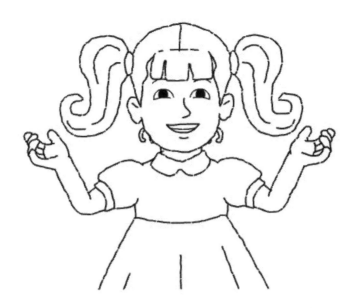

CHAPTER FOUR:
MY LITTLE PONY(TAIL)

I'm proud that you're practicing your de-tangling, but first things first: You have to master a ponytail. This is not only easy and soul building, but also a staple style for little girls across the globe. You wake up and your little girl's hair is a mess? Put it in a pony! You want a polished look, but are running super late for school? Pony time! You want to look like a hero who can do hair? Pony, pony, pony!

The trick with the ponytail is two fold: You want it to stay in, and you also want it to look symmetrical, so it doesn't appear as if your child tried to make a ponytail and now looks like she is auditioning as one of the orphans in a revival of *Annie*.

GET READY FOR YOUR PONY

The ponytail just requires your basic hair supplies—a brush or comb and some kind of tie for the top of the pony. Be sure you have secured the ponytail with a basic ponytail holder.

DADDY DO TIP

You can use plain old string if there is nothing else around, although in a pinch I prefer packing string. Dip the string in some water and squeegee it out. Finally, just tie it in a knot around the ponytail tie. As it dries, it will shrink and thus really lock in the ponytail. Of course, you can also invest in a big packet of coated ponytail holders, so the hair doesn't rip out. Remember that your girl will leave these everywhere, so buy an extra pack because it's easy to lose them. Goody Ouchless bands are great for this.

Please don't use that horrid rubber band that holds your Sunday paper together. Yes, it will hold your pony, but it will also rip your daughter's hair out when you try to take it out. Avoid future tears and find an alternative.

DADDY DO TIP

Make sure you also have some bobby pins on hand to secure any loose strands while doing a pony. If you have old bobby pins with the end worn off and If you want to go to the next level buy some clear nail polish and coat the ends of any old bobby pins. This way the little tip of the bobby pin won't scratch your girl's noggin.

YOU CAN DO IT

Remember that a ponytail is as basic as checking your tires before you go on a long drive. Keep in mind that if you can't properly fix your car, it won't work. It will break down and your life will become miserable. The same thing goes for a ponytail. If you don't do it properly, it will fall out or sag and your kid will be miserable until you fix it. The point is: Get it right the first time and avoid any whining or tears. Again, it just takes a little bit of practice. #practicepeople

WHAT KIND OF PONY

The first thing you'll do with your little girl is to determine where the pony should rest. Is it going to be a high pony, middle pony or low, side pony? There are so many variations and like picking the right lettuce there really is no absolute or perfect thing. Just determine your pony goal, which is the first step.

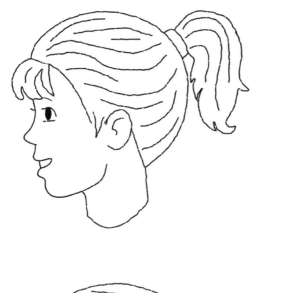
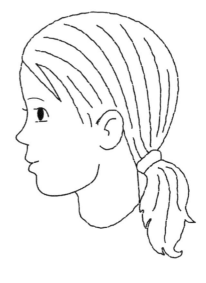
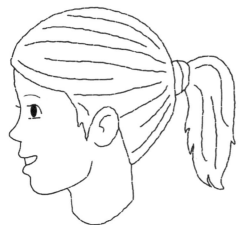
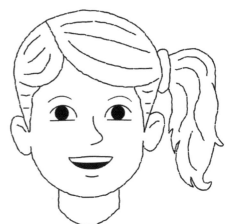

WE HAVE PONY OPTIONS!

 @DBANO @DEANBANOWETZ

 #DADDYDOS

For rookies, I'd suggest the basic middle pony. It's pretty, and pretty foolproof. If it's your first time, you might want to avoid the middle pony because you don't have the experience to center it. It will save a lot of embarrassment if you just start small until you get this pony thing down. Ready for a tutorial? Thought so.

DADDY DO IT!
THE PERFECT MIDDLE PONY

▢ Take a regular paddle brush and start at the side of the head.

▢ Brush a big portion of hair into your open hand.

▢ Let the hair fall gently into your hand. Brush it straight. Keep it in your hand.

▢ Take hair from the other side and brush it back to rest it in your hand.

▢ Now take the hair from the forehead, pull it back and let it join its friends.

▢ Make sure you haven't missed a spot. If so, scoop it up and put it into the pony.

▢ Group the strands in the upper middle of your daughter's head. Secure with ponytail holder.

VIDEO TUTORIAL!
See it at daddy.do/middle-pony-perfection

Note: If your daughter has short bangs, you can leave them alone as bangs with a pony is super cute. FYI: They also belong outside of the pony.

PONY TROUBLESHOOTING

Q: What if some of the hairs keep falling out and refuse to go into the pony?

A: Lightly mist them with water. It will help you keep them together and get rid of annoying fly-aways or use a bobby pin or a snap barrette depending on the length of the hair.

Q: What if my daughter seems like she's in pain when I make a pony?

A: This isn't good and you're pulling too hard. Don't pull too tightly. You don't want her hair plastered against her head. Save plastering for the walls in the dining room. You don't want to cut off her brain circulation either. It absolutely shouldn't hurt. If she says "ouch" then relax the pony a bit.

Q: I found tangles when I went to make the pony. Should I give up and join the Merchant Marines?

A: You must remove the tangles first. Go back to the tangle chapter, take action, and then when de-tangles. Start over from Pony step one.

Q: Do you personally prefer using a brush or a comb when making a pony?

A: I like to use a brush; it's more manageable.

Q: How do I secure the pony?

A: Get out your coated hairband and go over it two or three times to make sure it's secure. Then you're good to go! Whenever I do live TV shows I ALWAYS use ponytail ties just to make sure it is secure.

ACCESSORIZING YOUR PONY

After you secure your pony, your job might not be done. I know you're thinking, "Dean, you lied because you said this would be fast and easy." First, I'm hurt that you think this of me because I did not lie. Accessorizing a pony can take less than a minute. Think of it this way: You will spend less time accessorizing that pony than you do trying to adjust the seat in your car. Don't you have less than a minute for your child? I'm sorry, but I'm pulling out the big guilt here because an accessorized pony is a true dream come true. You can thank me later. It will take your pony esthetic to the next LEVEL!

DEAN'S RULE FOR DADDY DOING:

☐ **When using an accessory, the key to remember is that less is NOT more.** More is actually better.

☐ **Start small and add colorful or glittery bows to the pony.** Or you can tie the bottom of the pony with a pretty ribbon.

☐ **You might want to color coordinate the ribbon with the outfit.** There's nothing cuter than a polka dot dress with a matching polka dot ribbon.

☐ **You can make your own bows.** Buy the metal clasps and take a bit of fabric or tulle and make a pretty knot. Need help? Go to Michael's and ask for help.

☐ **You can buy adorable little pom-pom bows to put back there.** Girls love pom- poms and your Daddy coolness factor will quadruple.
☐ **Fourth of July time?** Buy one of those bouncy ponytail holders with streamers and stars coming out of it.

☐ **Glitter is great.** The more glitter on a bow the better. It's *bougie* which is my word, which means fancy. Now, let's try it in a sentence: "You are so bougie."

☐ **Christmas? New Year's? How about a bigger, glittery star on the pony?** Holidays mean you can go literally crazy with the accessories.

☐ **For Dads into sports, listen to Dean. I don't know JACK about sports;** however, I do know that if Dad is a Bears fan there is nothing wrong with an orange and blue ribbon on your daughter's pony on game day. Nothing says bonding like sharing the team's colors. You can also do your school's colors.

☐ **Do not raid your wife's hair accessory drawer for your daughter.** Your wife likes her stuff where it is and not in foreign drawers where she will never find these accessories again. (Kids have a rule that when they take out a bow, it falls to the ground and they leave it there or behind a bed where the dog starts to eat it.) Go to Target or Justice or Claires or anywhere and buy a few bows to surprise your daughter when you do her hair. You have gone from hero to King.

Enough with the ponytail for a second.

THE RAG ROLL SET THE NIGHT BEFORE

How about another option for going out hair? This requires a little more practice. If you want more *bougie* and you're going to an event, it's great to do a little hair project with your daughter. You can do a rag roll set the night before. At this point you might be saying, "Dean, are you speaking a foreign language here?" To do this, all you need to do is go into your manly workshop (or the store) and get shop cloth or regular strips of thin cotton fabric. Roll up the hair and tie it. Start at the ends making sure they are even on the cloth BEFORE you roll up the hair to the scalp. Then tie the ends in a bow. No one likes fishhook ends on hair. They only like it when they are BASS fishing. Make sure hair is 95% dry first.

DADDY DO IT!
THE RAG ROLL SET THE NIGHT BEFORE

▢ Split the hair in small sections.

▢ To secure, wrap hair around the fabric rolling it up to the scalp.

▢ Take the two ends of fabric and tie together to create the rag roll set.

▢ This will create amazing and erratic curls because in the morning you will take out the fabric and your child will have instant curls. Over the course of the day, the curls will loosen up. Secure with ponytail holder.

DOUBLE OR NOTHING

You can easily make double ponies, which is a great style if your daughter is going to day camp or even a swim class and needs her hair out of her face. Maybe she's a cheerleader or in dance class. It's a cute look that's also functional. If you want to be a cutting edge Dad, try it this way:

DADDY DO IT!
DOUBLE OR NOTHING

□ Make one pony at the crown by grabbing the hair from halfway up the head.

□ Secure with elastic band.

□ Take the hair underneath (or bottom half) and make a second pony.

□ The key is to add the tail of the top pony to your hand for the second pony so they are now attached. It looks like the first pony is going right into the second pony. instant curls. Over the course of the day, the curls will loosen up.. Secure with ponytail holder.

Is it okay to do a Pebbles pony? In my world, the Pebbles Flintstone top of the head pony is still okay. In fact, it's a great way to really deal with her long hair on a hot day.

DADDY DO TIP

There is no need to use hair spray on a ponytail. You want to have that swing factor. HOWEVER, a little blast of hairspray will lay down any fly aways that didn't make it into the pony.

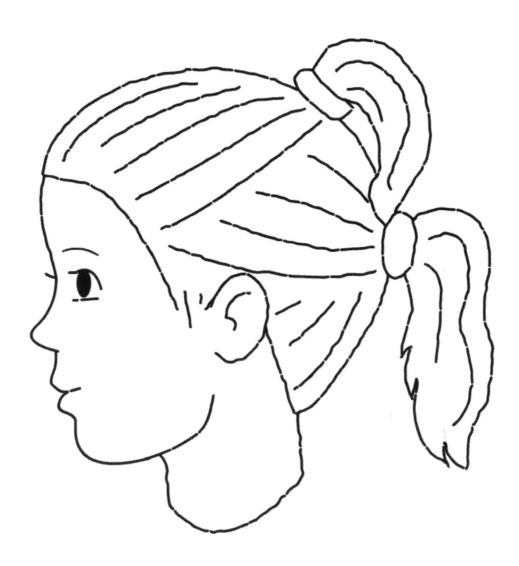

DOUBLE OR NOTHING!

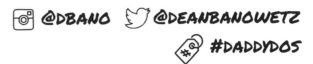 @DBANO @DEANBANOWETZ

#DADDYDOS

DEAN'S DIY RECIPE FOR A SILKY PONY

I have absolutely no problem with DIY beauty recipes if they work. If you want your daughter to have a sleek pony, you can grab a dime-sized dot of hair gel and run it over the pony. Let's say you live in a "gel-less" house. Go into the kitchen and put a ¼ of a teaspoon of real sugar (not fake) in your hand and about six small drops of water. Swirl with your other finger to break down the sugar until it's a bit syrupy. Swirl as you go along, so you don't drown the sugar in too much water. You want the consistency of a runny maple syrup. Rub the mixture between your hands and the over the hair that is on the scalp by the roots to create a sleek, shining look. This is the best homemade gel ever and works great on vacation if you forget your gel. The end of the ponytail should be free to move.

DADDY DO TIP

Stop, in the name of good hair. You can also get way ahead of yourself and make a bun with the pony. But first master your pony and that can only be done with practice. Make sure it's perfection before we move onto topknots and buns in the following chapters.

GETTING THE PONY TAIL THINGY OUT

I hear horror stories of giant tangles that start when a ponytail tie gets stuck in the hair. Dads will try to maneuver the little rubber band out while the kid stands there doing a crying jig. There is no need to have all this angst in your home. Let's say it's bedtime, a tired kid and a ponytail tie that won't come out, find a tiny pair of sewing scissors in the house (or other small scissors). Cut the tie so the hair will come right out. You're done. Avoid the ocean of tears.

IT'S GETTING HOT IN HERE

Since I want to talk about curling the ponytail – and this is the first time I've mentioned using actual powered tools on hair (sort of like power tools, but not really) -- it's time to talk turkey about how to stay safe around children and heat. First of all your daughter has young, silky hair that hasn't been colored (unless she lives in Hollywood and works in the motion picture industry…and then who knows?)

The first rule when using a curling iron or any other heat product on your child is to spray her hair with a thermal setting spray before you use the hot tool. I love the Aquage Thermal setting spray. You don't want to actually burn her hair, which would cause tears that might last weeks, and your better half locking you out of the house—perhaps permanently. Don't be afraid of using these tools. They can be very dangerous if not used in the right way.

First things first: You never want your child to touch them in any way. Little hands can easily get burned. Hot hair tools are not toys and you need to be firm with your child. The last thing you want EVER is for your child to plug one in and try it on a friend. Keep these tools out of the reach of your younger children. Tell your kids that they are not allowed to touch these things, as they are adult tools, much like the Chevy Tahoe parked in the driveway. Other tips for using hot tools:

☐ **Never use them in the tub or shower even if it says the product is a wet and dry tool.** Never ever ever! Someone could get electrocuted.

☐ **Don't leave the tool in the hair for too long.** Use it for a couple of seconds. Don't freak out if you see a little steam when you are using a hot tool. It is simple excess product on the hair. If you see smoke and HEAR sizzle then you are literally burning the hair. Get that heated tool away from her hair – stat!

☐ **If you smell the hair, it's burning.** That's a horrible smell and you'll know it. The smell always reminds me of butchering chickens on the farm and singeing the little hairs off. GAY-ROSS!

▢ **If your child's hair is thicker or course, you will leave the heated tool in for a second or two longer.** A second or two… not longer.

▢ **The finer the hair, the less time you leave in a hot tool.** This type of hair will burn easier. You don't want to see her hair stuck to the heated hair tool.

▢ **Remember that the first time you curl your daughter's hair it doesn't have to be perfect.** She's not in a Miss USA pageant. She doesn't even know Donald Trump. Just do a few curls to practice. As you feel more comfortable you can do more with hot tools. #MissAmericaRequiresTalent

▢ **Remember that hairdryers get so hot these days that they are also hot tools.** Dry your child's hair on a cooler setting even if it takes longer. It's easy to burn their hair, scalps and even their necks if you use Mom's salon professional hairdryer on a little head.

▢ **Use common sense and caution here.** You don't want to be known for the rest of your life as the "Burn Daddy."

▢ **Always read the users manual included for any heated tool.** #usecommonsense

You're going to be careful, but the more practice you get, the more comfortable you'll become.

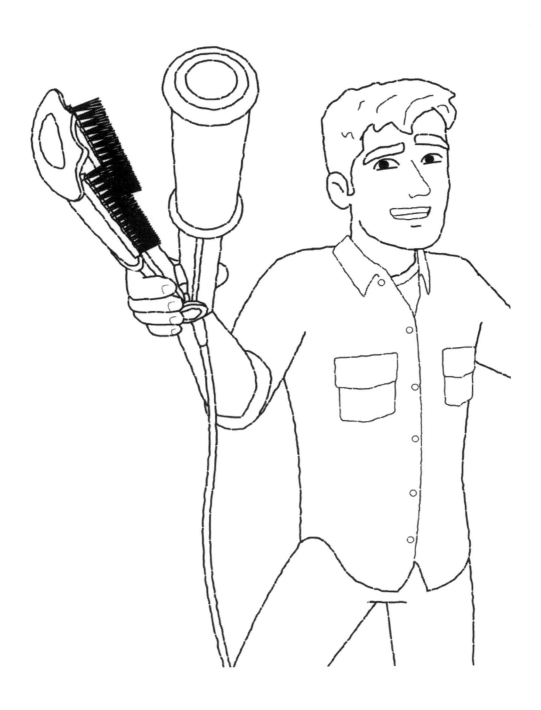

I LOVE USING THE #INSTYLER!

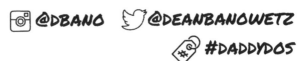 @DBANO @DEANBANOWETZ

#DADDYDOS

A FEW LAST WORDS ABOUT HOT TOOLS

As you're mastering hot tools, remember this rule: the longer you keep the heat on *doesn't* mean a better curl. If you really want to lock the curl in, drop the curl out of the curling iron after a few seconds. (This is how I get curls to stay longer when I am working on *Dancing with the Stars*). Put down the hot tool in a safe spot where you're not dropping it on your own leg. Now, take your fingers and wrap the curl around your fingers. Clip it with a bobby pin.

Let the curls stay clipped for several minutes until they are cool to the touch and then take out the pins. You'll have amazing curls and they will last much longer after trying this technique. Plus, the next time Mommy curls her hair and she asks about the pin trick, the female parent here might say, "What pin trick?" Big points for Daddy!

In summary:

☐ **Use a thermal protector on the hair before you use hot tools including blow dryers.** I love Biolage Thermal Spray.

☐ **Smell hair? You've left the hot tool in too long.** Not good.

☐ **Explore rag curls or even try sponge rollers (both are a whole lot safer) before going to hot tools.** It will make everyone's life much safer.

☐ **If you are looking for a hot tool I would suggest looking into purchasing an InStyler to lock in some curls.** It will become your new favorite tool.

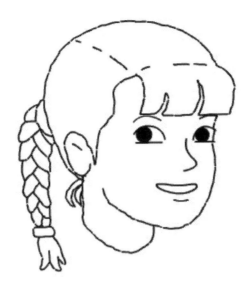

CHAPTER FIVE:
THE BEST BRAIDS EVER!

It's time to let your fingers do the talking. Before you try the actual braiding in this book, it's time to go to rookie hair camp where your head counselor Dean will take you through a few training exercises.

This might sound crazy, but I want you to try the following in your spare time – and you can do this in private without prying eyes. If someone catches you doing this exercise then simply put it away in your tackle box and talk about fishing hooks with worm guts attached to them or the films of Arnold Schwarzenegger. When in doubt, get macho. Nothing makes ladies run out of the room during inopportune moments like the mention of worm innards or quoting *The Terminator*.

LET'S START BRAIDING

Here is the great news: It's very easy to braid your daughter's hair. Men, it's important to wipe the entire idea of hair out of the picture here. Just imagine that you're dealing with the cables of a TV or stereo system. In your mind, you're fixing the cables so you get a great picture for the big game. Feeling motivated now? Let's go!

DADDY DO IT!
THE PERFECT DEAN BRAID - PRACTICE RUN

You need: One PS3 TV cord.

▢ Gather your imaginary daughter's hair (the wires) into a ponytail.

▢ From left to right, arrange the cable colors (white, yellow, red). Remember, these are cables not hair.

▢ Take the red cable and criss cross it over the yellow cable.

▢ Take your white and criss cross it over red.

▢ Take the yellow and criss cross it over white.

▢ Take the red and criss cross it over the yellow.

▢ Gather your imaginary daughter's hair (the wires) into a ponytail.

▢ REPEAT. Do red over yellow, white over red, yellow over white.

▢ Continue until you have no more cable left. Focus on the pattern.

▢ At the end, fasten all of the cables together with one tie.

▢ Now practice this over and over and over until you can do it in seconds.

▢ After you've mastered the cables and ONLY when you've mastered the cable braid then you can move on to the real hair cable braid!

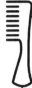

DADDY DO IT!
THE PERFECT DEAN BRAID - THE REAL DEAL

You need: Take the following out of your tackle box: Yellow, red, two black and white ponytail ties and your brush.

▢ Gather your daughter's hair into a ponytail with a black hair tie. Within that pony, break it into three sections.

▢ At the end of section one, put a white ponytail tie. Use a yellow pony tie for the second section, and a red pony tie for the thirds. Remember, these are no longer strands of hair. They are cables (in your mind). Now, breathe. Smile. Your kid is nervous.

▢ Take the red cable and criss cross it over the yellow cable.

▢ Take your white and criss cross it over red.

▢ Take the yellow and criss cross it over white.

▢ Take the red and criss cross it over the yellow.

▢ Now… go red over yellow, white over red, yellow over white. Continue until you have no more cable left.

▢ Stay focused on the pattern. At the end, put all of the cables together and take a black ponytail tie and put it just above the red, yellow and white ties.

▢ Take the colored ties out. Save them in your tackle box for your next training.

▢ Drink a beer. You earned it.

VIDEO TUTORIAL!
See it at daddy.do/perfect-dean-braid

Imaginary conversation after you make this perfect braid:

Wife (to you):
"Did Sally braid her own hair?"

You:
"No, I did."

Wife (look of shock registering while she wonders if you were kidnapped by aliens who gave you a hairdresser probe while experimenting on you):
"How did you do it?"

You:
"It was easy. Go relax, honey."

Bonus: You are having sex tonight.

It's safe to say here—after you've broken your braiding cherry—that this hairstyle is beyond huge. Now you have a basic braid in your trick bag and you should be feeling confident. I'm sure your daughter looks adorable. Extra points if your girl has really long hair. I'm proud of you because you've done a whole braid without f-ing it up.

Now, it's time to get a bit more advanced in our braiding. Turn the page for your next adventure.

DADDY DO IT!
ADVANCED MANLY BRAID TRAINING

☐ Take 20 pieces of yarn and cut identical 8 to 10 inch strips.

☐ On your workbench counter, tape the strands down in a neat row using duct tape to make sure they are secured.

☐ Start in the middle and grab three strands of yarn.

☐ Pick them up and crisscross them over each other.

☐ Pick up the next strands and crisscross them. You are learning how to braid. Breathe. This is not brain surgery.

☐ Continue to work on your crisscross technique.

☐ The key is to pick up another string as you go from side to side

VIDEO TUTORIAL!
See it at daddy.do/manly-braid-training

Do this when your daughter or partner is not around, so you don't look like a total freak.

Spoiler: This is the beginning training for a French braid.

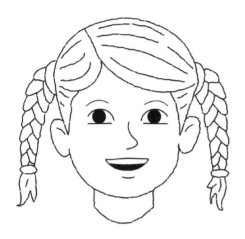

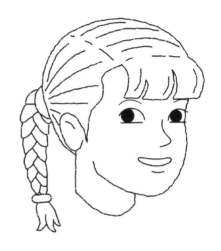

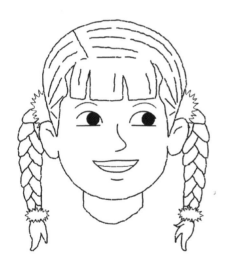

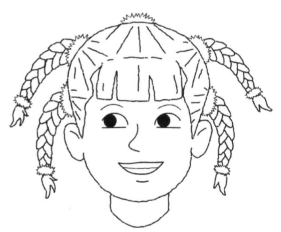

**BRAIDED
PIG TAILS!**

@DBANO @DEANBANOWETZ

#DADDYDOS

If you want to do really great hair then put the time in with this exercise. When you feel confident enough go find one of your daughter's dolls—the one with the long hair. When you're all alone and everyone is out of the house practice braiding on the creepy doll.

Take this seriously. It is your pre-game.

I know this isn't how you usually spend your weekend, but this is a worthwhile way to kill 15 to 20 minutes. If someone walks in on you while you're playing with the doll's hair then simply call your daughter over and finish the story. Just say, "And then the prince marries the princess and all is happy in the end." Lie to your wife and say you're perfecting your storytelling abilities. She'll be so shocked that she won't even remember that the guy who tosses her over his shoulder has actually braided that American Girl doll's hair.

Kids are often too smart for this lie. It follows that if a kid actually walks in on you just say, "Honey, her neck was kind of squeaky and I wanted to make sure your brother didn't rip her head off. These dolls are expensive and money doesn't grow on trees." The minute you mention money, your daughter's eyes will glaze over and she will want to leave the room without any more nosy questions asked.

Your daughter's Barbie is also a great tool here during your practice sessions. Split her hair into four sections and make a quick ponytail. Think of your work with Barbie like taking the back off of your TV or defusing a bomb during any action film. Pretend you actually are Liam Neeson in any one of his later-in-life films where bombs and babes over 30 are involved. Think to yourself that this isn't Barbie hair, but yellow, red and white cables. You will pull the safest cable (section of hair) into a pony and thus are defusing a bomb (in your mind).

Now that you've practiced, it's time to get to some of the real styles that you will perfect.

ADDING ACCESSORIES TO YOUR BRAID (OH YES YOU CAN!)

Braids were made for accessories including cute, decorative hairpins and even bows. It's all about placing it where you want this tool to hold the actual hair. Why settle for a plain ponytail tie at the end of your braid? Learning what to do with the braid you created is a lot of fun. Think of your original braid as the foundation for slightly more complex (but truly easy) things you can do with your daughter's hair.

DADDY DO IT!
A BASIC BRAID

☐ Brush the hair smooth and put the hair into a ponytail with a hair band (any color)

☐ Section that ponytail into three different ponytails this time using the **red**, **white** and **yellow** hair bands

☐ Take **yellow** and move it to the center crossing OVER the **white**

☐ Take **red** and move it to the center crossing OVER the **yellow**

☐ Take **white** and move it to the center crossing OVER the **red**

☐ Take **yellow** and move it to the center crossing OVER the **white**

☐ Take **red** and move it to the center crossing OVER the **yellow**

☐ Repeat this pattern continuing all the way down the hair and tie off the end with a **black** band (remove **red**, **white** and **yellow** bands)

VIDEO TUTORIAL!
See it at <u>daddy.do/basic-braid-by-dean</u>

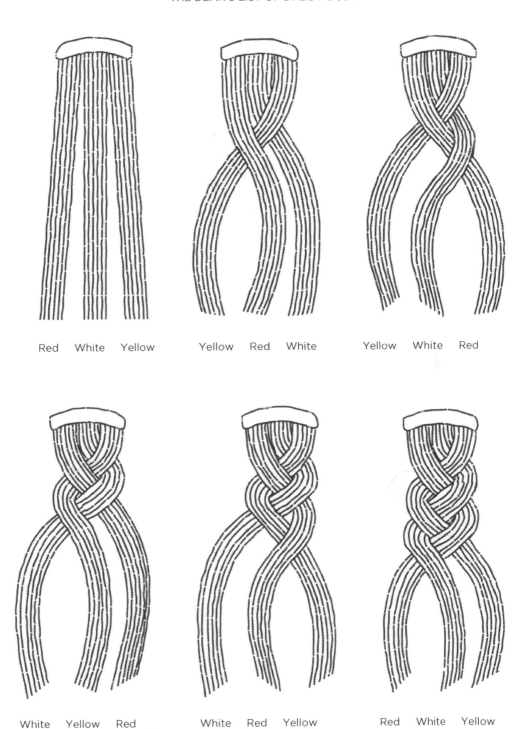

| Red | White | Yellow | Yellow | Red | White | Yellow | White | Red |

| White | Yellow | Red | White | Red | Yellow | Red | White | Yellow |

BRAIDING HOW-TO!

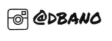 @DBANO 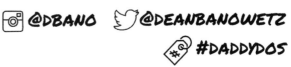 @DEANBANOWETZ #DADDYDOS

DADDY DO IT!
A FRENCH BRAID

☐ Before braiding, brush hair smooth. Take a section at the top of the head and divide the hair into three equal strands.

☐ Cross the **yellow** strand over the **white** section, and then repeat this action with the **red** side, smoothing hair as you go.

☐ Before repeating the crossover action with the **right** section, gather some of the additional hair from the head's **right** side, and adding it to this section.

☐ Cross this larger strand of hair over the **middle** stand of hair.

☐ Gather a section of hair the same size as the **right** side from the head's **left** side, and then add to strand and cross over middle strand.

☐ Repeat steps 4 and 5 all the way down the head until you've gathered all additional strands. Finish at the bottom with a regular braid.

☐ Tie off the end with a hair band.

VIDEO TUTORIAL!
See it at <u>daddy.do/a-very-french-braid</u>

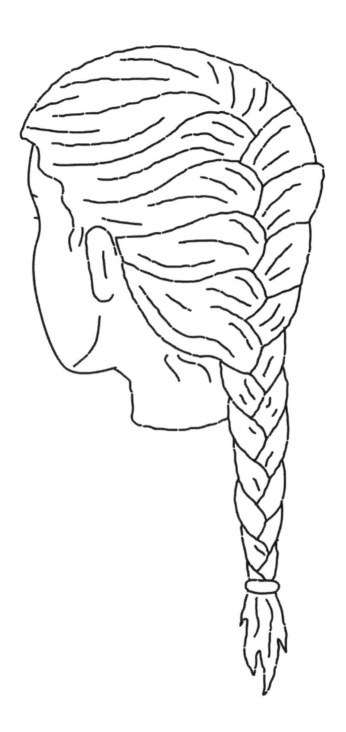

FRENCH BRAID!

 @DBANO @DEANBANOWETZ

#DADDYDOS

DADDY DO IT!
A FISHTAIL BRAID

☐ Before braiding, brush hair smooth.

☐ Divide hair into two large sections, parting straight down the middle.

☐ Pull a thin strand of hair from the outside of the **left** section. Pull it over the top of the **left** section, and add it to the **right** section. Try to use the same thickness for each strand throughout or your braid will look uneven.

☐ Repeat on the **right** side. Pull a skinny strand of hair from the outside of the **right** section, pull it over the **right** section, and then add it to the **left** section.

☐ Keep alternating sides, weaving over and under, until you reach the bottom of the braid.

☐ Tie off the end with a hair band.

☐ The smaller the section, the more it will look like a fishbone; the larger the section, the less time it will take and the less it will look like a true fishbone. Start with larger sections. When you have it down, start taking smaller and smaller sections.

VIDEO TUTORIAL!
See it at <u>daddy.do/a-fishtail-braid</u>

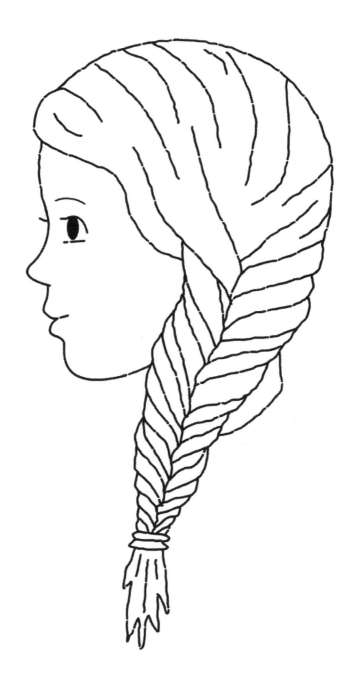

FISHTAIL BRAID!

@DBANO @DEANBANOWETZ
#DADDYDOS

DADDY DO IT!
A ROPE BRAID

▫ Before braiding, brush hair smooth.

▫ For a tighter, more structured rope braid, start by putting the hair in a ponytail. For a messier look, skip to the next step and start the braid at the nape of her neck.

▫ Separate the hair into two equal sections. Now, twirl each section around your fingers, or pinch the top of the section, twist, move down another inch, twist again, and so on. Both sections should be twisted in a clockwise or rightward motion.

▫ Cross the **right** section over the left section.

▫ Keep braiding all the way down the hair.

▫ Tie off the end with a hair band.

DADDY DO TIP
Take the braid and use bobby pins to fasten it up.
Use the same color pins as your daughter's hair.
There is nothing worse than blonde hair and black
pins. #ThanksKimiMessina

DADDY DO TIP
It is easier to braid with slightly dirty hair because it
has less "slip." So, let your child skip a hair washing
the night before you know you're going to braid.

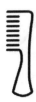

DADDY DO IT!
A FRENCH ROPE BRAID

☐ Before braiding, brush hair smooth.

☐ Gather a small section at the front hairline and divide into two equal sections.

☐ Twist each strand to the right, or clockwise. For a French Rope, you'll twist the hair, as you go, so don't worry if you only have the base of the strand twisted for now.

☐ Cross the twisted **right** strand over the twisted left strand.

☐ Grab the section of hair directly beneath where you started the braid. Then twist the new section around the strand on the **right**. It might take a few twirls for you to get them into one cohesive twist.

☐ Cross the larger **right** section over the smaller **left** section.

☐ Grab the section of hair directly beneath the last one you took.

☐ Add the new section around the strand on the **right**. Again, it might take a few twirls for you to get them into one, cohesive twist. Repeat adding new sections and twisting until you reach the desired length.

☐ Tie off the end with a hair band.

☐ Practice over and over.

VIDEO TUTORIAL!
See it at <u>daddy.do/french-rope-by-dean</u>

Let's say your daughter has her big dance recital and your partner (the one who does good hair) has to go out of town. This is not the time to pack up the kids and move to Alaska. They still have dance recitals in the tundra. If you want to be a really cool Dad, master the basic braid and then take a glance at the dress your daughter will wear for her dance routine.

If her outfit is purple, go out and buy a big purple ribbon and even some thinner ribbons (about a quarter of an inch wide), too. You can often find these ribbons at stores including Target, Walmart and Justice. Note: If you go to Justice, prepare yourself to hear so many boy band songs that you will feel as if you should form a boy band. Suddenly, you're answering your cell phone humming, 'Baby, baby baby...." But we digress.)

When you put the pony in, clip the thinner ribbon to a safety pin and close the safety pin. In the center of that pony, you will stick the safety pin through and pull the ribbon through the ponytail tie. Now, take the safety pin off and pull it through to the end. You've literally created another strand to braid here. Instead of letting that new purple ribbon strand hang, incorporate it into one of the red, yellow OR white cable sections. Pretend it's just another part of that section of hair – I mean, another cable. Continue to braid as you bring this ribbon into the braid. When you reach the end of the section, tie with an elastic hair tie. Then tie the ribbon ends together in a bow. It will give it a cute ribbon braided loop. (If you choose to do a braided bun – and more on buns later – you can work it through the bun). After this not-so-complex move, you might have to call your buddies and go to the local bar for some wings. I mean, you color coordinated the ribbon to go with an actual dance outfit. This is major! I think you should do a shot or go shoot hoops!

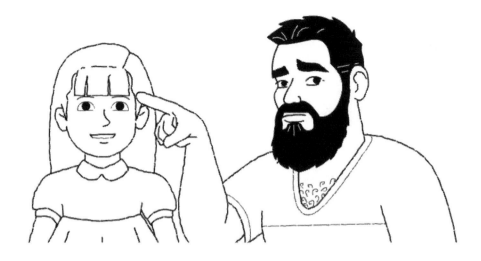

CHAPTER SIX:
BANG YOUR HEAD

There are times when any father is tempted to take a scissors to their child's hair, and most of the time as a top hairdresser to the stars, I want to scream, "Little child, run fast, run far, run to your Uncle Dean's house where there will be milk, cookies, and tastefully cut, perfect 'dos!" We've come to the point in the book, however, where I believe I'll have to let go and allow you Dads to cut your child's bangs. I'm not letting you cut her entire head of hair! The bangs are quite enough.

I do have to say that I love bangs on girls and they even help to conceal any irregular hairlines. Bangs also disguise high and low foreheads. If you have one of those high Christina Ricci foreheads and want to cover it up, just cut some bangs. Another great reason to cut bangs is that they keep the hair out of your girl's face when she's dancing, playing soccer, riding bikes, or chasing down bullies or boys. Bangs are great for kids who swim or do gymnastics, as they're a way to manage to have long hair that doesn't interrupt the activity at hand.

Are you considering bangs for your child? The first thing I tell adults is to think long and hard about it before doing it. I know I just said I love bangs, but they are a hair commitment. In other words, it will take FOREVER to grow them out. If your child hates them on day one, FOREVER will seem like forever plus eternity. Bangs are a decision that requires a consultation with your partner. You don't just "do bangs." You talk about getting bangs first with everyone involved and all parties get a vote. There might even be a lengthy period of debate. Go with the flow. You've only got one vote.

It also helps to remember that bangs require frequent trims, so you must commit to the idea of keeping her bangs fresh and exciting. One note: When you're a kid, face shape really doesn't matter when it comes to bangs. If your child has a round face, you can frame it with bangs and that will look super cute as well.

DADDY DO TIP

Make sure to get your bangs cut first by a qualified hairdresser. You don't want your child sitting in your bathroom or kitchen upset as her long hair hits the floor. And you don't want to start out with bad bangs that become shorter and shorter and weirder and weirder as you try to fix them. Get professional help. As a hairdresser, I'm happy to take the five minutes to cut a child's bangs. You could probably just take your child into your hairdresser and ask if during a break he or she will do some bangs. A hairdresser will also shape or thin out bangs so they look gorgeous. Later on, if the bangs need a trim you can probably pop back into your hairdresser for a quick reshaping. Or I'll allow you to trim them at home if you pay close attention in this chapter.

WANT TO DO BANGS AT HOME OR TRIM THE BANGS YOU ALREADY HAVE?

Then listen up. The first step is to determine what kind of bang you want it to be… shorter, longer, wispy or perhaps fuller. You'll want to clip the hair from the other areas out of the way. Remember that less IS more when trimming your child's bangs. In other words, don't get cray-cray here. Just do a little trim, and for God's sake leave enough hair for your hairdresser to fix it if this becomes a 911 moment.

DADDY DO IT!
CUTTING CUTE BANGS

Before you begin:

□ Don't use your household scissors, which I'm sure are dull. Go to the drugstore and get professional hair cutting scissors. They only cost about ten bucks.

□ Do not use tape. Tape stretches the hair.

□ I would never EVER cut bangs when they're wet. They will shrink up and you'll end up with some wacko, hack job bangs. In fact, they could snap up about an inch, depending on the tension (how tight you pull the bangs down) when cutting

Here we go:

□ Hold 100% dry hair in a comb.

□ Pull hair away from the face with your hand. Make tiny cuts.

▫ Don't cut straight across. Those tiny chipping cuts (angling your scissors) are more forgiving.

▫ Use the eyebrows as a guideline.

VIDEO TUTORIAL!
See it at <u>daddy.do/bang-trim</u>

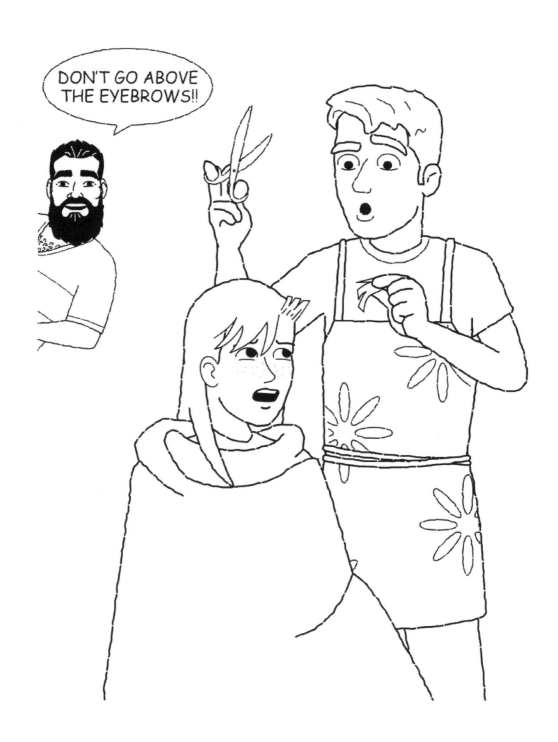

REALLY?
I SAID...

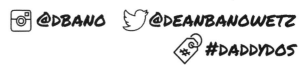

DADDY DO TIP

If bangs are so long they're falling into the eyes, they need a trim. But let me remind you, baby steps. Less is more. You can cut more tomorrow.

DADDY DON'T TIP

NEVER GO ABOVE THE EYEBROWS. I'M SCREAMING THIS TO YOU! You're going much too short if you go above the brows. If your child wants those cute short-short bangs, go see a pro. Remind your child it will take forever and another forever to grow those out.

Let's say, hypothetically, of course, you didn't listen to any of the above and started hacking at your daughter's bangs. Now they're way too short and you're afraid to tell her to open her eyes. You know at that moment when she sees your creepy short bangs, she will ask to be put up for adoption. If you went too short, STOP! Put down your tools. Take a step away from the child. Grab the car keys. Get in the car. Go see a real hairdresser for a fix. The more hair you leave, the easier the fix. The more you keep cutting, the worse it gets.

ANOTHER THOUGHT ON BANGS

Many adults have had professional photos taken of themselves at the local J.C. Penney when we were kids (and often victims of botched bangs). Many of these photos could double for prison pictures. I do believe our parents took us for these photos after cutting our bangs as a way to blackmail us when we were older. Now that there's Facebook, Twitter, Snapchat, Instagram, Vine, YouTube and Periscope, the blackmail options never go away. Blackmail for life. In fact, our parents often pull out those pictures when we get engaged, when we get our doctorate in nuclear science or at our weddings or various family holidays. Be a progressive parent. Don't let bangs become your future blackmail over your own child.

If you jack up your kid's bangs, it might even cause a divorce or you'll sit in the hair penalty box or the "THINK ABOUT IT" corner for a few weeks. If you're bad at hair cutting just don't do it. It's not a learning experience that you need.

If the bangs you have cut came out cute, then your wife might even want you to trim her bangs. You will definitely get lucky that night. She might even let you take a couple of buddies to a strip club. There might even be a NASCAR weekend in your future. So if you're handy with a scissors, it is worth a try. Just remember if you screw up your partner's bangs, you will be living an existence I call botched hair hell on earth. It might be easier to just drive him or her to the hairdresser and avoid total relationship banishment.

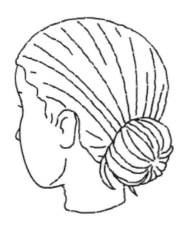 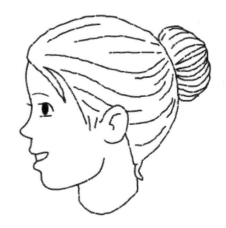

CHAPTER SEVEN: BUNS OF STEEL AND CINNAMON

Congratulations! You've reached this part of the book without having any kind of nervous breakdown. I'm guessing that your little daughter is running out of the house looking cuter than the average second grader while insisting, "My Dad totally rocks." Your partner's jaw has repeatedly been picked up off the floor as you've commanded the bathroom to create the world's most adorable ponytails and have even trimmed her bangs when in a pinch. When you braided, you actually had to tell your partner to lay down with a cold compress. He or she was in shock.

There have been no projectile tears from either partner or child, which is a plus. You're ready to take Uncle Dean out for a beer, which is appreciated, but not necessary. Now it's time to really butch up and get creative with hair. You're going to get off your buns and learn how to make a bun.

I know that many of you are shaking your heads, thinking I have lost my mind, but that's hardly the case. Making a bun is actually easier than jumpstarting a car or making one of those complicated Boy Scout knots. Plus, there is nothing that looks clean and classic like a wonderful bun. Let's get to work!

There are several kinds of buns, and I'll detail them in order of what you should try first. Just remember that your crowning achievement is putting smiles on your little girl's face.

DADDY DO IT!
A MESSY BUN

▢ Brush hair smooth to prep for bun.

▢ Pull hair back using just your hands. Hold the hair where you want to have the bun.

▢ Make a ponytail with a hair band.

▢ Create the messy bun by taking the tail and wrapping it around the base of the ponytail, covering the band. Use two or three bobby pins or whatever is needed to secure the tail around the base.

▢ Finish the bun by spraying a bit of hairspray.

VIDEO TUTORIAL!
See it at <u>daddy.do/sexy-messy-bun</u>

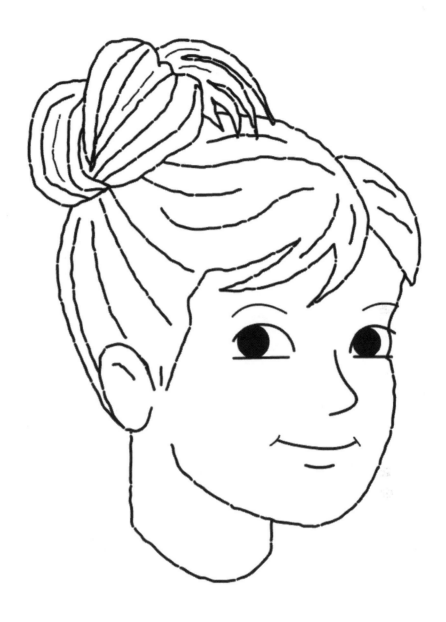

**A MESSY
BUN!**

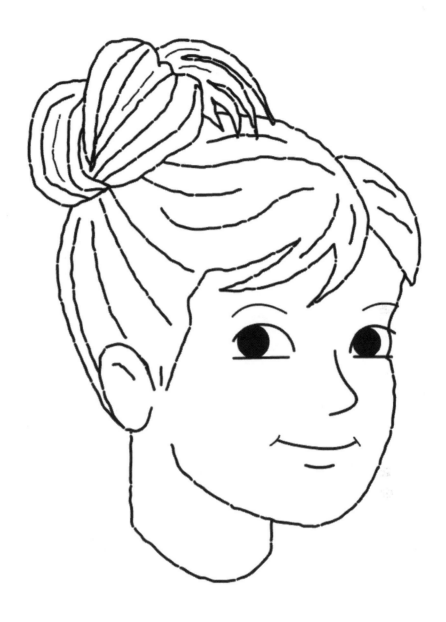 @DBANO @DEANBANOWETZ

#DADDYDOS

DADDY DO IT!
A SLEEK BUN

☐ Brush hair smooth to prep for Topknot.

☐ Pull hair up high into a high ponytail

Twist hair into a knot. Take the handful of hair and twist it in the same direction, creating a rope-like piece. Then, wrap it onto itself to make a knot-like spiral.

☐ Wrap a hair band around topknot.

☐ Finish the bun by spraying a bit of hairspray.

VIDEO TUTORIAL!
See it at <u>daddy.do/sleek-bun-by-dean</u>

Turn the page for an example (you can also color, of course).

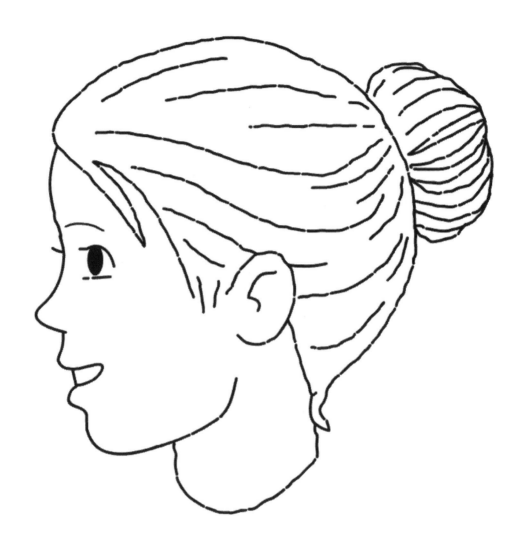

KEEPIN' IT SLEEK!

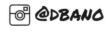 @DBANO 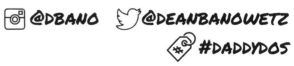 @DEANBANOWETZ

#DADDYDOS

DADDY DO IT!
A TOPKNOT

☐ Brush hair smooth to prep for topknot.

☐ Pull hair up high into a high ponytail.

Twist hair into a knot. Take the handful of hair and twist it in the same direction, creating a rope-like piece. Then, wrap it onto itself to make a knot-like spiral.

☐ Wrap a hair band around topknot.

☐ Finish the bun by spraying a bit of hairspray.

VIDEO TUTORIAL!
See it at daddy.do/top-knots

Can't visualize it? I've got you covered on the next page, boo.

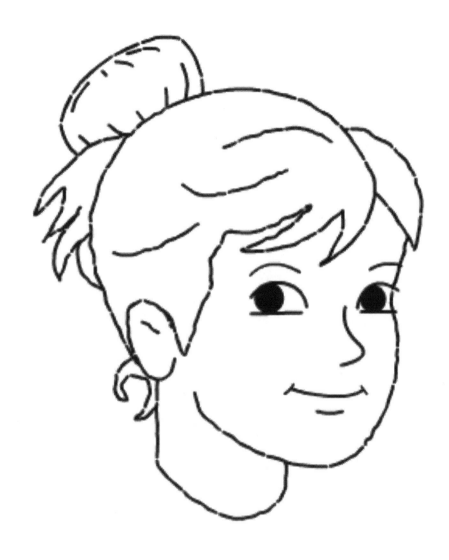

A KNOT ON THE TOP!

[image] @DBANO   [image] @DEANBANOWETZ

[image] #DADDYDOS

Word on the street is that you've become a bun master. In that case, feel free to have fun with these more advanced techniques:

DADDY DO IT!
A BRAIDED BUN

☐ Brush the hair smooth to prep for bun.

☐ Pull the hair back. A braided bun can be placed at any location on your head. It can be created using a brush for a very professional and sophisticated look, or finger-pulled back for a more relaxed appearance. Use a ponytail to secure the location on your head.

☐ Braid the ponytail.

☐ Create the bun. Starting at the base of your braid, wrap it around the ponytail tie into a spiral shape. When you get to the ends, tuck them beneath the base of the bun. Secure your hair with a few bobby pins, making sure that your hair will not fall out.

☐ Finish the bun by spraying a bit of hairspray.

VIDEO TUTORIAL!
See it at daddy.do/a-braided-bun

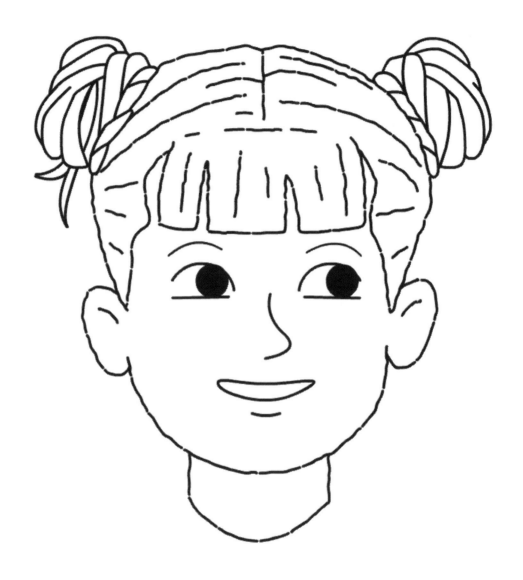

BRAIDED BUN MAGIC!

 @DBANO @DEANBANOWETZ #DADDYDOS

DADDY DO IT!
A SOCK BUN

☐ Brush the hair smooth to prep for bun.

☐ Pull the hair back. Select the place on your head you would like to create your sock bun and make a ponytail.

☐ Prep the hair sock by cutting a hole in the toe end of a sock and rolling it up into a doughnut shape.

☐ Take the sock and slide it onto your ponytail all the way to the base.

☐ Spread the hair over the doughnut, making sure the sock is fully covered, and then wrap a hair band around the base of the bun.

☐ Wrap the ends around the base of the bun, then tuck them under and pin them in place.

☐ Finish the bun by spraying a bit of hairspray.

☐ Make sure if you're working with dark hair to use a dark sock.

VIDEO TUTORIAL!
See it at daddy.do/sock-bun-by-dean

You know the drill. See it on the next page!

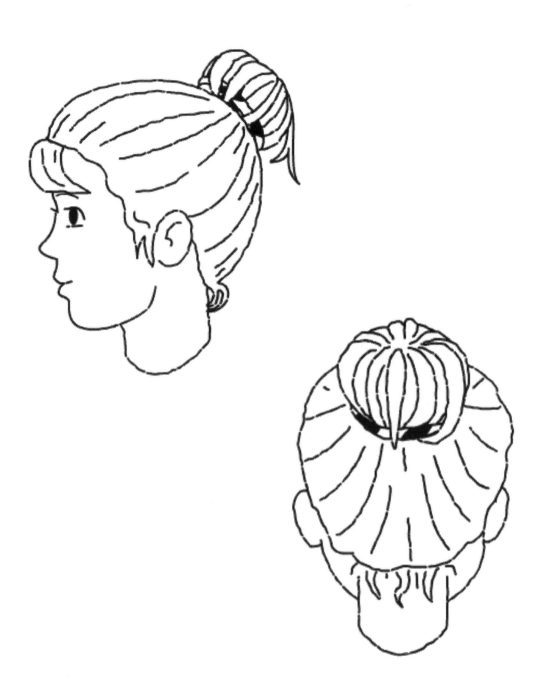

SOCK BUN RIGHT HERE!

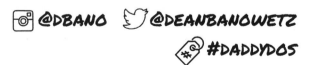

@DBANO @DEANBANOWETZ

#DADDYDOS

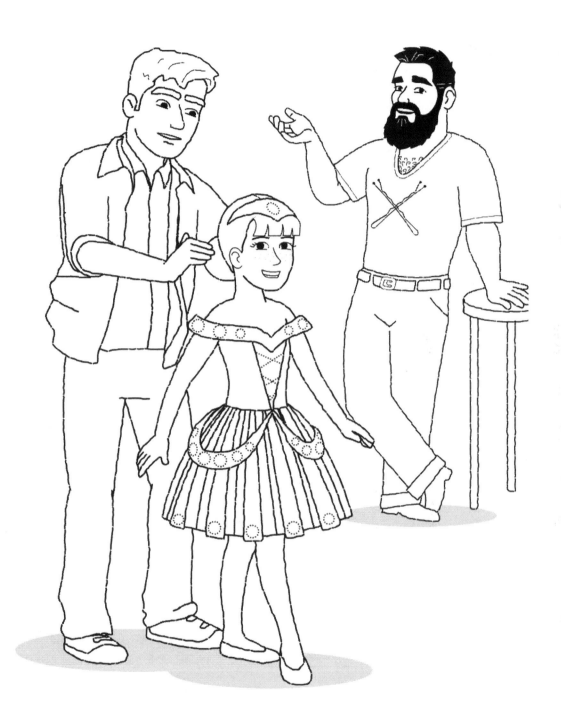

BRO YOU DID IT!

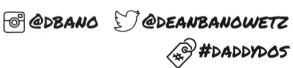

@DBANO @DEANBANOWETZ

#DADDYDOS

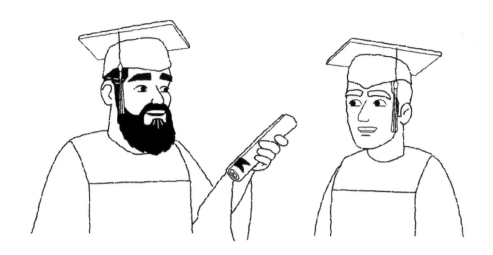

CHAPTER EIGHT: EXTRA CREDIT DADDY DOS

Think of this chapter like grad school. You've mastered the pony, the braid and the bun. Now it's time to explore some other options to make your little girl look fabulous.

HAIR LENGTH AND TRIMS

Let's start with how long you want your daughter's hair to grow. Just remember that the longer it gets the more tangled it will be over time. It's crucial to not just allow your daughter's hair to grow and grow. Have your child's hair cut every four weeks. Remember that their hair grows faster than adults, just another perk of youth. You can trim the ends, or take them in to a quick cut place to keep them trimmed. Those ends get really dry and that can become a split-ends nightmare.

Remember, if you go to a regular hairdresser, you can ask them to do a "bang drive-by" or "ends drive-by" on your child, which basically means you bring them in for about five minutes for a quick trim. It's a real lifesaver and will help your child develop great habits, while also looking neat and clean. Regular trims will also make styling much easier for you.

WHAT IF YOUR KID PITCHES A FIT?

There are girls (and boys) who love pampering and others who toss a hissy when it's time for a haircut. The whole thing about haircutting (in my opinion—back off Dr. Phil) is that you gotta pull out the bribes. Of course, there are levels of bribes. You might choose ice cream, a new Barbie or a trip to the islands. It just depends on how your family does bribes. If you do the trip then please adopt me. I'm available.

First and foremost, you need to have a hairdresser the kid likes and trusts. You might not want to take your child to that crazy Led Zeppelin rocker dude. There are a lot of different salons these days that cater to kids, and make it fun with funky chairs and kiddie music, plus candy as a treat. It makes me sad that I didn't get to go to one of them when I was younger. My dad just lined all of us up and buzzed our hair GONE. You never cried or you got a spanking. I hate spankings. Just take your kid to a cool place, smile, and bribe them. Easy! A trip to Yellow Balloon for a no drama haircut? It's a small price to pay.

Remember that you're going to be hair cutting every four weeks, so make sure these bribes are affordable. Also let your hairdresser know the deal, especially if the child is afraid or hates going there. When I worked at my salon in Iowa, I'd keep little toys and treats for the kids in a special drawer. Or the parent can give the hairdresser a treat to bestow on the child for being good during their haircut. I remember a little boy, Kenny, who hated going for haircuts. His mom gave me a plastic plane to hide in one of my drawers. I promised Kenny if he didn't cry and sat still, I'd have a special treat for him after I was done. Kenny behaved and then became my new best friend after I gave him that plane. He even started asking Mom when we were going to see his new buddy Dean again. Last week, I gave Kenny a Toyota Prius and Taylor Swift's home phone number—just kidding. But you get the idea.

YOUR HAIRDRESSER AND YOUR CHILD

The one gripe kids have when it comes to hairdressers is when they go silent. Kids don't feel comfortable around silent people. I talk to kids the entire time when we're doing a cut. Some kids talk to me, but many will just sit there and feel good that I'm talking. Other kids don't give a rat's ass about the gibberish, but I'm sure they would be a little freaked if I was just this silent big guy hovering over them with a scissors.

I will ask the kids what celeb they want to look like—if there is one. One little girl in my chair was obsessed with Pink's haircut and her mom gave the A-OK to cut the child's hair like the famous rocker. We shaved the sides and kept it longer on the top. Adorable doesn't begin to describe it because this little girl had great 'tude. The cut made her feel even more empowered. The next time, the mom told me, "My daughter is beyond sassy now." Both Mom and I were so glad, because this girl wasn't just connected to her true self, she was empowered by her beauty at this young age. Now, that's a great feeling!

If your kid starts crying in the hairdresser's chair (and I've seen it all), I keep talking to them. I'll even talk slowly like a teacher. With boys, a lot of times the clippers freak them out. I'll pretend the clippers have transformed into an airplane landing on their heads. The thing is, your hairdresser should make the entire situation seem less intimidating. If he or she doesn't do that, it might be time to find someone new for your child.

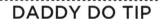

DADDY DO TIP

It's really helpful to bring a photo of EXACTLY what you want to your hairdresser. This includes bringing in a photo for what you want your child's hair to look like because hairdressers aren't mind readers!

SHOULD I COLOR MY KID'S HAIR?

I'd never do all-over color on a child. Some parents prefer to do a few highlights, but I'd say never more than a few foils. Kids have a lifetime to dye their hair, and there is no point of ruining the natural shine of their beautiful youthful locks. And you don't want your six-year-old to look like a Goth princess with roots as it grows out – even if you are a Goth princess and want people to know this is your child. The point is, hair color and children don't usually mix. Sure, a little hint of pink or purple that washes out in a few weeks as a quick highlight can be fun. Just make sure your child won't hate it in 24 hours.

COMPLICATED CUTS

I'm so sick of the Bieber cut for boys. You can tell he was counseled on the haircut by a committee who thought, "This is cool hair." Don't be hell-bent on a certain celeb style. Those people have hairstylists at their beckon call. You don't want your child to have a complicated cut that will probably soon go out of fashion. Then you're stuck with the complex growing out period. Believe me, it's better to have a real person hairstyle that's easy to do. Kids need to be quick and easy when it comes to hair care. If daily hair care takes more than 5 to 10 minutes, it's too complex.

HOT WEATHER HELP

In the summer, I like to give boys a fresh buzz cut and girls can do little bobs. It's great to get the hair away for all the summer activities like sports and swimming. By the way, the bob is also a great year round style for girls with finer hair. It will look thicker shorter. If your child is upset about getting shorter hair then do it gradually with several smaller cuts, which helps them get used to it. If your little girl is still married to the long hair then spend the summer up in a pony or a braid and call it a day.

FUN WITH BANDANAS

I love a little bandana on girls, which is s great way to pull all of her hair up. Think of it like doing a high pony. Swoop the bandana around the nape of her neck and pull upwards into a pony. Tie it yourself. A square knot that you learned as a kid works great and looks fantastic.

HEADBANDS R US

A headband is also a great, quick and easy fix. Just slide it back and allow your daughter to find the best spot. When it comes to headbands, girls know what to do. I'd suggest pulling the bangs out for an uber cute look. But if the bangs are annoying her, pull them back, too.

DADDY DO TIP

Many Dads think that headbands are just for girls with long hair, but not true. They look adorable on super short hair too.

NO PONYTAIL TIE!

Let's say you're a camping family and you forgot your Dad hair toolbox. Shame, shame, shame, but the day is not lost. Your daughter is sick of her hair in her face, but you don't have anything out there to secure a ponytail. Just take an old T-shirt and cut a strip off the bottom. Tie up that pony! If you rip the strip of T-shirt off with your bare hands then you really are Superman Dad.

DADDY DO IT! HALF UP/HALF DOWN

One style I love on girls if half up, half down. Start at the top of her ears and with your fingers work your way back, separating the hair. Take this top portion and put in a ponytail tie to anchor it. Add any accessory like a flower bow or a pretty barrette over the tie. If you're camping (again) or need a fast 'do in a pinch, I love this style to get the hair out of the face. Again, if faced with no ponytail holder, a zip tie from a food bag will work in a pinch.

TRY A MULTIPLE PONY

Start with the half up, half down do. And then go back to the middle of the ear and slide in another ponytail. Put that ponytail in with the second. Do the exact same thing under the ear. You can take the rest of the hair and put it into a pony.

> ### DADDY DON'T TIP
> Do not use any wire in a ponytail. It's just too dangerous and could be used as a weapon against her brother later on. You don't want to turn dinner into a scene from *Game of Thrones*.

LOW PIGTAILS

If the hair is short, I love a high ponytail. Low pigtails are cute if you wrap them with little bows You can even do that with a younger toddler, but make sure they don't eat the ponytail holders or bows. I've found that bows are cute for baby pictures, but take them out before they can choke on them.

TRY A PONY FLIP

You can do a pony flip with a loose pony. I usually like medium to low pony flips. You reach down through the ponytail between the scalp and the ponytail tie and grab the pony. Pull it up all the way through and twist the pony. The pony flip is great. You can make it as dressy as you want and put a beautiful bow on it. It will look amazing.

DO A PUSH BACK

This is a nice, kicky little style. Just push some hair back around the temple areas and clip on both sides with a snap barrette. This is a quick fix at the soccer game when you need that hair immediately out of the face. This is also popular when the hair is growing out including when you want to turn growing bangs into all one-length hair.

STYLES FOR THE LITTLE GUYS IN YOUR LIFE

Now that you've become the hair master in your household, your partner is going to look at you and say, "Can you cut Tommy's hair too?" It's true that your work is NEVER done. These are some styles I'm going to suggest to my friend Simon Cowell once his little boy is old enough to have enough hair. Or maybe I'll just tell Simon that I'll come over to do the job. Since I can't go to every household in America, it's up to you Dads to learn how to give your little boys a great haircut. It's simple. It's easy. And your son will be glad to get it over with! In a pinch, you could try, or better yet just take them to a professional. Just take this handy book with you to the salon for the hairstylist.

DADDY DO IT! FOR HIM
"TEXTURED TOM"

▢ Use a #4 sized clipper on the back and sides.

▢ Use a #6 or #7 on the top then blend. (AKA scissor-over-comb on sides and back and finger length on top)

▢ Apply flexible to firm hold hair wax or pomade by using your fingers to the of the head and piece it up.

DADDY DO IT! FOR HIM
"DASHING DOUG"

□ Taper the neck up and around the ears into about an inch and a half on the top of the head.

□ When hair is still wet part it to the side with a comb and then style with a product that has some hold.

DADDY DO IT! FOR HIM
"SPIKEY SCOTT"

□ Use a #2 sized clipper on the sides and back, a #3 or #4 on top, and then blend.

□ Apply firm hold gel when hair is wet if needed.

DADDY DO IT! FOR HIM
"MESSY MARV"

□ Tapered up around the ears and neck and the top left long.

□ While hair is still wet arrange hair into place with fingers.

□ Let air dry.

□ Spray texturizing spray throughout if wanted.

DADDY DO IT! FOR HIM
"PIECE-Y PAUL"

□ Keep interior layers short for texture. Leave bangs and perimeter longer.

□ Apply light hold foam throughout hair when wet.

□ Let air-dry.

See these styles for yourself. Flip over!

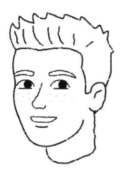

Textured Tom

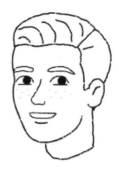

Dashing Doug

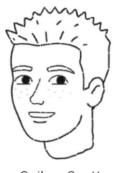

Spikey Scott

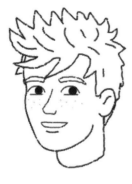

Messy Marv

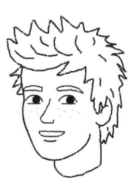

Piece-y Paul

DADDY DOS FOR HIM!

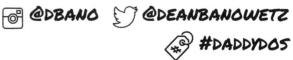 @DBANO @DEANBANOWETZ #DADDYDOS

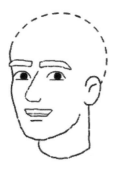

Textured Tom

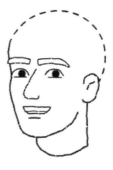

Dashing Doug

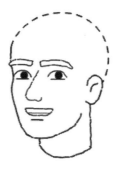

Spikey Scott

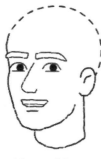

Messy Marv

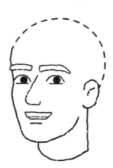

Piece-y Paul

YOUR TURN TO DRAW SOME DOs!

@DBANO @DEANBANOWETZ #DADDYDOS

DADDY DO IT! FOR HIM
"BEACHY BRODY"

☐ Use a razor to cut the shape (early Justin Bieber haircut)

☐ While still wet use fingers to arrange hair by pushing top hair forwards and bangs to the side.

☐ Let air-dry.

☐ Apply light-hold pomade and pinch the tips of hair.

DADDY DO IT! FOR HIM
"SURFER STEVE"

☐ Keep the nape and ear area clean but leave the sides around and inch and the top around two to three inches long

☐ Towel dry then air dry.

☐ Apply wax throughout hair with fingers and spike the hair on top back.

DADDY DO IT! FOR HIM
"WHISPY WESTON"

☐ Use clippers with a low guard size around neck and ears; then blend to longer pieces on top.

☐ Apply a little pomade on dry hair.

DADDY DO IT! FOR HIM
"CURLY CURTIS"

☐ Keep hair a couple inches long all over to show natural curl.

☐ Apply soft hold gel when wet and comb hair forward.

☐ Scrunch with fingers.

DADDY DO IT! FOR HIM
"MOHAWK MATT"

☐ Keep hair short around the temples and ears and blend to long down the middle of the head.

☐ Let air-dry.

☐ Spray some hairspray for texture.

Now, let's get back to the girls . . .

GREAT STYLES FOR MULTI-CULTURAL HAIR

DADDY DO IT!
BANTU KNOTS

□ Prep the hair by wetting and brushing through hair.

□ While still partially wet, separate hair into multiple sections. The exact width will vary depending on how short or long your hair is, as well as the look you want to go for if you plan to do knot-outs. Typically speaking, if you have short hair, you should use smaller sections, while women with long hair can opt for larger sections.

□ Apply a curl cream or similar setting product. Stick with a product that has light to medium hold to create knots and knot-outs that hold their form without becoming stiff. Twist the product into each section of hair.

□ Twist a small coil at the base of your scalp. Twist each section of hair for a few turns in between your fingertips, as though screwing in a screw or turning a doorknob. Only wind the hair enough to create a short spring-like coil against your scalp.

□ Wrap the rest of the hair around this section. Gradually wind the remaining hair in the section around the base coil, bringing the hair closer to your head with each wrapped layer.

▫ Set in place. If the coils are tight enough, you can usually tuck the ends under the coil to hold them in place. If the coils feel a little too loose, however, you can use hairpins or small elastic ponytail holders to hold the end of the knots in place.

▫ Repeat the knotting procedure on the remaining sections. Each section of hair needs to be twisted into a small coil. Wrap the remainder of each section around its corresponding coil and tuck or pin the ends in place.

VIDEO TUTORIAL!
See it at <u>daddy.do/bantu-knots-by-dean</u>

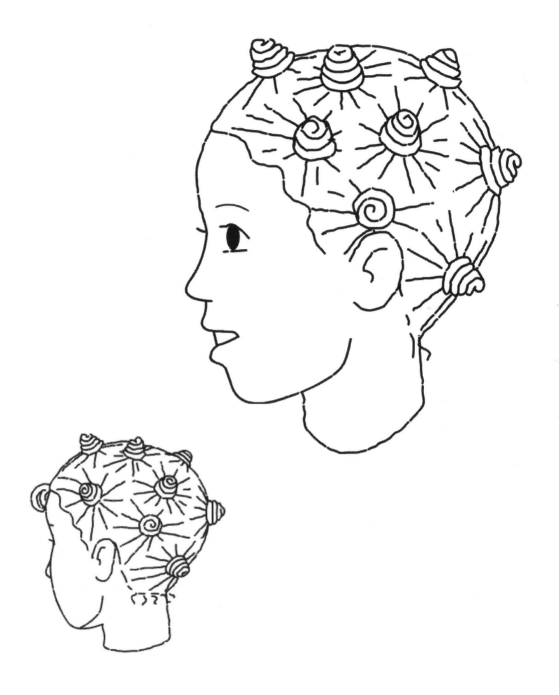

BANTU BABY!

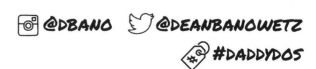

@DBANO @DEANBANOWETZ

#DADDYDOS

DADDY DO IT!
STRAND TWIST (ROPE BRAID)

▫ Before braiding, brush hair smooth.

▫ For a tighter, more structured rope braid, start by putting the hair in a ponytail.

▫ For a messier look, skip to the next step and start the braid at the nape of your neck.

▫ Separate the hair into two equal sections. Now twirl each section around your fingers, or pinch the top of the section, twist, move down another inch, twist again, and so on. Both sections should be twisted in a clockwise or rightward motion.

▫ Cross the right section over the left section.

▫ Keep braiding all the way down the hair.

▫ Tie off the end with a hair band.

VIDEO TUTORIAL!
See it at daddy.do/strand-twist-by-dean

DADDY DO IT!
BRAID OUT

☐ Prep hair by brushing and washing hair.

☐ Part the hair in four quarters. First, part down the middle of the head, so there are two big halves. Secondly, part across, horizontally, so that there are two sections in each half part, four total on the head.

☐ Clip each section.

☐ Apply leave-in moisturizer to each of the four, separated sections. I find that combing the product through works best on very, very, VERY thick hair. Be sure to pay attention to the roots and the ends.

☐ When all parts of the hair are amply moisturized, grab oil and rub it on the hands as if rubbing someone down. LOL! Just kidding. Anyway, rub the oil on the hands and in between fingers. Greasy hands make for even distribution when braiding the hair.

☐ Loosen each of the four sections (one by one) and put four or five braids in each.

☐ Do Step 4 as needed for each section.

☐ When all sections are plaited up, slap on a satin bonnet.

VIDEO TUTORIAL!
See it at <u>daddy.do/braid-out-by-dean</u>

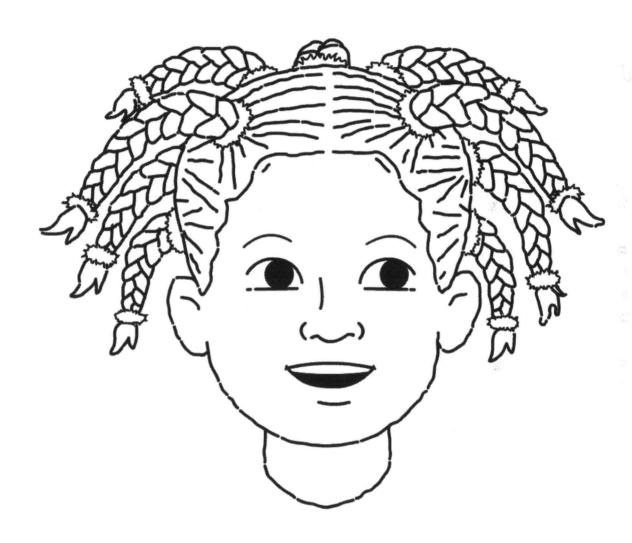

BRAID IT
OUT!

@DBANO @DEANBANOWETZ
#DADDYDOS

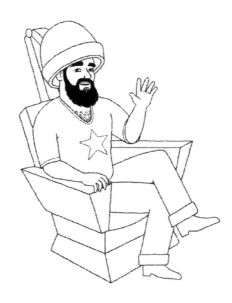

CHAPTER NINE: BEAUTY SCHOOL

People are always asking me for my best beauty tips for both adults and the kids. Here are some of my top suggestions:

☐ **Learning the structure of your hair is important.** Remember that when their hair is wet, it is fragile. Don't pull on it hard or it will rip and snap. I tell all of my clients, big and small, to always use a wide toothed comb to detangle wet hair. Proceed carefully. Comb and do not rip.

☐ **The basic hair care regime is to wash and then condition.** I think the real first step to successful hair is to make sure you comb hair out prior to ever getting it wet. It will be so much better and easier to wash.

☐ **You should wash your hair in water that's never too hot or too cold.** Tepid is the best. Kids basically hate hot water and you could burn them. Make sure to test the water in the shower before you tell them to get in. Remember that a child's sensitivity to heat is much greater than ours. You can stand that hot shower; she cannot. Yes, it does burn her.

▢ **It's great to buy a baby shampoo.** Kids will turn savage if they have burning shampoo in their eyes and they will blame you forever.

▢ **There are all sorts of DIY hair care recipes out there for both kids and adults.** I've heard of using egg white and even mayo or baby powder to absorb the oil if you can't wash. Remember that eggs can be dangerous if residue is left in the tub because they're slippery. They can even turn into salmonella poisoning, so I'd avoid using eggs. Mayo just seems messy. A sprinkle of baby powder will help dry up oil. Make sure to brush it out, so you don't walk around with white fluff in your hair.

AND NOW A FEW DADDY GROOMING TIPS:

I can't help it, but I want to spread beauty everywhere. Since you've taken such great care of your little girl, it's time for a little papa pampering. A few last words for you fabulous daddies from your best friend Dean:

▢ **When you cut your hair have the hairdresser cut your eyebrows.** You don't want to braid them.

▢ **You wouldn't be happy if your little daughter had hair growing out of her ears.** She feels the same way about the fur in your lobes and nose. Removing that hair is basic grooming 101. You don't have to be Beckham, but good grooming is a must for all men.

▢ **Get your hair cut every four weeks.** You will always look good. Some men prefer more regular cuts. I cut Simon Cowell's hair every ten days. The point is, if you wait too long you will get split ends. And you don't want to look like a shaggy mess.

▢ **You don't have to blow dry your hair.** Just towel dry it out dry. You can also use a dime-sized drop of gel to control it. Just air dry and call it a day.

▢ **Don't use too much product.** You don't want to be an oil slick. The same goes for not washing your hair every single day. Remember, you don't want hands to glide off your head.

▢ **The three products I believe every man needs are a basic hair gel, a finishing pomade or putty, and hair spray.** That's what I use on men whose hair I cut.

▢ **Spend three more minutes in the shower and use conditioner.** Also use it to soften your beard. It will make shaving so much easier for you. Plus, I hate shaving cream. I just use shampoo and conditioner in the shower to shave. It's so much easier on your facial skin than some harsh shaving cream with menthol.

▢ **Guys, wash your hair well after a workout.** After a workout, you release hormones that can even clog your pores and cause balding. So don't just jump into a shower and avoid your hair. It's stinky, plus you could become a baldie over time – and not that much time. Wash out what is clogging your scalp and thus causing your hair to fall out.

▢ **If you are balding, I recommend getting a shorter cut, which will conceal it.** You can also explore other options. I've had four hair transplants done on my head (shoutout to bosley.com). Most say that transplants look horrible. Do I look horrible? No! It's really important to get an initial consultation. If you can't afford transplants or don't want to do it, you can also look into a hairpiece. Some pieces do an amazing job. This is not the time to skimp on price. A cheap piece looks like a cheap piece. In other words, you get what you pay for here.

▢ **To avoid baldness, do a nightly scalp massage.** Even Jon Bon Jovi reportedly does it. Just rub your fingers in circular motions gently on your scalp. Don't do it on wet hair because that is fragile hair. Do it when your hair is dry. A scalp massage increases oxygen rich blood and brings it to the surface to feed the hair. There are also drugs that help retain your hair. Ask your doc. If you use the shampoos to cope with balding make sure you're consistent. You can't use them "sometimes" because they won't work that way. Check out Bosley Professional Strength Shampoo and Conditioner.

☐ **Take Vitamin A, D and E, which are crucial for skin, hair and nail health.** I'm always really aware of my vitamins.

☐ **By the way, bald is really hot on a lot of guys.** Embrace it. Love it. Get rid of all the hair and don't just leave a '70s patch. So get rid of that horseshoe of hair and commit to bald. My favorite product is the Headblade. A little shadow however looks hot. Remember to put sunscreen on your shaved head because nasty burns happen fast. Or wear a hat.

☐ **Have fun with hair**—your own, and the hair you create for you daughter!

Until next time,
Your Do Master, Dean

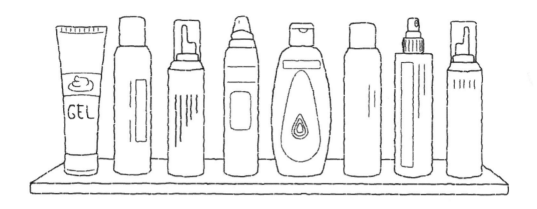

APPENDIX: TOP PRODUCTS FOR THE KIDS

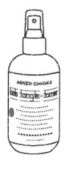

JOHNSON'S BABY SHAMPOO

Baby's delicate eyes need special care during bath time. JOHNSON'S® baby shampoo is as gentle and mild to the eyes as pure water. This baby shampoo's NO MORE TEARS® formula cleanses gently and rinses easily, leaving your baby's hair soft, shiny, manageable and clean while smelling baby-fresh.

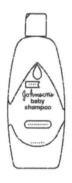

MIXED CHICKS KID'S TANGLE-TAMER

Worried about what to do the next day with your little one's nest? Mixed Chicks Kid's Tangle-Tamer light, moisturizing formula revives bedhead and gives wild hair a fresh look.

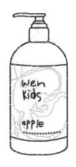

WEN KIDS™ APPLE CLEANSING CONDITIONER

This menthol-free formula is made exclusively with rice protein and contains no nuts, no wheat and no soy ingredients, making it safe to use even for those with many common allergies.

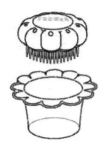

TANGLE TEEZER FLOWER POT PRINCESS PINK

A pretty flower-shaped Tangle Teezer brush which is easy to hold and perfect for children. Comes with a flower pot case that can be used to store hair clips and bands.

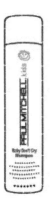

PAUL MITCHELL BABY DON'T CRY® SHAMPOO

Gently cleanses and soothes hair and scalp. Mild cleansers and a neutral pH create a tearless formula. A unique blend of extracts helps to hydrate and prevent moisture loss, while chamomile and cornflower extract calm and soothe.

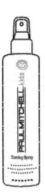

PAUL MITCHELL TAMING SPRAY® OUCH-FREE DETANGLER

Easily detangles dry or damp hair. Leaves hair fresh and full of body. Smoothes static and helps control children's "morning hair."

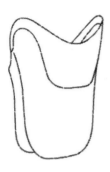

NUBY TEAR FREE RINSE PAIL

The Tear Free Rinse Pail is designed to make bath time easier and more enjoyable. It features a comfortable grip for Mom or Dad, a deep base for easy filling in shallow water and a unique tear free edge that can be gently placed against your baby's skin to help prevent water from running into your baby's eyes.

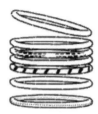

GOODY OUCHLESS ELASTICS

Only Goody Ouchless elastics are made with SmartStretch Core™. This improvement helps each one hold its shape longer without stretching out while giving you the same gentle and comfortable hold.

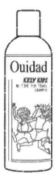

OUIDAD KRLY KIDS NO TIME FOR TEARS SHAMPOO

KRLY Kids No Time for Tears Shampoo is a super-gentle, tear-free formula that cleanses while helping delicate curls retain moisture. Proteins and amino acids restore internal weight so curls are moisturized, tangle-free, manageable, and healthy.

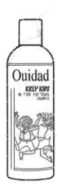

OUIDAD KRLY KIDS NO MORE KNOTS CONDITIONER

KRLY Kids No More Knots Conditioner is a detangler and nourishing conditioner that softens curls and protects against frizz and split ends. A gentle duo of proteins and amino acids penetrate hair strands, giving curls substance and encouraging separation and easy detangling.

SUNDAY AFTERNOON SUN HATS

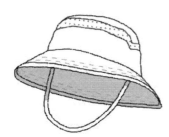

The need for children's sun protection is unprecedented; early education and use of natural sun care, including sun protective wear is critical for their future health. Sunday Afternoon Sun Hats offer a wide down sloping brim, excellent ventilation.

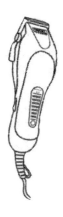

WAHL LITHIUM ION CLIPPERS FOR KIDS CUTS

Powered by Lithium Ion technology, the clipper outperforms standard Wahl rechargeable clippers by providing up to two times the run time, clocking in at one hour and forty minutes on a full charge.

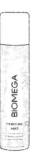

BIOMEGA MOISTURE MIST CONDITIONER

Revitalizes fine, limp or thinning hair with a volumizing infusion of lightweight Omega-nutrients and Gugo Bark Extract. It detangles and conditions hair without weighing it down.

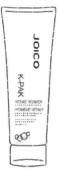

JOICO K-PAK INTENSE HYDRATOR

There's dry hair… and there's hair that's so parched, so thirsty, so starved for moisture that only a serious drink could bring it back to life. Intense Hydrator is the cocktail of choice: a profoundly nourishing treatment (at a gentle 3.5 PH level) offering immediate hydration to hair that's gasping for air.

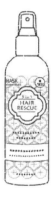

HASK ESSENTIALS 5 IN 1 HAIR RESCUE

Repair That Hair is formulated with a specialty blend of ingredients developed to pack your hair with moisturizing agents that are lost due to environmental and styling damage.

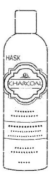

HASK PURIFYING CHARCOAL SHAMPOO

Charcoal, derived from coconut shells, combined with lemon and grapefruit oils, thoroughly cleanses and clarifies while helping to eliminate impurities from your hair and scalp. Gentle enough for daily use and safe for color-treated hair.

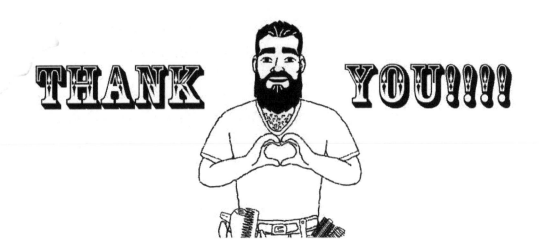

THANK YOU!!!!

A very special thanks goes to a few people. Here they are:

▢ My mom Marcella, #SallyorSal, who always encouraged me when I was in beauty school and still does with everything I do in my life.

▢ All of my siblings Judy (#1), Alice (#2), Dee (#3), Lloyd (#4), Steve (#5), Allan (#6), Mary (#7), Marv (#8), Dick (#9), Debra (#10), Annette (#11), Leon (#12), (I'm #13), Randy (#14) and Patti (#15).

▢ Kyle Assenmacher, #10.2, my one and only godson, and all my nieces and nephews…

▢ A special thanks to #12 for telling me to go to beauty school and giving me pep talks of encouragement. He has always been who I look up to and want to be like.

▢ I look to a lot of my celebrity clients who I admire for their constant support and loyalty:

  ▢ Leeza Gibbons who has always told me I am the perfect husband because I anticipate what is needed and I know when to embrace the silence. She inspires me to try new and different things regardless of fear. She is my #1 fan and the woman who, just by knowing her, makes me want to be a better person.

▫ Simon Cowell who is one of the most amazing men I have met who has taught me the importance of loyalty in the business. He has allowed me to explore the globe going to new and beautiful places; something I never thought would happen to a farm boy from Iowa.

▫ Melanie Griffith is one of the kindest and most generous people I know. I love her passion for life and adventure.

▫ Lori Greiner for her constant friendship and encouragement to take the leap and make it happen. She is always ready to chat about what I want to do with my life and how I can change the world around us with hair.

▫ Noah Galloway, who I instantly bonded with on the set of *DWTS*. As a U.S. vet who has overcome so much in his life, I admire how he lives his life to the fullest and inspires others daily!

▫ Ryan Seacrest, who I styled and groomed for 10 years, has taught me more about being an incredibly hard worker, a meticulous thinker about my business, and how to make sure everything fits together in perfect harmony.

▫ Carlos and Alexa Pena-Vega—this amazing couple have been a constant source of joy in my life since meeting them years ago. They are always encouraging me to take the leap to my next adventure and are always super supportive. I have learned valuable traits from them, live your life with love and compassion tackle life with a positive attitude and kind intensions. All things are possible with hard work and guidance from above.

▫ All my hair people who I have worked with over the years who have taught me to see the world a little differently through hair: Meagan Herrera-Schaaf, Cory Rotenberg, Don Wismer, Luis Alverez, Suzanne Weerts, Ryan Randall, Roni Roehlk, Linda Flowers, Sydell Miller, Mitch

Stone, Ann Bray, Milton Buras, Mary Guerrero, Kimi Messina, Jen Guerrero, Sean Smith, Gail Ryan, Sharon Blain, Vivienne Mackinder, Nicolas French, Sara Jones, Vince Davis, Ann Mincey, Michael Maron, Joe Santy, Stephanie Wiley, Maren Lonergan, Yuko Koach, Melissa Jaqua, Melanie Verkins, Nancy Stimac, Cheryl Marks, Jerilynn Stephens, Dev Rice, Pat O'Keefe, Ralph Abalos, Rachel Dowling, Alyn Topper, Kay Majuerus, Lotus Corricelli, Sallie Nicole, Cortney Ajamian, Lyndsey Palumbo, Keyonna Tillman, Karen Kaalberg, Lawrence Davis, Derrick Spruill, Renee Vaca, Miss Deb, Margaret Dempsey, Kear Lonergan, Okyo Sthair, Trista Bremer, all my 706 Union hair and make up friends I get to work with everyday, and many, many more.

□ My core group of non-doing-hair friends who don't judge me and make my world a better, happier, safer place to be: Scott Carter, Leann Donovan, James Aquilina, Doug Rago, Glenn Soukesian, Dave Lawrence, Mike Catlett, Mark Keppy, Julie Kozak, Keith Crary, Amy Scribner, Stacie Krajchir, Kamy Bruder, Trish Suhr, Heidi Clements, Kyle Kleibeoker, Phil Pallen, Jeff Hall, Charles F. Reidelbach, Hillary Bibicoff, Cindy Pearlman, Arline Kramer, Doloras Cardelucci, Rhonda Roeder Evans, Deaquinita Hill, Sean Nadeau, Robin Radin and many more.

□ My heart and soul are one with Claire Kaye, the best beauty PR person I've ever met. Claire has believed in me more than I have believed in myself. She is a constant source of knowledge and wisdom; the 1st person I call whenever something is happening in my life. Claire, I love you and am so happy you are in my life.

□ My manager Cat Josell who has been my biggest cheerleader and supporter in life. I appreciate all you do and look forward to doing so much more in the future. Get me my own show!!!!!! :)

□ Lisa Gregorisch Dempsey, a prolific TV executive I met at "EXTRA" who has always encouraged me to think big and jump in feet first! It is all about the Four Agreements!

◻ Winn Claybaugh and all the Paul Mitchell Schools throughout the United States. I love being a part of this learning culture! Winn thank you for always being there to listen to my ideas and helping me fulfill my dreams. You are amazing and I love and appreciate you very much! Everyone needs a hair daddy!! Thanks for being a great mentor!

◻ Sara Jones for believing in me from the beginning. She hired me for my first professional hair gig. She has been a personal and professional friend ever since #Joico

◻ My Instyler leaders Dave, Mark, Karl, Marty Jon, Stephanie and everyone on the team, thank you for having faith in me its a pleasure to collaborate with all of you.

LOOK FOR DEAN'S NEXT BOOKS

THE DEAN'S LIST OF...

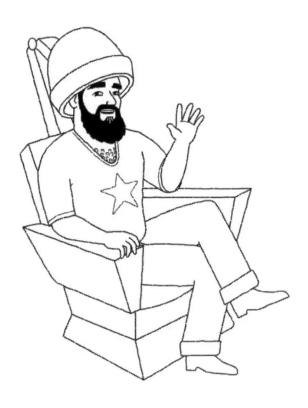

41615797R00101

Made in the USA
Middletown, DE
18 March 2017